Mental retardation

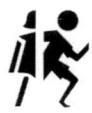

Fondazione Pierfranco e Luisa Mariani ONLUS
viale Bianca Maria 28
20129 Milan, Italy

Telephone: +39 02 795458
Fax: +39 02 76009582
Publications coordinator: Valeria Basilico
e-mail: publications@fondazione-mariani.org
www.fondazione-mariani.org

Mental retardation

Edited by

D. Riva, S. Bulgheroni and C. Pantaleoni

Mariani Foundation Paediatric Neurology Series: 18
Series Editor: Maria Majno

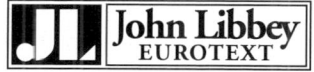

ISSN: 0969-0301
ISBN: 978-2-74-200687-8

Cover illustration: design by Costanza Magnocavallo.
Technical and language editor: Oliver Brooke.
(Third book of the series dedicated to *Developmental cognitive neurosciences* – the previous were vol. 13 and vol. 16.)

Published by

Éditions John Libbey Eurotext
127, avenue de la République, 92120 Montrouge, France.
Tél.: 33 (0)1 46 73 06 60; Fax: 33 (0)1 40 84 09 99
e-mail: contact@jle.com
http//www.jle.com

© 2007 John Libbey Eurotext. All rights reserved.

Unauthorized duplication contravenes applicable laws.

Il est interdit de reproduire intégralement ou partiellement le présent ouvrage sans autorisation de l'éditeur ou du Centre Français d'Exploitation du Droit de Copie, 20, rue des Grands-Augustins, 75006 Paris.

Contents

Chapter 1	Cognitive and behavioural assessment in children with mental retardation *Sara Bulgheroni, Chiara Vago, Arianna Usilla and Daria Riva*	1
Chapter 2	Neurodiagnostics for children with mental retardation *Chiara Pantaleoni, Morena Doz, Sara Bulgheroni, Chiara Vago and Stefano D'Arrigo*	13
Chapter 3	Mental retardation and epilepsy *Thierry Deonna and Eliane Roulet-Perez*	19
Chapter 4	Mental retardation in patients with neuromuscular disorders *Eugenio Mercuri, Marika Pane, Sonia Messina and Angela Beradinelli*	33
Chapter 5	Mental retardation in paediatric disease *Angelo Selicorni, Marta Cerutti, Cecilia Vellani, Melissa Bellini and Donatella Milani*	49
Chapter 6	Laboratory: instructions for proper use of genetic tests *Angelo Selicorni, Cecilia Vellani, Marta Cerutti, Melissa Bellini and Donatella Milani*	63
Chapter 7	X-linked mental retardation: a diagnostic, clinical and molecular update *Rossella Caselli, Filomena T. Papa, Francesca Ariani, Ilaria Meloni and Alessandra Renieri*	79
Chapter 8	Phenotypes of Smith-Magenis syndrome *Stefano D'Arrigo, Sara Bulgheroni and Chiara Pantaleoni*	93
Chapter 9	Rett syndrome and its variants *Michele Zappella*	101

Chapter 10	Phenotypes in chromosome 15-linked syndromes *Agatino Battaglia*	111
Chapter 11	The psychopathological structure of the child with mental retardation *Pietro Pfanner and Mara Marcheschi*	119
Chapter 12	Psychiatric comorbidity in intellectual disability (mental retardation) *Carlo Cianchetti, Marta Meloni and Giorgio Gaspa*	127
Chapter 13	Pharmacological treatment of psychiatric comorbidities in mental retardation *Gabriele Masi and Cinzia Pari*	141
Chapter 14	Neuropsychological rehabilitation in children with cognitive impairment *Chiara Gagliardi, Sara Martelli and Renato Borgatti*	153
Chapter 15	An educational approach in mental retardation: how to build an individualized education plan (IEP) *Stefania Bargagna, Margherita Bozza, Francesca Liboni and Anastasia Dressler*	161
Chapter 16	Medical treatments for mental retardation: the neurobiological bases for new therapeutic approaches *Alessandro Zuddas, Nicoletta Adamo, Cristina Peddis, Giulia Congia and Tatiana Usala*	169
Chapter 17	The Feuerstein method: an effective tool for rehabilitation in mental retardation *Antonia Madella Noja*	183
Chapter 18	Understanding alterations during human brain development with molecular imaging: a guide to new treatment approaches for mental retardation *Diane C. Chugani*	191
Chapter 19	Mental retardation: definition and classification systems *Daria Riva, Arianna Usilla, Chiara Vago, Federica Aggio and Sara Bulgheroni*	203
Chapter 20	Neuropsychological profile of Williams syndrome *Stefano Vicari*	211
Chapter 21	Neuropsychology of mental retardation: fragile X syndrome as paradigm of the cognitive-behavioural phenotypes *Daria Riva, Arianna Usilla, Chiara Vago, Federica Aggio and Sara Bulgheroni*	223

Chapter 1

Cognitive and behavioural assessment in children with mental retardation

Sara Bulgheroni, Chiara Vago, Arianna Usilla and Daria Riva

*Department of Developmental Neurology, Fondazione IRCCS Istituto Neurologico 'C. Besta',
via Celoria 11, 20133 Milan, Italy*
neuropsicologia@istituto-besta.it

Summary

For a diagnosis of mental retardation based on the international classification systems, a person's intelligence and adaptive skills must have been significantly below average during the developmental period. Establishing this diagnosis generally calls for the administration of standardized tools for assessing intelligence and adaptive behaviour, and an evaluation based on the analysis of documents and interviews with observers, demonstrating that the disability existed before the person was 18 years old.

In both clinical practice and research, cognitive and behavioural assessment of children with mental retardation relies on standardized tools capable of identifying strengths and weaknesses both in comparison with a normative reference group and in ipsative comparisons which evaluate each person as their own 'control'.

The importance of a thorough functional assessment stems from the need to avoid confining the assessment to indices derived from intelligence scales. These are not enough in themselves to support any diagnostic conclusions unless there is good consistency between the concurrent validity criteria and external validity criteria (such as other formal and informal test results, information on the individual's environment, and reports from parents and teachers). That is why the standardized scales used for assessing cognitive efficiency and psychomotor competence are combined with methods for investigating adaptive behaviour and tools for evaluating emotional and behavioural disorders, which are often associated with mental retardation.

The clinical judgement is also fundamental when it comes to decision-making or integrating the data emerging from multidimensional assessments with the contextual information available.

Introduction

The cognitive and behavioural assessment of mental retardation for diagnostic purposes calls for the use of powerful psychometric tools that focus on the domains identified in the definition of the diagnostic category of mental retardation. According to the *Diagnostic and Statistical Manual of Mental Disorders*, fourth edition, text revision (DSM-IV-TR) (American Psychiatric Association. 2000), mental retardation is an extremely heterogeneous condition characterized not only by significant limitations in intellectual functioning (criterion A), but also by concomitant impairment in adaptive functioning skills (criterion B), and by onset before 18 years of age (criterion C). The American Association on Mental Retardation

(AAMR) accordingly defines mental retardation as a particular state of functioning that begins in childhood and is characterized by significant limitations both in intellectual functioning and in adaptive behaviour, as expressed in conceptual, social, and practical abilities (AAMR, 2002).

A reliable and valid assessment of intellectual and adaptive functioning demands the use of tools with good psychometric properties and standardized on a large sample of individuals with and without disabilities. On the basis of these standardized measurements, significant limitations are defined operatively as a performance that comes at least two standard deviations below the mean. The clinical diagnosis calls for an increasingly strict approach to individual cases, effectively combining clinical judgement with the use of standardized procedures for collecting objective and repeatable data, in line with the evidence-based medicine approach.

As a first step, it is important to have tests that are standardized on a typical population to compare the performance of individuals with mental retardation with a control group matched for both mental age and chronological age in order to determine whether an ability is spared, is a relative strength, or is at expected levels. Unfortunately, we have no clear-cut boundaries separating these three concepts. By definition, 'spared' implies that children with mental retardation perform at or near the same level as typical children of the same chronological age. A 'relative strength' is observed when the group performs significantly above mental age levels but below chronological age levels. Finally, one might find neither sparing nor relative strength but a performance that is appropriate given the group's overall level of mental age.

A second step involves a more in-depth profile analysis using ipsative methods – that is, considering each person as their own control. The self-as-control strategy compares the scores of children across cognitive and behavioural domains to reveal strengths and weaknesses characterizing the functioning of the subject studied.

Profile analysis of intelligence and adaptive scales begins with an assessment of the scatter in the various scores. Only if the difference between the maximum and minimum scores is significant do we compare the score obtained in each subtest with the others and with the mean of all subtest scores. From a clinical standpoint, only abnormal differences between standard scores are of interest – that is, differences that are statistically significant and also have a low likelihood of recurrence (less than five per cent) in the normative population.

Another requirement for a valid tool in the diagnosis of mental retardation is that it must have been standardized on a population with mental retardation. This procedure ensures that the tool has diagnostic sensitivity and specificity, and also provides reference data relating to the general population with mental retardation so as to determine whether cognitive and behavioural strengths or weaknesses are unique to the subject under consideration or common to the majority of people with mental retardation.

Intelligence

Intelligence has been defined as 'a general mental faculty that includes capacity for reasoning, problem solving, abstract thinking, programming and learning from experience, and that reflects a more ample capacity for understanding the surrounding environment' (Gottfredson, 1997). Nowadays, empirical data seem to be unequivocally in favour of the idea that intellectual functioning can be explained only in terms of a general intelligence factor (Carroll, 1997). This does not mean that intelligence can be brought down to a unitary capacity, but rather that the majority of the differences between different higher cognitive skills can be explained by such common general intelligence factor.

Most theories on multiple intelligences have not been validated by standardized, quantifiable measurements, and even Sternberg (1988) and Greenspan (1997) failed in their attempts to apply tasks for the purpose of quantifying the construct of the tripartite models and developing an adequate measure of intelligence.

Evaluating intelligence is of fundamental importance in the diagnosis of mental retardation because all the definitions refer to significant limitations in intellectual functioning as one of the essential diagnostic criteria.

There is a general problem with regard to the validity and specificity of standardized intelligence scales for the purpose of diagnosing mental retardation – that is, whether it is really appropriate to judge a person with suspected mental retardation using tools that assure the best psychometric properties when they are administered to people whose scores come within two to three standard deviations from the mean. No tools have been designed specifically for use with people whose test performance is very low or very high, although the diagnosis of mental retardation, by definition, presupposes more extreme results such as could well give rise to greater measurement errors.

In the light of this, there is reason to doubt the practical utility, for diagnostic purposes, of a cut-off that is weak from a psychometric standpoint. Every time decisions are made relating to a diagnosis of mental retardation. We have to bear in mind that an IQ of 70 should be considered not as a precise cut-off but as a confidence interval defined by at least one standard error of measurement (SEM) (that is, scores from 66 to 74, with a 66 per cent probability of inclusion) or 2 SEM (scores from 62 to 78, with a 95 per cent probability of inclusion). As seen previously, both the American diagnostic systems refer to a significantly lower than average intellectual functioning as a determining feature of mental retardation. The DSM-IV-TR defines an IQ of 70 or less as significantly lower than the mean, adding a reference concerning the measurement error and giving the example of an IQ of 70, measured using the Wechsler scales, being considered as representative of a range of scores from 65 to 75. After allowing for measurement errors, the AAMR sets the cut-off at around 70–75 (AAMR, 2002).

It is also important to remember that lower than average intellectual functioning is a necessary but not sufficient criterion for establishing a diagnosis of mental retardation – a concomitant assessment of adaptive behaviour is always required. The strong correlation between IQ and adaptive behaviour scores in population with mental retardation, and particularly in individuals of preschool age and with severe disabilities, initiates in practice a redundant process that ensures a stronger, more precise diagnosis.

Another crucial point concerns the choice of the intelligence test, because the IQ scores obtained with different tools are not necessarily equivalent. Which tool is most suitable will be a matter of clinical judgement, depending on the personal characteristics of the individual being assessed.

Although the reliability of IQ scores in estimating the general intelligence factor has been the object of much controversy among researchers, this variable remains the measure of human intelligence that continues to be awarded the most credit in the scientific community (Gottfredson,1997).

The Wechsler scales are the tools most often used in the clinical setting to assess intelligence. The Wechsler Preschool and Primary Scale of Intelligence (WPPSI) (Wechsler, 1967; Orsini & Piconi, 1993) is designed for children aged from 3 years 6 months up to 6 years 6 months, while the Wechsler Intelligence Scale for Children-Third edition (WISC-III) (Wechsler, 1991; Orsini & Piconi, 2006) can be used from 6 years to 16 years 6 months. Wechsler (1944) considered intelligence as 'a global, unitary entity' and designed a scale for 'assessing an

3

individual's capacity to act intentionally, think rationally, and interact effectively with his/her environment'. Within this relatively broad concept of intelligence, 12 subtests (six verbal and six performance) each measure different facets of intelligence, such as verbal and arithmetical reasoning abilities, judgement in practical situations, attention to visual details, visual perceptual organization, constructive praxia, and visual-motor planning.

The WISC-III retains the structure and content of the earlier Wechsler Intelligence Scale for Children-Revised (WISC-R), but it improves the sensitivity and validity of the subtests. The work of revision and restandardization updated the normative data and extended the tool's range of applicability to individuals with moderate mental retardation (lower limits for Verbal IQ = 39, Performance IQ = 36, and Full scale IQ = 30), and also reinforced the factorial structure with the introduction of four factorial quotients known as 'Verbal Comprehension', 'Perceptual Organization', 'Processing Speed', and 'Freedom from Distractibility'. It is worth noting the decision to emphasize the confidence intervals in the score sheet, suggesting a more critical and careful approach to the interpretation of the profile of functioning.

The Leiter International Performance Scale – Revised (Leiter-R) (Roid & Miller, 1997) is an intelligence scale that demands no use of language by the examiner and the individual being tested. This tool aims to measure fluid intelligence, which is believed to be uninfluenced by education, social background, or family experiences. It is divided into two batteries: 'Visualization and Reasoning' and 'Attention and Memory', the first being specifically for the assessment of non-verbal intellectual abilities. The work done to revise the scale has given rise to a tool characterized by better normative data and psychometric properties, thanks to its standardization on a random stratified sample of 1769 people aged between 2 and 21 years.

In the context of psychological testing, the Leiter-R scale is currently considered a tool with several significant strengths:
- it is suitable for a wide range of ages (children, adolescents, and young adults from 2 to 20 years 11 months) and it facilitates longitudinal assessments;
- it entails straightforward administration and scoring methods;
- it is particularly useful with special clinical populations – for example, patients with pervasive developmental and communication disorders, severe motor impairment, brain trauma, attention deficit disorder, and so on;
- it provides not only quotients and standard scores describing the individual's performance compared with the normative group, but also growth scores that supply a dynamic measure sensitive to even minimal changes in the individual's performance (most standardized scales are unable to document any such improvements, particularly in groups of individuals with severe functional impairments, in whom the application of psychometric tools carries the risk of suffering from a floor effect and producing measurements that are scarcely sensitive and discriminatory).

The hierarchical interpretation of non-verbal cognition begins globally with an IQ assessment on the full scale to estimate the global intellectual factor g. The composite scores combining the results of two or more subtests are then computed to measure different aspects of the same construct in the sense that they can predict a common indicator of performance. The three composite scores in the Visualization and Reasoning battery are: (1) fluid reasoning, which assesses competence in terms of deductive reasoning, seriation, and the generation of rules; (2) fundamental visualization, which explores the basic visualization abilities, such as visual discrimination, contextual understanding, and attention to visual details without involving memorizing or conceptually reorganizing the stimuli; (3) spatial visualization, which investigates the capacity for inductive reasoning and the ability to perceive and preserve the spatial orientation, shape, and position of objects.

IQ and composite scores must always be considered in conjunction with other indicators. These are: the percentile rank of the score; the descriptive classification labels for Leiter-R non-verbal IQ scores (that is, the average); the confidence interval within which the value lies for different error probabilities.

Finally, the raw score obtained at each test, the sum of the raw scores obtained in the subtests contributing to the composite scores, and the short and full IQ scores can be converted into a growth score that is an estimate of the person's growth level on the criterion-referenced scale.

The growth scores also include an estimate of the difficulty of each item, facilitating the interpretation of each individual's performance. Instead of being compared to other children, the subject's skill level is defined by the tasks they can typically handle successfully. As the child's overall abilities and task performance abilities are placed along a linear scale, it is possible to determine what kind of tasks are too hard, too easy, or just about at the right difficulty level for the child on each domain of cognition sampled by the Leiter-R subtests. This knowledge should assist in determining strengths and weaknesses in the diagnostic phase and thus planning intervention programmes. One way to use the growth scale is to focus on the skills that are reflected in items between 0 and +20 points below the ability of the child – as an 'instructional range'. In the instructional range, items are not too difficult for the child, and yet require additional practice to achieve a mastery level for the specific ability (90 per cent probability of success).

The growth scale ability scores can be converted into equivalent age scores (range 2 years to 20 years, 11 months) which can be used mainly to explain growth scores that are not self-explanatory. If you want to determine a mean test age for the child, arrange the scores for the subtests in order and identify the central value.

A valid and reliable assessment of intelligence is generally not possible in infants and young children because traditional IQ test instruments are not applicable under 3 years of age. It is nonetheless important to identify and report cases with global developmental delay – that is, children with a performance two standard deviations or more below the mean on an age-appropriate, standardized, norm-referenced developmental scale (Shevell *et al.*, 2003). For instance, the Griffiths Mental Development Scales (Griffiths, 1984; Griffiths, 1996) measure development trends that are significant for intelligence, or indicative of mental growth in babies and young children from birth to 8 years of age. There are two sets of scales for two different age groups, 0–2 years and 2–8 years.

A major revision of the Griffiths 0–2 scale was undertaken in 1996 and the revision of the extension kit (2–8 years) was published in May 2006 and also became available in Italy in June 2007, published by Organizzazioni Speciali. The revision process fulfilled the following aims: to update the norms; to improve scoring standards, making them explicit and less open to subjective evaluation; to improve the administration instructions (including the provision of practice items on selected items); to improve the visual and aesthetic impact of the test materials; to include additional new items to assess previously untapped areas of development and to remove items that do not add value; and to replace outdated training aids. The basic qualities of the Griffiths scales, particularly their child-friendly nature, have been preserved. Designed to assess psychomotor development in children from 0 to 8 years old, they provide a general developmental quotient (GQ) by investigating the child's capabilities on six different scales:

- The *locomotor scale*, which evaluates postural-kinetic organization.

- The *personal/social scale*, which investigates the level of bodily and personal awareness, the degree of independence in daily activities, and interpersonal relational capacity with both adult figures and peers.
- The *hearing and language scale*, which considers expressive and receptive language competence.
- The *hand and eye coordination scale*, which investigates practical-manipulative organization in single and two-handed tasks, and visual-motor integration in spontaneous and copied graphic activities.
- The *performance scale*, which evaluates the speed and accuracy of execution in practical building tasks of increasing complexity and perceptive and visual-spatial organization.
- The *practical reasoning scale* (administered from 3 years onwards), which assesses auditory sequential short term memory, the ability to solve practical comparisons, and the acquisition of elementary arithmetic notions and automatic series.

The division into subscales enables to determine whether children have difficulty in specific developmental settings and, for each setting, which items they cannot deal with successfully. This is very useful both for diagnostic purposes and for programming teaching and rehabilitation measures. The revised Griffiths 0–2 scale provides IQs, percentile ranks, and standard and age-equivalent scores.

A feature of the original Griffiths Mental Developmental Scales (2–8 years) was the use of standard deviations for each scale, based on a simple ratio transformation of the raw data – mental age divided by chronological age. As the GQ and each scale have slightly different means and standard deviations, direct comparisons between Griffiths subscale scores, and between Griffiths and other scores, are prone to misinterpretation.

As suggested by Ivens & Martin (2002), a possible solution is to develop category ranges for Griffiths scores that are equivalent to those used by other popular tests, with a mean of 100 and an SD of 15, such as the Wechsler Scale. Descriptive terms for the score ranges, such as 'borderline' or 'low' for scores of 70–79, and 'normal' or 'average' for scores of 90–109, refer implicitly to this shared standard. Table 1 shows the downward extension of these ranges, with the Griffiths scale score bands for the DSM-IV-TR mental retardation ranges.

Table 1. Griffiths scale score band equivalents for DSM-IV-TR ranges of mental retardation

	DSM-IV-TR levels of mental retardation (standardised score range)			
	Profound < 20–25	Severe 20–25 to 35–40	Moderate 35–40 to 50–55	Mild 50–55 to 70
Total scale (GQ)	< 32–36	32–36 to 45–49	45–49 to 58–62	58–62 to 75
Locomotor	< 13–19	13–19 to 30–35	30–35 to 46–51	46–51 to 68
Personal-social	< 14–19	14–19 to 30–35	30–35 to 46–52	46–52 to 68
Hearing and speech	< 5–11	5–11 to 23–29	23–29 to 41–47	41–47 to 64
Hand and eye coordination	< 17–23	17–23 to 33–38	33–38 to 49–54	49–54 to 69
Performance	< 8–14	8–14 to 25–31	25–31 to 43–48	43–48 to 65
Practical reasoning	< 7–13	7–13 to 24–30	24–30 to 42–48	42–48 to 65

DSM-IV-TR, *Diagnostic and Statistical Manual of Mental Disorders*, fourth edition, text revision; GQ, general developmental quotient.

Adaptive behaviour

Adaptive behaviour is defined as 'the effectiveness or degree with which the individual meets the standards of personal independence and social responsibility expected for his or her age and cultural group' (Widmann & McGrew, 1996). This entails a set of conceptual, social, and practical abilities that people learn in order to function in their daily lives (AAMR, 2002).

Adaptive behaviour is a multidimensional construct with a hierarchical structure that is context-specific – that is, it depends on the expectations of the environment – and age-specific, in the sense that it is develops rapidly in the early years of life and reaches a point of maximum competence in adolescence/adult age, then declines with old age.

The revised AAMR definition also emphasizes the expression, or performance, of main adaptive abilities, not just their acquisition. The causes of limited adaptive abilities can thus be expected to include the following: not knowing how to perform certain abilities (acquisition deficit); not knowing when to use the abilities acquired (performance deficit); and other motivational factors affecting the expression of these abilities (performance deficit).

In individuals with a limited intellectual capacity, both acquisition deficits and performance deficits may be attributable to mental retardation. In line with this approach, the majority of tools for studying adaptive behaviour measure the level of typical performance in the individual's habitual activities rather than what they might do given the opportunity or sufficient motivation.

It is important to bear in mind that a definition of significantly impaired adaptive functioning requires a performance at least two standard deviations below the mean in at least one domain or in the total score, using a tool that measures all three domains.

If a person obtains a score that does not reach the cut-off but comes within one standard deviation of the cut-off score, it is best to double check the score for reliability or to reassess the individual concerned using another tool. If an individual reveals no significant impairment in their adaptive behaviour acquisition or performance scores, or both, then they cannot be diagnosed as mentally retarded.

The measure most often used to assess adaptive behaviour is the Vineland Adaptive Behaviour Scales (Sparrow et al., 1984), a semistructured, respondent-based interview for parents or carers. In cases in which no detailed psychometric testing has been undertaken (for example, in individuals with severe or profound mental retardation, sensory or motor impairments, and so on), the Vineland scales may be used as a screening tool to assess the developmental level.

The Vineland scales are available in three different versions: an expanded form (540 items), which affords a detailed analysis of the construct under consideration; a survey form (261 items), which is shorter and useful for a quick preliminary assessment; and a classroom edition, for use in evaluating the adaptive behaviour of students.

The Vineland scales provide a comprehensive assessment of adaptive behaviour in terms of interaction between individuals and their environment, and the activities of daily living they must be able to handle in order to be sufficiently independent and to cope with the tasks deriving from their role in society, so as to comply with what their environment expects of an individual of their age and cultural context. The scales provide an ecological assessment, indicating strengths and weaknesses in different adaptive skills, and offering step-by-step guidelines for planning an individual programme. As this tool is not very sensitive to minimal changes, the authors recommend follow-up assessments, not only for trends in the global scores of the scales but also to identify any changes in single crucial items.

Each item is scored as follows: 2 = activity usually or habitually completed successfully; 1 = activity only sometimes successful or only partially successful; 0 = activity never completed because the subject is too young or immature, the activity is beyond their capabilities, or physical or sensory deficits prevent its completion; N or 'lack of opportunity' = the activity is not performed because of an external contingent impediment; NS = a skill in which the interviewer does not know how the subject would perform.

The Vineland scales allow the evaluation of four distinct domains, comprising specific subdomains: (1) communication (receptive, expressive and written); (2) daily living skills (personal, domestic and community); (3) socialization (interpersonal relations, play and leisure time, and coping skills); and (4) motor skills (gross and fine) – only applicable to children less than 6 years old or with severe motor deficits.

In relation to the structure of the Vineland scales in the population with mental retardation, De Bildt *et al.* (2005) confirmed that a single central concept seems to underlie the scales, rather than three mutually interdependent concepts, and they found that the arrangement of subdomains into domains is easily recognizable in people with mild and moderate levels of intellectual deficit, but less well recognized in those with severe/profound deficit. Children and adolescents with lower IQs seem to show behaviour that can be divided into a more technical domain of *daily living skills* and one that could be interpreted as *contact behaviour*, instead of the original three domains.

It has also been demonstrated that the Vineland scales possess a good discriminant validity regardless of the level of mental retardation. Balboni *et al.* (2001) highlighted specific adaptive behaviour patterns in three groups of individuals with mental retardation and communication, social behaviour, or motor ability disorders, compared with age- and IQ-matched subjects with mental retardation but no such associated disorders.

The expanded form of the Vineland scales has recently been standardized on 1197 Italian children with disabilities aged 6 to 18 years (Italian adaptation by G. Balboni & L. Pedrabissi, 2003). Italian standardization shows two statistical limitations. First, the expected level of adaptive functioning for disabled subjects is calculated on the sample as a whole, disregarding the degree of disability. Only qualitative descriptors (that is, below average, average, above average) are provided for groups divided according to chronological age and the degree of mental retardation. Second, the reference data available on the typical population only enable age-equivalent scores to be obtained, not quotients of deviation comparable with those obtained by the intelligence scales.

Behavioural or emotional problems

In accordance with most studies (for a review see Dykens, 2000), the international classification systems report that the prevalence of psychopathology and severe behavioural or emotional dysfunction in subjects with mental retardation is nearly four times higher than in the general population. *Diagnostic overshadowing* is nonetheless still common – that is, clinicians tend to attribute maladaptive behaviour of individuals with mental retardation to their more limited intelligence rather than to concomitant psychopathology or mental illness (Reiss & Szyszko, 1983; Jopp & Keys, 2001).

Given that a single tool may be of limited use in helping to understand behaviour in mental retardation, clinicians and social science researchers advocate a mixture of methods. It has became almost a mantra that behavioural assessment should involve multiple assessments and multiple reports (across multiple settings and over multiple time points) (Hodapp & Dykens, 2005).

The *questionnaire* is probably the most often used tool as it constitutes an initial general screening procedure for maladaptive behaviour. Like all approaches, parent-reporting questionnaires have both strengths and weaknesses. On the strengths side, they are completed by parents or caregivers, avoiding the problem that individuals with mental retardation are often unreliable at reporting on their own behaviour or feelings. Moreover, unlike clinicians or even teachers, parents interact with their children across multiple settings and over the child's entire life, thereby providing a broader view of their child's behaviour. However, parent-reporting measures have their weaknesses as well. Given the specific skills tapped, parents are unlikely to have the necessary specific conceptual understanding of the distinctions required to score items describing unusual behaviour shown by individuals with mental retardation. Clinicians must also be wary of parent-reporting on maladaptive behaviour items because a child's maladaptive behaviour often correlates positively with parental stress (see Hodapp, 2002, for a review), making it hard to say whether the child's severe behaviour problems are eliciting more stress in parents, or whether stressed parents are attributing worse behaviour problems to their children.

Achenbach's Child Behaviour Checklist (CBCL) has been helpful for examining maladaptive behaviour, particularly in the light of its broad-band factors (internalizing-externalizing) and its narrow-band factors (withdrawal, somatic complaints, anxiety/depression, social problems, thought problems, attention problems, delinquent behaviour, and aggressive behaviour), as well as its many individual items (for example, overeating, fearful, and so on) (Achenbach, 1991; Achenbach & Rescorla, 2000; Frigerio *et al.*, 2004; Frigerio *et al.*, 2006). Unfortunately, the CBCL has only been standardized on typical populations.

Among the checklists that have been standardized for mentally retarded populations, one of the most widely used is the Developmental Behaviour Checklist (DBC) (Einfeld & Tonge, 2002), a 96-item checklist completed by parents or caregivers to assess a broad range of behavioural and emotional problems in children aged 4–18 years with mental retardation. The items were derived from 664 clinical records with detailed descriptions of behavioural concerns. The five original empirically-derived subscales – disruptive/antisocial, self-absorbed, communication disturbance, anxiety, and social relating – showed a good internal consistency and inter-rater and test-retest reliability. The DBC's criterion and concurrent validity are also satisfactory and the tool has proven specific and sensitive in distinguishing psychiatric disorder cases from non-cases, even if it is not necessarily compatible with DSM-IV-TR psychiatric diagnoses.

When moving from describing maladaptive behaviour to establishing a psychiatric diagnosis, however, a more specific, psychiatric interview seems necessary. The *diagnostic interview* has a high degree of validity with regard to the method (or setting) adopted, but is not always very reliable. Its reliability depends on the degrees of freedom allowed – that is, how strictly the interview is structured. Of course, the training of the clinicians administering the test, and their capacity to enter into the individual and investigate the most salient behavioural aspects in greater depth are fundamental issues. Even here, however, several problems arise. With the exception of some instruments specific for autism (for example, the Autism Diagnostic Interview – Revised), clinicians have been forced to rely on tools providing typical measures of psychiatric diagnoses. As some investigators have argued that the symptoms of several underlying psychiatric conditions may need to be weighted differently in mental retardation (for example, vegetative signs of depression), there is a need to establish more reliable and valid for groups with mental retardation.

Conclusions

Now that standardized, reliable, and valid tools have been developed to assess different domains, strength and weakness profiles can be established in each domain for children with mental retardation compared to typical children matched for mental age and chronological age, and in comparison with other people with mental retardation. These profiles can be conveyed in a uniform language of standard scores, percentile ranks, or equivalent-age scores.

Using psychometric measures for clinical purposes allows an invaluable standardized approach to diagnosis, but it does not do away with the need to consider broad clinical issues. A systematic, direct observation of each individual is fundamental, including their social and conversational interactions (appropriate to their developmental level). Given the within-subject variability existing even in the population with mental retardation, only an accurate assessment of each individual can lead to better diagnostic process and individualized intervention strategies.

References

Achenbach, T.M. (1991): *Manual for the Child Behavior Checklist 4/18 and 1991 profile*. Burlington, Vermont: University of Vermont, Department of Psychiatry.

Achenbach, T.M. & Rescorla, L.A. (2000): *Manual for the ASEBA preschool forms and profiles*. Burlington, Vermont: University of Vermont, Department of Psychiatry.

AAMR American Association on Mental Retardation (2002): *Mental retardation: definition, classification and system of support*, 10th ed. Washington DC: Library of Congress.

American Psychiatric Association (2000): *DSM-IV-TR: Diagnostic and statistical manual of mental disorders, 4th ed., text revision*. Milan: Masson.

Balboni, G., Pedrabissi, L., Molteni, M. & Villa, S. (2001): Discriminant validity of the Vineland scales: scores profiles of individuals with mental retardation and a specific disorder. *Am. J. Ment. Retard.* **106,** 162–172.

Carrol, J.B. (1997): The three-stratum theory of cognitive abilities. In: *Contemporary intellectual assessment: theories, tests, and issues*, eds. D.P. Flanagan, J.L. Genshaft & P.L. Harrison, pp. 122–130. New York: Guilford Press.

De Bildt, A., Kraijer, D., Sytema, S. & Minderaa, R. (2005): The psychometric properties of the Vineland adaptive behavior scales in children and adolescents with mental retardation. *J. Autism Dev. Disord.* **35,** 53–62.

Dykens, E.M. (2000): Psychopathology in children with intellectual disability. *J. Child Psychol. Psychiatry* **41,** 407–417.

Einfeld, S.L. & Tonge, B.J. (2002): *Manual for the Developmental Behaviour Checklist*, 2nd ed. Victoria: Monash University.

Frigerio, A., Cattaneo, C., Cataldo, M.G., Schiatti, A., Molteni, M. & Battaglia, M. (2004): Behavioral and emotional problems among Italian children and adolescents aged 4 to 18 years as reported by parents and teachers. *Eur. J. Psychol. Assess.* **20,** 124–133.

Frigerio, A., Cozzi, C., Pastore, V., Molteni, M., Borgatti, M. & Montirosso, R. (2006): La valutazione dei problemi emotivo comportamentali in un campione italiano di bambini in età prescolare attraverso la *Child Behavior Checklist* e il *Caregiver Teacher Report Form*. *Infanzia e Adolescenza* **5,** 24–37.

Gottfredson, L.S. (1997): Mainstream science on intelligence: an editorial with 52 signatories, history, and bibliography. *Intelligence* **24,** 13–23.

Greenspan, S. (1997): Dead manual walking? Why the 1992 AAMR definition needs redoing. *Educ. Train. Ment. Retard. Dev. Disabil.* **32,** 179–190.

Griffiths, R. (1984): *The abilities of young children. A comprehensive system of mental measure for the first eight years of life*. High Wycombe: The Test Agency.

Griffiths, R. (1996): *The Griffiths mental development scales: from birth to 2 years. Manual*. High Wycombe: The Test Agency.

Hodapp, R.M. (2002): Parenting children with mental retardation. In: *Handbook of parenting*, 2nd ed., ed. M. Bornstein, pp. 355–381. Hillsdale, New Jersey: Erlbaum.

Hodapp, R.M. & Dykens, E.M. (2005): Measuring behaviour in genetic disorders of mental retardation. *Ment. Retard. Dev. Disabil. Res. Rev.* **11,** 340–346.

Ivens, J. & Martin, N. (2002): A common metric for the Griffiths scales. *Arch. Dis. Child* **87,** 109–110.

Jopp, D.A. & Keys, C.B. (2001): Diagnostic overshadowing reviewed and reconsidered. *Am. J. Ment. Retard.* **106,** 416–433.

Orsini, A. & Picone, L. (1993): *WPPS: contributo alla taratura italiana*. Firenze: Organizzazioni Speciali.

Orsini, A. & Picone, L. (2006): *WISC-III: contributo alla taratura italiana*. Firenze: Organizzazioni Speciali.

Reiss, S. & Szyszko, J. (1983): Diagnostic overshadowing and professional experience with mentally retarded persons. *Am. J. Mental Defic.* **87,** 396–402.

Roid, G.H. & Miller, L.J. (1997): *Leiter International Performance Scale-Revised*. Wood Dale, Illinois: Stoeling (Italian translation by Organizzazioni Speciali, 2002).

Shevell, M., Ashwal, S., Donley, D., Flint, J., Gingold, M., Hirtz, D., Majnemer, A., Noetzel, M. & Sheth, R.D. (2003): Practice Committee of the Child Neurology Society. American Academy of Neurology and the Practice Parameter: evaluation of the child with global developmental delay. Report of the Quality Standards Subcommittee of the Practice Committee of the Child Neurology Society. *Neurology* **60,** 367–380.

Sparrow, S.S., Balla, D.A. & Cicchetti, D.V. (1984): *Vineland adaptive behavior scales*. Circe Pines, Minnesota: American Guidance Service. Italian adaptation by G. Balboni & L. Pedrabissi (2003): *Vineland adaptive behavior scales. Revisione della Vineland Social Maturity Scale di A. Doll. Forma completa*. Firenze: Organizzazioni Speciali.

Sternberg, R.J. (1988): *The triarchic mind: a new theory of human intelligence*. New York: Penguin Books.

Wechsler, D. (1944): *The measurement of adult intelligence*. Baltimore: Williams & Wilkins.

Wechsler, D. (1967): *Wechsler preschool and primary scale of intelligence*. San Antonio, Texas: Psychological Corporation, Harcourt Brace.

Wechsler, D. (1991): *Wechsler Intelligence Scale for Children-Third edition*. San Antonio, Texas: Psychological Corporation, Harcourt Brace.

Widmann, K.F. & McGrew, K.S. (1996): The structure of adaptive behaviour. In: *Manual of diagnosis and professional practice in mental retardation*, eds. J.W. Jacobson & J.A. Mulick, pp. 97–110. Washington, DC: American Psychological Association.

Chapter 2

Neurodiagnostics for children with mental retardation

Chiara Pantaleoni, Morena Doz, Sara Bulgheroni, Chiara Vago and Stefano D'Arrigo

Department of Developmental Neurology, Fondazione IRCCS Istituto Neurologico 'C. Besta', via Celoria 11, 20133 Milan, Italy
pantaleoni@istituto-besta.it

Summary

Mental retardation, or psychomotor developmental delay in younger children, is the common denominator of the majority of paediatric neurological diseases. It may have genetic causes or be due to central nervous system malformations, or to early pre-, peri-, or postnatal exogenous lesions. According to the numerous publications, the estimated likelihood of establishing the aetiology in cases of mental retardation varies considerably, from 10 per cent to 81 per cent.

This study concerns a series of 147 patients. A diagnosis was obtained in 51 per cent of these (57 per cent in the cases of psychomotor delay and 44 per cent in the cases with mental retardation). In relation to the severity of the deficiency, a diagnosis was reached in 48 per cent of the mildly retarded, 40 per cent of the moderately retarded, and 59 per cent of the severely retarded patients.

The diagnostic process is based primarily on a strict methodology, the first stage of which entails an accurate recording of the patient's clinical history, focusing on identifying risk factors in the child's family and personal history. It is essential that all children with psychomotor delay or mental retardation undergo a neuroradiological assessment, preferably brain magnetic resonance imaging. The other instrumental test that we consider useful in all patients is an electroencephalogram. In relation to genetic laboratory investigations, every patient should undergo standard karyotyping, molecular analyses for fragile-X syndrome, examination for subtelomeric rearrangements, and finally comparative genomic hybridization (array-CGH), the latest cytogenetic-molecular technique.

Introduction

Mental retardation, or psychomotor developmental delay in younger children, is the common denominator of the majority of paediatric neurological diseases. It may have genetic causes (particularly numerical or structural chromosome anomalies or single gene mutations), or be due to central nervous system (CNS) malformations, or to early pre-, peri-, or postnatal exogenous lesions (van Karnebeek *et al.*, 2005a), but the defect underlying the condition often remains unknown (Wilska & Kaski, 2001). According to numerous reports, the estimated likelihood of establishing the aetiology in cases of mental retardation varies considerably, from 10 to 81 per cent. Such a wide variability can be attributed to numerous factors, including the heterogeneity of the reported case series, the severity of the mental retardation in the sample studied, the extensiveness of the instrumental investigations undertaken, and technological advances in the available tools and in genetic and radiological techniques in particular (Shevell *et al.*, 2003).

Our aim in this paper is to present a personal case series of patients with mental retardation or psychomotor delay and to discuss the diagnostic significance of the instrumental investigations conducted.

Methods

This study involved a series of 147 patients consecutively referred to the Developmental Neurology Department of the Istituto Neurologico C. Besta during the year 2005. The patient selection criterion for this study was a diagnosis at presentation of psychomotor delay or mental retardation.

On arrival, a clinical history was obtained in all patients, who then underwent general clinical assessment and neurological examination. A developmental scale or intelligence test (Griffiths Developmental Scale, Leiter-R, WIPPSI, WISC-R) was administered to all children to assess, confirm, and quantify the suspected diagnosis. Subjects with an IQ of 85 or more were excluded from the study.

Based on the information collected at this stage, specific instrumental investigations were prescribed case by case, including routine blood chemistry tests (white blood cell count, red cell count, platelets, glucose, nitrogen, electrolytes, aspartate transaminase, alanine transaminase, creatine phosphokinase, phosphocreatine, total proteins, and coagulation tests); brain magnetic resonance imaging (MRI); electroencephalography (EEG), both awake and asleep; multimodal evoked potentials, electromyography/electroneurography; metabolic and genetic screening; and a muscle biopsy.

Results

The sample consisted of 147 patients, amounting to 37.8 per cent of all those referred to the department during 2005. The male to female ratio was 1.6:1 (62 per cent male and 38 per cent female). Patients with psychomotor delay (aged less than 5 years) accounted for 54.4 per cent of the sample, while 45.6 per cent were mentally retarded. Mental retardation was mild in 39 per cent, moderate in 22 per cent, and severe in 39 per cent.

A diagnosis was obtained in 51 per cent of the cases (in 57 per cent with psychomotor delay and in 44 per cent with mental retardation). A diagnosis was reached in 48 per cent of the mildly retarded patients, in 40 per cent of the moderate retarded group, and in 59 per cent of the severely retarded group.

The diagnoses were distributed as follows: genetic syndromes (31 per cent), infantile cerebral palsy (29.7 per cent), pervasive developmental disorder (13.6 per cent), CNS malformations (8.1 per cent), metabolic-degenerative diseases (8.1 per cent), neuromuscular diseases (6.7 per cent), and neurocutaneous syndromes (2.8 per cent).

Discussion

The diagnostic process is based primarily on strict methodology, the first stage of which entails an accurate recording of the patient's clinical history, focusing on identifying risk factors in the child's family and personal history (van Karnebeek et al., 2005b). It is worth emphasizing the importance of tracing the family tree back at least three generations, and assessing other family pathologies and the recurrence of miscarriages. In the child's personal history, it is essential to consider any pre- or perinatal problems and to inquire about threatened miscarriages and maternal intercurrent diseases, the use of medications, exposure to environmental risks, instrumental assessments (serology, ultrasound, amniocentesis), weight gain, and the onset and features of fetal movements. Concerning delivery and the perinatal period, it is important to record gestational age, duration of labour, neonatal anthropometric measurements, Apgar score, any need for intensive care, suckling characteristics, and whether there was jaundice, tremor or convulsions.

On the subject of the child's personal history, it is necessary also to consider how the pathological elements emerged during the child's psychomotor development, and whether the signs recorded remained stable or improved with the progressive acquisition of new capabilities. This information helps to orient the diagnosis towards 'static' forms, whereas progression of the symptoms and the loss of previously acquired capabilities points to a diagnosis of progressive degenerative or metabolic forms.

Then comes the clinical assessment, which primarily involves a general examination to record the auxological variables and a study of the growth curves, with a precise identification of both major malformations and minor anomalies (dysmorphisms), of which there must be at least three to be deemed significant. This last feature demands careful observation and measurements, taking care to refer the findings to standards of normality (Jones, 1997). However, while it is important to define any dysmorphisms accurately, it is equally useful and sometimes diagnostic to make a global assessment of the phenotype, the Gestalt, which can sometimes suggest a first diagnostic hypothesis. Of course, such a hypothesis must then be validated or rejected by a more in-depth assessment. It is worth emphasizing that collections of photographs, possibly including the other members of the child's family, can prove helpful when it comes to reassessing the case over time.

In a more strictly neurological context, it is important to search carefully for signs of CNS and peripheral nervous system involvement and to carry out a clinical evaluation of the child's visual and auditory functions. The clinical neurological assessment can be supported by tools for evaluating the child's cognitive state – scales that allow a qualitative and quantitative definition of any cognitive deficiencies. Depending on the child's age, there are various tests for assessing global cognitive function, which can be expressed as an intelligence quotient (IQ), development quotient, or mental age. To define the behavioural phenotype, clinical observations (based on serial observations of the child in different environmental settings) can be supported by standardized tests that enable a qualitative and quantitative evaluation of the behavioural disorder.

Having completed the clinical assessment, we can proceed with the instrumental investigations suggested by our clinical suspicions. In our opinion, it is essential for all children with psychomotor delay or mental retardation to undergo a neuroradiological assessment, preferably brain MRI. This test is a fundamental starting point, in combination with the clinical findings, to orient the diagnostic process: it enables to identify alterations indicative of pre- and perinatal brain damage, malformational/dysplastic conditions, and changes suggestive of metabolic or degenerative disease (Battaglia, 2003). That is not all. MRI is also useful when it identifies no pathological signs, as this enables us to rule out a number of disorders and thus concentrate on other possible conditions.

In a recent complex study by the American Academy of Neurology, a thorough meta-analysis was conducted on 160 previously published retrospective and prospective reports on the diagnosis of psychomotor delay (Shevell *et al.*, 2003). In evaluating the diagnostic weight of the single investigations, the Academy adopted a cut-off of one per cent for diagnostic significance (or diagnostic yield). Brain MRI was attributed a value of 48 per cent, so this assessment method was strongly recommended, particularly (but not exclusively) in the case of neurological signs. As Moeschler emphasized in 2006 – in a paper from the American Academy of Pediatrics that analysed the Shevell study – there was no mention of the diagnostic value of a negative MRI, but this is nonetheless considerable because it enables us to rule out with a fair degree of certainty any traumatic, malformational or degenerative anomalies of the CNS and so concentrate on the conditions in which such anomalies are not involved (Moeschler *et al.*, 2006).

The other instrumental test that we consider useful in all patients with psychomotor or mental retardation is EEG. There is no consensus in the literature concerning this test; however, Shevell awards the test a diagnostic power of 0.4 per cent – that is, below the cut-off point for significance. In our opinion, EEG is a non-invasive, easily conducted, and essential test because, in addition to providing information on the brain's functional organization, it can also identify any epileptiform anomalies (even in the absence of clinical symptoms) and any patterns suggestive of specific conditions which may correlate with certain syndromes or cerebral degeneration and malformation processes.

On the other hand, we agree with Shevell that investigations into the child's metabolism should be reserved for patients whose clinical data and MRI are specifically suspect (Shevell *et al.*, 2003). In particular, clinical data suggestive of such a diagnosis include affected blood relatives in the family tree, familial recurrence, stoppage/regression of psychomotor development, feeding difficulties and growth disorders, and hepatosplenomegaly (Papavasiliou *et al.*, 2000). When clinical data are suggestive of a metabolic condition, the diagnostic yield of such tests rises, according to Shevell, to five per cent, while general screening in all patients – including blood gas analysis, blood ammonia, blood and urinary amino acids, and urinary organic acids – would have a diagnostic yield of around one per cent. As for genetic laboratory investigations, every mentally retarded patient should undergo standard karyotyping with a resolution of at least 500 bands. It is worth making the point here that, given the rapid evolution of cytogenetic techniques, it may be a good idea to repeat these tests if 5 years have elapsed since they were first done. However, cytogenetic analyses such as high resolution karyotyping with pro-metaphasic banding above 850 bands, fluorescent in-situ hybridization (FISH), and karyotype analysis on skin fibroblasts, are only recommended to confirm a clinical suspicion (Chelly *et al.*, 2006).

Molecular analyses on samples of DNA or RNA to detect gene defects responsible for the disorder should again be prescribed only on the strength of a clinical hypothesis (Reymond & Tarpey, 2006). The only exception to this rule, in our opinion, concerns the molecular analysis for fragile-X syndrome, which is mandatory in all cases of mental retardation not otherwise classified, irrespective of the patient's sex, unless the patient has microcephaly, which rules out the diagnosis. The significance of molecular investigations for fragile-X syndrome increases from 2.6 per cent to 7.6 per cent, according to Shevell, if clinical preselection of patients is conducted on the strength of the following variables: a family history of mental retardation; distinctive facial features (high forehead, prognathism, large ears); joint hyperextensibility; soft and fleshy skin on the palms of the hands; macro-orchidism; and a peculiar behavioural phenotype characterized by initial shyness and lack of eye contact followed by excessive friendliness and verbosity (Shevell *et al.*, 2003).

According to recently published data, subtelomeric rearrangements are responsible for approximately five per cent of cases of mental retardation (de Vries *et al.*, 2003). Testing for this condition is recommended in the presence of several factors: a family history of mental retardation; delayed intrauterine growth; postnatal growth anomalies (excessive or insufficient growth); at least two dysmorphic facial features, and one or more extra-facial dysmorphic features; and congenital malformations. The latest cytogenetic-molecular technique is comparative genomic hybridization, or array-CGH (Shaw-Smith et al., 2004). This method enables a simultaneous and highly specific assessment of several chromosome regions and thus identifies cryptic chromosome imbalances of the order of a few dozen kilobases in a single experiment. This investigation is currently only available at a few laboratories, but will hopefully soon become more readily accessible, as early results carry the promise that it will make a significant contribution to the diagnostic process.

References

Battaglia, A. (2003): Neuroimaging studies in the evaluation of developmental delay/mental retardation. *Am. J. Med. Genet. C Semin. Med. Genet.* **117**, 25–30.

Chelly, J., Khelfaoui, M., Francis F., Cherif, B. & Bienvenu, T. (2006): Genetics and pathophysiology of mental retardation. *Eur. J. Hum. Genet.* **14**, 701–713.

de Vries, B.B., Winter, A., Schinzel, A. & van Ravenswaaij-Arts, C. (2003): Telomeres: a diagnosis at the end of the chromosomes. *J. Med. Genet.* **40**, 385–398.

Jones, K.L. (1997): Normal standards. In: *Smith's recognizable patterns of human malformation*, ed. K.L. Jones, pp. 747–770. Philadelphia: W.B. Saunders Co.

Moeschler, J.B., Shevell, M. & the Committee on Genetics (2006): Clinical genetic evaluation of the child with mental retardation or developmental delays. *Pediatrics* **117**, 2304–2316.

Papavasiliou, A.S., Bazigou, H., Paraskevoulakos, E. & Kotsalis, C. (2000): Neurometabolic testing in developmental delay. *J. Child Neurol.* **15**, 620–622.

Reymond, F.L. & Tarpey, P. (2006): The genetics of mental retardation. *Hum. Mol. Genet.* **15**, 110–116.

Shaw-Smith, C., Redon, R., Rickman, L., Rio, M., Willatt, L., Fiegler, H., Firth, H., Sanlaville, D., Winter, R., Colleaux, L., Bobrow, M. & Carter, N.P. (2004): Microarray based comparative genomic hybridisation (array-CGH) detects submicroscopic chromosomal deletions and duplications in patients with learning disability/mental retardation and dysmorphic features. *J. Med. Genet.* **41**, 241–248.

Shevell, M., Ashwal, S., Donley, D., Flint, J. Gingold, M., Hirtz, D., Majnemer, A., Noetzel, M. & Sheth, R.D. (2003): Practice parameter: evaluation of the child with global developmental delay: report of the Quality Standards Subcommittee of the American Academy of Neurology and The Practice Committee of the Child Neurology Society. *Neurology* **60**, 367–380.

van Karnebeek, C.D., Scheper, F.Y., Abeling, N.G., Alders, M., Barth, P.G. Hoovers, J.M., Koevoets, C., Wanders, R.J. & Hennekam, R. (2005a): Etiology of mental retardation in children referred to a tertiary care center: a prospective study. *Am. J. Ment. Retard.* **110**, 253–267.

van Karnebeek, C.D., Jansweijer, M.C., Leenders, A.G., Offringa, M. & Hennekam, R. (2005b): Diagnostic investigations in individuals with mental retardation: a systematic literature review of their usefulness. *Eur. J. Hum. Genet.* **13**, 6–25.

Wilska, M.L. & Kaski, M.K. (2001): Why and how to assess the aetiological diagnosis of children with intellectual disability/mental retardation and other neurodevelopmental disorders: description of the Finnish approach. *Eur. J. Paediatr. Neurol.* **5**, 7–13.

Chapter 3

Mental retardation and epilepsy

Thierry Deonna and Eliane Roulet-Perez

Neuropaediatric Unit, CHUV, rue du Bugnon 46, 1011 Lausanne, Switzerland
Thierry.Deonna@chuv.ch

Summary

In all chronic neurodevelopmental disorders of childhood (mental retardation, autism, cerebral palsies), epilepsy is a frequent occurrence. However, the type of epilepsy, the nature of the association between epilepsy and the basic disability, and the importance of epilepsy in the overall functional handicap of the child can be very different. Many clinical studies on this topic – particularly in autistic disorders – have recently appeared and the same general logical questions apply to children with mental retardation who are not autistic (Roulet-Perez & Deonna, 2006).
It is also useful to draw on the experience of the minority of normal children with epilepsy but whose seizures (or bioelectrical disorder as seen on electroencephalography) affect their cognitive functions or behaviour, whether transiently or more rarely permanently. Although this is a rare occurrence in the absence of progressive underlying brain disease, these situations may be very informative about the possible direct causal or aggravating role of epilepsy in developing mental function.
In this chapter we review the different aetiologies of associated mental retardation and epilepsy, including recently recognized genetic and metabolic disorders. The special diagnostic and therapeutic problems of epilepsy in the presence of a cognitive handicap and their implications for management are particularly emphasized. Finally, the issue of prognosis and drug withdrawal is discussed.

Introduction

It is surprising that most modern textbooks on childhood epilepsy do not have a chapter specifically devoted to the frequent and most important topic of mental retardation and epilepsy, despite its great practical importance, though there are notable exceptions (see Sillanpää, 2004). This probably reflects an overnarrow view, predominant among epileptologists and centred on epileptic syndromes and antiepileptic therapy, with less emphasis on the complex interrelations between epilepsy and mental handicap and the consequences of epilepsy in the life of these children.

Any professional dealing regularly with children (or adults) suffering from mental handicap will be faced with the reality of epilepsy. Epilepsy occurs in about one-third of all people with severe intellectual disability and in about one-sixth of those with mild intellectual disability. The same pathology is most often responsible for both epilepsy and intellectual disability, which are two independent manifestation of the basic condition. When there is associated cerebral palsy, the likelihood of epilepsy is greater, because cerebral palsy is often the result of acquired focal or multifocal prenatal, perinatal, or early postnatal destructive lesions of the brain, mainly cortical, which can be highly epileptogenic. These basic facts should not obscure other more challenging considerations: there are children with severe mental retardation or specific mental retardation syndromes in whom epilepsy is not at all a frequent occurrence. On the other hand, there are children with severe epilepsies who have and retain normal cognitive function. Finally, some epilepsies may, though rarely, be a cause of acquired mental handicap or significantly aggravate a pre-existing one. These examples show that the relation between mental retardation and epilepsy has many different facets which need to be examined separately.

Aetiological aspects

As mentioned above, among the different brain pathologies that cause mental retardation some are much more commonly associated with epilepsy than others (Table 1). Epilepsy can start very early, be quite severe, and have special clinical and electroencephalographic (EEG) characteristics. We will review these conditions.

Table 1. Aetiological categories of linkage between epilepsy and mental retardation

Chromosomal disorders associated with epilepsy
Special brain malformations associated with epilepsy
Acquired brain damage with resulting mental retardation and epilepsy
Epileptic syndromes with mental regression ('epileptic encephalopathies')
Some partial epilepsies with cognitive regression (CSWS)
Metabolic diseases with epilepsy as the initial or main symptom

Chromosomal disorders and epilepsy

There are several 'classical' and an increasing number of newly recognized chromosomal disorders causing mental retardation in which epilepsy is a constant or at least a very frequent feature, often but not always from very early on in life. Table 2 has been constructed from the detailed review of this topic carried out by Battaglia & Guerrini (2005). It is important to note that some of the disorders listed have quite specific seizure and EEG characteristics – for instance, non-convulsive status epilepticus in ring-chromosome 20 (Roubertie *et al.*, 2000), which are usefully detailed in this review. These may be clues to the underlying genetic disorder. In the practical management of the child (special seizure manifestations, drug response, prognosis, and so on), it is important to know the clinical characteristics of the epileptic syndrome and the reader should refer to this review when managing a mentally handicapped child with a genetic syndrome of this type.

From Table 2 it is clear that epilepsy is an important feature of aberrations affecting different chromosomes, implying that the ultimate mechanisms of epilepsy must be multiple. The best known and most severe epilepsies are those seen in mutations affecting chromosome 15 (typically Angelman syndrome), which carry genes involved in inhibitory γ-aminobutyric acid (GABA) neurotransmission.

The recent recognition that epilepsy may be caused by a chromosomal anomaly in the absence of dysmorphism and in children with a normal intellect (at least initially) is quite challenging

Table 2. Chromosomal syndromes associated with epilepsy (constructed from a review by Battaglia & Guerrini, 2005)

Syndrome	Chromosome
Del 1p36 syndrome	1
Del 4p (Wolf-Hirschhorn) syndrome	4
Trisomy 12p syndrome	12
Ring-chromosome 14 syndrome	14
Angelman syndrome	15
Inv-dup or Idic(15) syndrome	15
Ring-chromosome 20 syndrome	20
Trisomy 21 (Down's) syndrome	21
Fragile-X syndrome	X
Klinefelter (XXY) syndrome	XX

and has been only rarely studied, apart from the now well recognized ring-20 syndrome. Macleod *et al.* have recently reported 10 young children with normal phenotypes and severe epilepsy requiring several drugs (Macleod *et al.*, 2005). Three had normal development before the onset of epilepsy (all three had ring-X 20) and seven had a mild developmental retardation: ring 14 (one child); ring 20 (four children); 47XXY (two children); and others (three children). The genetic diagnosis had been delayed and these particular causes of epilepsy are probably underrecognized. Hints for a diagnosis of a chromosomal disorder were refractory seizures, multiple seizure types, and an interictal EEG showing spike and slow wave abnormalities. The fact that some children had normal or only mildly delayed early development and later deteriorated with the onset and severe evolution of epilepsy suggests a direct contributory role of the epilepsy itself or its treatment.

Brain malformations and epilepsy

Severe diffuse brain malformations such as holoprosencephaly, lissencephaly, and pachygyria are almost always associated with epilepsy in addition to severe mental retardation. In others, such as double cortex syndrome (band heterotopia), tuberous sclerosis, and hypothalamic hamartoma, epilepsy may be very severe and in itself contribute significantly to the mental handicap, which is not always severe or may even be absent, at least initially.

Acquired brain damage with resulting mental deficiency and epilepsy

In a small percentage of children, mental retardation is caused by a postnatally acquired brain disease with epilepsy as a sequel. Epilepsy is occasionally very severe or resistant, especially in multifocal destructive cortical lesions (for example, post-meningitic, post-encephalitic, or post-traumatic) and may be the main disability. The damage caused by cerebral malaria is a common example in developing countries.

Acquired prenatal destructive vascular or inflammatory disorders (for example, toxoplasmosis) can be the cause of mental deficiency and epilepsy, but usually with major motor signs as well (cerebral palsy).

Metabolic diseases with epilepsy as initial or main symptom

Epilepsy is an early and often severe manifestation of many brain diseases caused by genetic neurometabolic disorders. There is often severe and progressive mental deterioration, almost always with abnormal motor signs, although epilepsy may be the first sign of the disease (for example, in Lafora disease and ceroid-lipofuscinosis). The question is whether apparently idiopathic generalized seizures can be a unique early sign or a manifestation of a treatable metabolic disease in children with mild developmental delay. Glucose transporter deficiency type 1 (GLUT-1 deficiency) may be one of these conditions (Wang et al., 2005). Characteristics are intractable seizures starting in early infancy, acquired microcephaly, and developmental delay. However 'formes frustes' with less severe epilepsy and no microcephaly do exist. They have not been reported in detail yet and are a diagnostic challenge (Roulet-Perez, 2007).

Epileptic encephalopathies

These are conditions in which deterioration results mainly from epileptic activity with the exclusion of progressive neurodegenerative diseases (Dulac, 2001). They typically include West syndrome (infantile spasms with hypsarrhythmia), Lennox-Gastaut syndrome, myoclonic-astatic epilepsy, and severe myoclonic epilepsy of infancy (SEMI or Dravet syndrome). Investigators sometimes include Landau-Kleffner syndrome and partial epilepsies with continuous spikes and waves during slow sleep (CSWS), or even extend the concept to Rasmussen's encephalitis and Sturge-Weber syndrome.

Without entering into this debate, the fact that some epilepsies – either clinically very severe or with continuously abnormal epileptic activity on EEG – can be the cause of cognitive regression and permanent mental defect is the main justification for the term 'epileptic encephalopathy'. It has the merit of alerting physicians to the important and sometimes preventable mental consequences of these epilepsies and other practical implications for management.

Acquired cognitive impairment as a result of epilepsy

With some chronic epilepsies the child may have initially normal mental development, but then shows cognitive stagnation and with the passage of time brain function enters the mentally retarded range. If the epilepsy is very severe the child may even present with mental regression (dementia), but after a period there is stabilization and the child is left with mental deficiency and the same general learning/behavioural/adaptation problems as one with a fixed congenital mental handicap of similar severity. This is relatively rare in the general population of children with mental retardation and epilepsy, but it is important to discuss it here in some detail. First, it is a potentially treatable cause of mental retardation. Second, it obliges one to consider the possible additional direct or indirect effects of epilepsy on cognitive functions in any mentally retarded child who develops epilepsy, or in whom known epilepsy worsens.

Fig. 1 shows schematically the various different evolutionary patterns of cognitive function over time in a child suffering from an epilepsy which directly affects brain areas that influence cognitive function, or in which other indirect consequences of the epileptic disease may lead to mental retardation. Note that the child may have a normal or nearly normal early development, or may already be mentally retarded, with the epilepsy only aggravating a pre-existing handicap. Such long-term evolutionary patterns – which can differ markedly and which are only rarely documented in a prospective fashion over many years – are well known to

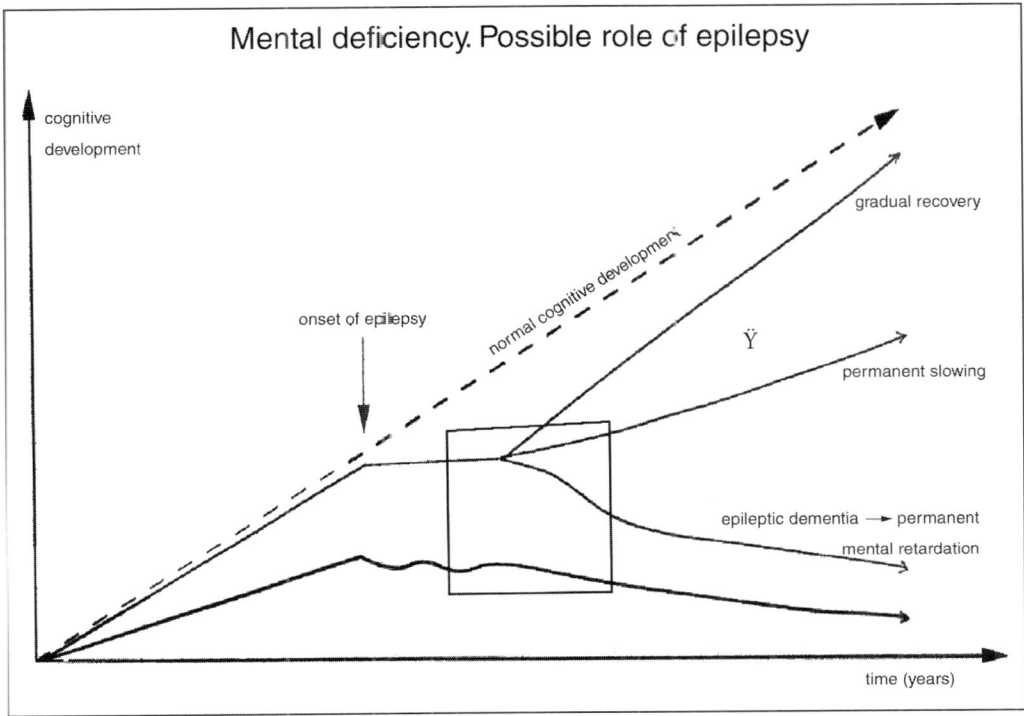

Fig. 1. Schematic diagram of the possible effects of epilepsy on cognitive development.

experienced clinicians working in residential institutions or special schools for children with severe epilepsy (Chaudhry & Pond, 1961; Besag, 1987). Cognitive stagnation, intermittent or permanent regression, or gradual late improvement – sometimes remarkable and unexpected – can all be seen. Many different factors may account for these variable outcomes. We will focus only on those children in whom disease evolution is directly or indirectly related to the epileptic disorder, and not those rare cases in which epilepsy is symptomatic of a progressive brain disease (unusual neurometabolic disorder, tumour, chronic viral infection, and so on). One should always keep this latter possibility in mind, even in children in whom the initial work-up did not reveal any recognizable and potentially progressive brain disease.

Fig. 2, which is an enlargement of what is represented in the square shown in Fig. 1, attempts to analyse in a different fashion the evolution of cognitive function over time. The development of a child who maintains stable cognitive functions despite epilepsy (that is, who learns at a level that can be expected from his basic abilities) is represented by the horizontal upper line of the graph. Any decrease – short or more protracted, temporary or permanent (graphically shown by the downward 'drop' of the baseline) – can be considered an effect of the epilepsy in a global sense. Note that the time scale may be weeks, months, or years in this scheme. The term 'state-dependent' has been coined to refer to these fluctuating, variably prolonged, and severe reductions in cognitive performance which should alert the physician to look actively for a potentially treatable factor related to the epilepsy. These can go unrecognized or be misinterpreted. Subtle clinical epileptic activity during the day (for instance non-convulsive status epilepticus) or during the night, the effects of epileptic discharges (especially during sleep, the so-called continuous spike-waves during sleep or CSWS), and the side effects of

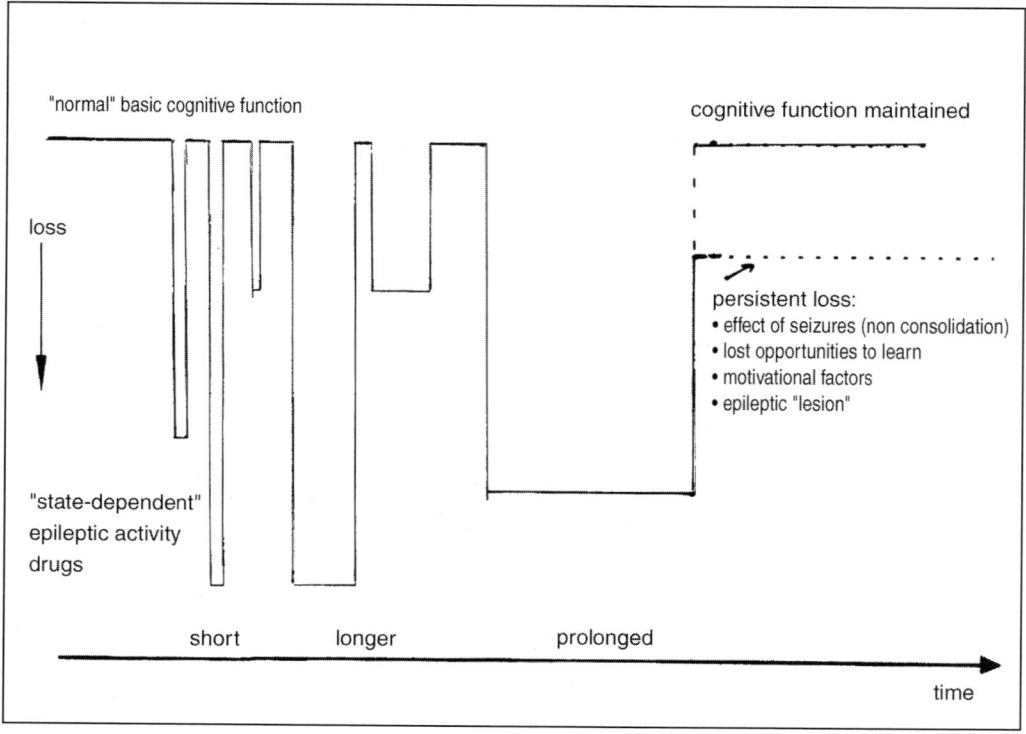

Fig. 2. Intermittent and persistent acquired cognitive 'epileptic' dysfunction. (This is an enlarged view of what is included in the square in Fig. 1.)

antiepileptic drugs (even with normal serum drug levels and particularly with polytherapy) are the main possibilities. The many possible ramifications of the neurobiological factors related to epileptic disease and the potential psychological factors are beyond the scope of this chapter (see Deonna & Roulet-Perez, 2005).

In recent years, awareness that some epilepsies can manifest mainly or exclusively as an acquired and sometimes insidious cognitive disorder ('cognitive epilepsies') – namely acquired epileptic aphasia (Landau-Kleffner syndrome) or partial epilepsy with continuous spike-waves during sleep, sometimes with severe mental deterioration and 'psychosis' – has contributed to a new concept of the relation between cognitive function and epilepsy. Intense focal or multifocal EEG epileptic activity during the day such as focal sharp waves (FSW) and continuous activity during sleep (CSWS), with usually neither frequent nor severe epileptic seizures, is the hallmark of these syndromes. Importantly, these epilepsies often have a relapsing-remitting course during the most formative childhood years, with a variable or only temporary response to antiepileptic drugs. During the 'active epilepsy' period, loss of language, severe attention deficit disorder, cognitive arrest, various perceptive disorders, and behavioural problems with psychotic features can all occur, depending both on the function of cortical areas specifically involved and on the secondarily diffuse epileptic activity during sleep. When the prefrontal areas are involved, behavioural and cognitive disturbances can be extremely severe and long lasting and if untreated (or resistant to therapy) can be the cause of permanent mental retardation. These 'acquired epileptic frontal syndromes' (Roulet-Perez, 1993) show that the effect of partial epilepsy on cognition and behaviour is fundamentally different depending on whether or not it involves cortical areas which have a crucial integrative function, such as the prefrontal cortex. These cases probably constitute only a minority of all the children in whom epilepsy and mental retardation co-occur, but increasing recognition of such syndromes, more routine use of sleep EEG, and magnetic resonance imaging (MRI) of the brain indicate that these situations are not particularly rare and may be underdiagnosed. They can occur in children without visible brain lesions (idiopathic or cryptogenic cases) as well as in children with various focal brain lesions (symptomatic cases), including or even sometimes limited to the thalamus.

We exclude from this discussion those young children with the epileptic encephalopathies (Lennox-Gastaut syndrome, myoclonic-astatic epilepsy, Dravet syndrome) with refractory severe multiple seizure types, status epilepticus, or needing several antiepileptic drugs, in which these factors (and possibly the natural history of the basic brain disorder) play a role.

Sequelae of major status epilepticus

Mental deficiency as a sequel of major status epilepticus is exceptional in children with 'epilepsy only'. When it occurs, there was either previously unrecognized brain pathology or an acute insult to the nervous system which was the cause of the status epilepticus. In epileptic encephalopathies (see above), episodes of status epilepticus can aggravate the basic, often progressive, mental handicap.

Since the advent of MRI, bilateral damage to the hippocampus – a structure highly sensitive to the effect of prolonged seizures, especially in young children with repeated febrile status epilepticus – has been described. This hippocampal atrophy may occur first on one side and later on, during another episode of status epilepticus, on the other side as well. If this and adjacent crucial structures are affected on both sides, major regression combining severe mental retardation and autistic behaviour may ensue (DeLong & Heinz, 1997). This may be an under-recognized cause of acquired mental retardation/autism in early severe epilepsies, differing from the typical hypoxic-ischaemic damage which can occasionally result from prolonged major seizures.

Diagnosis of epilepsy in mental retardation

The importance of recognizing the numerous paroxysmal 'non-epileptic' neurological disorders is rightly stressed in basic modern neuropaediatric teaching because the list of such often bizarre symptoms is very large. In the past, an erroneous diagnosis of epilepsy was often made, with dire consequences. As epilepsy is the most common type of paroxysmal disorder with neurological symptoms, it is always the first diagnosis to be considered, and certainly more so if such an episode occurs *de novo* in a child with mental retardation, where epilepsy is known to be so frequent. If a mentally retarded child has already been diagnosed as having epilepsy, it is natural to think that any new paroxysmal manifestation is epileptic without thinking further. However, the same exercise of analysing paroxysmal symptoms in each new or repeated circumstance is necessary. We recall several instances in which syncope, a migraine attack, an acute dystonic phenomenon, a complex tic, or a cataleptic attack (Coffin-Lowry syndrome) was mistaken as epilepsy in a mentally retarded child.

There are specific reasons why the positive diagnosis of epilepsy may be difficult. First, the child may be unable to express particular sensory, vegetative or motor symptoms which can be so useful in the diagnosis of epilepsy. If the seizure manifestations have a cognitive component (loss of vigilance, arrest of purposeful activity, loss of language, or a global temporary decrease in cognitive performances), this will be less noticeable in a child with a basic low level of function. This is also true of the behaviour in the postictal state, when confusion or mental slowing can often suggest that a preceding seizure has occurred but was not witnessed.

On the other hand, the inner sensations or other symptoms (vegetative, fatigue) that may be experienced during the seizure or more often in the postictal state (and their sudden onset) which cannot be explained by the patient may cause an emotional reaction with a marked change in behaviour (panic, regression, aggression, irritability) which can be extreme and more severe than the seizure itself.

Finally, when the symptoms are indisputably epileptic, it remains to classify the seizure type, to see whether it corresponds to a known epileptic syndrome and if it can be attributed to the basic brain disease which caused the mental handicap. One should remember that idiopathic-genetic childhood epilepsies are very frequent and may occur in a child with mental retardation (for instance, petit mal epilepsy, Rolandic epilepsy, juvenile myoclonic epilepsy). This has obvious prognostic and therapeutic implications. The diagnosis may be complicated by the fact the EEG, which is so important in the diagnosis of specific epileptic syndromes, may be difficult to obtain or may give incomplete information (no sleep reached, no photic stimulation done, and so on).

Stereotypies and self-induced syncopes in mentally handicapped children

Epilepsy and stereotypies frequently co-occur in mentally retarded children as two different phenomena without any causal link, especially in retarded children who are autistic as well. Occasionally, complex partial seizures ('epileptic automatisms' or 'epileptic stereotypies'), which are manifestation of epilepsy of frontal origin can present with stereotyped movements ('clapping', 'applause', 'turning in a circle', and so on) which are mistaken for a 'common' non-epileptic stereotypy. The problem is likely to arise in young children with developmental delay and autistic behaviour, in whom these seizures may aggravate the overall functioning or even be its major cause (for details of these manifestations and the difficulty in their diagnosis, see Deonna *et al.*, 2002). Stereotypies may appear *de novo* in children who have mental regression following major status epilepticus, or during periods of intense epileptic activity on the EEG in children with 'non-convulsive status epilepticus', or during the active phases of Lennox-Gastaut syndrome in which children may have a temporary cognitive and behavioural regression for days or weeks), or briefly in a postictal state. These probably represent a release of lower motor programmes.

Rett syndrome is a typical example of a severe mental retardation syndrome in which there are constant multiple motor and more complex behavioural stereotypies and a high incidence of epilepsy. Affected girls often have bouts of intermittent crying and panic and episodes of hyperpnoea followed by apnoea and staring, both very disturbing and sometimes difficult to differentiate from epileptic manifestations which these girls also have, and which may be resistant to antiepileptic therapy.

Self-induced syncopes or presyncopes can be seen as the consequence of a respiratory stereotypy with self-induced apnoea after a forced expiration or Valsalva manœuvre. Abnormal gesturing can be followed by a brief loss of tone and unconsciousness and if more severe can lead to convulsive syncope. The differential diagnosis from epilepsy can be very difficult because these children may also have an independent true epilepsy (Gastaut *et al.*, 1982).

Management

Psychological impact of newly diagnosed epilepsy in a child with mental retardation

When epilepsy starts in a child with known mental retardation and after the family has started to adjust to the tragic reality and the many problems related to the handicap, the occurrence of epilepsy is felt to be a new disaster. There is fear that a seizure will compromise or limit the painstakingly acquired basic skills, independence or school knowledge, or worse, aggravate the basic handicap. Fortunately, this is not the case in the great majority of children and that should be emphasized.

The difficulty in having the child 'accept' and take regular daily medication and the fear that side effects will aggravate his mental functioning are also frequently in the parents' or caretakers' mind. Some institutions also have an *a priori* policy of avoiding any drugs acting on the nervous system. An opposite view is that the epilepsy was an unrecognized feature of the handicap and possibly a causal one, generating the hope that antiepileptic treatment will facilitate learning. Although this may exceptionally occur (see below), it should be stressed that this is not the main aim of therapy.

The special impact of epilepsy in various chronic neurological disorders

The special impact of epilepsy in various chronic neurological disorders is summarized in Table 3. Co-morbidity of mental retardation with autism or cerebral palsy, or both, is frequent. Autonomy, social relations, and work opportunities and abilities may depend as much on these associated handicaps as on the degree of mental handicap, especially in mildly or moderately retarded persons. Are the life consequences of epilepsy or the impact on the family any different in each of these handicaps? Frequent epileptic seizures in a mentally handicapped child can limit the amount of independence that parents and caretakers are willing to give but are so important to acquire. Seizures may temporarily disrupt the limited amount of attention motivation, and reasoning ability of which the child is capable at his best. This can be true but may be only anticipated or feared by the parents, adding to the overall burden of epilepsy. In children with cerebral palsy, seizures may worsen the already limited but useful walking capacity (increased ataxia, focal postictal weakness, fatigue, and so on) and lead to loss of independence. The risk of falls with severe injuries in such children is a special worry, although surprisingly this seems to occur relatively rarely (Vallenga *et al.*, 2006) except in children with refractory epileptic drop attacks. In autistic children, in whom a major problem is coping with novelty and adapting to changing circumstances, the experience of seizures themselves, the medical appointments, and the special investigations (EEGs for example) are difficult to tolerate and can aggravate the behavioural problems.

Table 3. Special impact of epilepsy in chronic neurological disorders

Main handicap	Special impact of epilepsy
Cerebral palsy	Impact on motor functions (falls, dysequilibrium, increased paresis)
Mental deficiency	Loss of independence, psychological consequences (possible cognitive decline)
Autistic disorders	Exacerbation of behaviour problems (change in routine, medical interventions)
Sensory handicaps (deafness, blindness)	Communication about symptoms; cerebral compensation (atypical brain organization)

Quality of sleep, mental retardation and epilepsy

Good sleep is fundamental for optimal cognitive functioning, and sleep disturbance is a cause of irritability and emotional distress in anyone. In children with diffuse brain disease, stable sleep organization is often delayed and remains abnormal, being complicated by secondary bad sleep habits. Epilepsy, which often occurs during sleep, can aggravate the situation in several ways by disturbing the quality of sleep and decreasing the optimal level of daytime functioning. Attention to all the factors that can aggravate the quality of sleep and all the possible remedies to improve or normalize sleep are an integral part of epilepsy management, but this is especially important in mentally handicapped children in whom basic sleep function is so often compromised.

Problems of antiepileptic therapy in mentally retarded children

The indications for starting continuous prophylactic antiepileptic therapy in newly diagnosed epilepsy, and which specific drug to use, should follow the same principles as in any other child. However, several considerations are especially important in the context of mental retardation. There will be a tendency to think that, even if the child has had only one or few seizures, these will be likely to recur when there is a chronic brain disease. However, some mentally retarded children may have occasional seizures, not necessarily severe and only occurring in certain circumstances known to lower the seizure threshold; in these circumstances chronic therapy may not be necessary. If treatment is indicated, the potential cognitive and behavioural side effects may be more likely to occur in children with a low 'cerebral reserve', in whom it is difficult to determine whether the observed changes are an effect of medication in the presence of many other possible explanations. However, some of these epilepsies may be severe and require more than one drug to achieve control, which in fact is sometimes not possible (refractory seizures). There is a danger of overmedication and therapeutic escalation, without obvious benefit or even with aggravation of the condition, especially in institutions. A impressive study was done in a large institution in the USA comparing the number of antiepileptic drugs given to each epileptic mentally handicapped child over three different time periods (1981, 1987, and 1991). A very significant percentage of children taking two or three drugs decreased gradually and the number with only one drug increased over this decade, without negative consequences (Pellock & Hunt, 1996). These data reflect the modern trend to minimize polytherapy in epileptic children in general, the availability of more effective drugs, and the recognition of the risk of severe side effects without significant gain in seizure control.

Despite these caveats, one should be aware that in some children with mental retardation epilepsy itself can have significant cognitive and behavioural consequences. This is particularly true in partial epilepsies of frontal origin or other partial epilepsies with continuous spike-waves during slow wave sleep. Such epilepsies may start in a previously normal child who becomes mentally handicapped, or in children with mild or moderate mental retardation (for instance, those with unilateral polymicrogyria) who progressively deteriorate up to a certain point and then remain stable. However, they may go through temporary phases of active epilepsy with new regression. Other children with non-convulsive status epilepticus – in the frame of Lennox-Gastaut syndrome or other syndromes – may go through variably long periods of obtundation, apathy, and loss of skills. This additional loss may not be immediately striking in a severely handicapped child but the gradual loss, for instance, of walking balance or self-help skills (eating, toilet training), which may be intermittent at onset, can cause major deterioration in the quality of life, not to mention the emotional welfare.

Epilepsy management, especially important in these circumstances, is difficult when adolescents or young adults no longer live with their parents. Frequent contact with a single caretaker is necessary to evaluate different therapeutic trials. EEG controls and blood drug monitoring are sometimes required and every hospital visit can be a nightmare. Liaisons with institution nurses and direct discussions between neurologists or neuropaediatricians and families or residential staff are a great help in such cases.

Management of acute seizures has been greatly facilitated by the use of a buccal or nasal powerful short-acting diazepine preparation (midazolam) administered in the institution or day care centres (Harbord et al., 2004)

Clinical evaluation of the role of epilepsy on cognitive function

When a child with epilepsy has cognitive, behavioural, or learning problems, the question of a possible direct role of epilepsy or of the side effects of antiepileptic therapy is always raised at one time or another. This is difficult to answer even in a child who has normal intelligence unless striking fluctuations in competence are seen in direct relation to clinical seizures or EEG epileptic activity, or immediately after introduction or increase in therapy. In a child with a low cognitive level and limited performance – often associated with difficult behaviours – fluctuations are not readily noticed and it may take a long time before the aggravating effect of epilepsy is recognized. The tendency to attribute all problems to the basic underlying brain pathology is also natural. Mood changes, unexplained apathy (sudden fatigue), intermittent 'disconnection', new problems with sleep or difficult awakenings (from unrecognized nocturnal seizures) can be indirect clues as to the possibility of a direct role of epilepsy.

Prognosis of epilepsy and the issue of drug withdrawal

A tendency to full remission or a significant decrease in the frequency and severity of seizures is a general trend of all childhood epilepsies, with few exceptions. However, this is highly variable, depending on many factors, but mainly on the type of epileptic syndrome and the specific aetiology. The prognosis and the possibility of drug withdrawal after a seizure-free period should be considered individually, as in any child with epilepsy – whether symptomatic or idiopathic. The old idea that symptomatic epilepsy from focal brain damage or more diffuse brain disease causing mental retardation is lifelong and will need continuous anti-epileptic therapy has been clearly contradicted by long-term follow-up studies of children with either cerebral palsy or mental retardation, in whom complete remission after a 5-year seizure-free period ranges up to 50 per cent or more. It is particularly interesting to look at the most severe childhood epilepsies with early onset and poor control, such as the Lennox-Gastaut syndrome (LGS) or specific genetic conditions like Angelman syndrome, to take just two examples in which long-term studies have been rare. In LGS, whether symptomatic or cryptogenic (Goldsmith et al., 2000), full remission is unlikely, although it should be noted that the duration of follow-up was only slightly over 3 years. In the longest reported follow-up study (average 16 years) (Yagi, 1996), 'characteristics symptoms of LGS continued in one third, and various abortive forms of LGS were seen in the other two thirds, although LGS did not evolve into a localization-related epilepsy during the survey period'.

In a recent impressive study of 23 patients with Angelman syndrome – one of the most severe of the genetic syndromes associated with epilepsy – half the subjects were followed to the age of 20 years and five for over 30 years (Uemura et al., 2005). Fig. 3, drawn from this article, shows the individual evolution with persistence of seizures, seizure freedom, and episodes of status epilepticus. At a glance one can see that several cases became seizure-free after years of continuous epilepsy and status epilepticus. In summary, even in the most severe early epilepsies with mental retardation, remission may occur at a late stage.

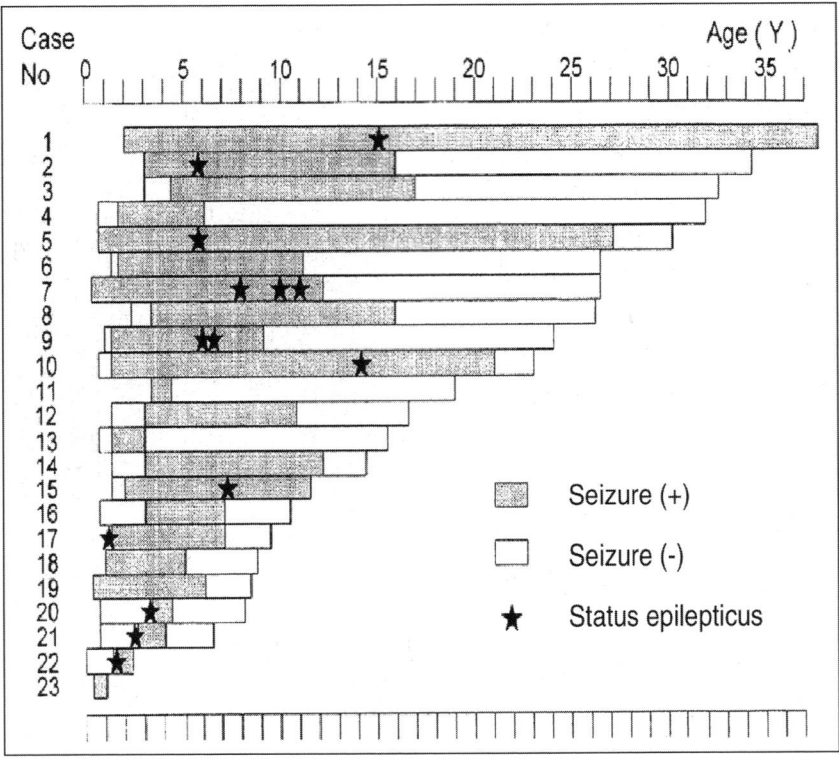

Fig. 3. Angelman syndrome. Clinical course of seizures in each patient (reproduced from Uemura et al., 2005, with permission).

A different situation arises in those rare children with localization-related refractory epilepsy caused by cerebral dysplasias or destructive lesions resulting from brain trauma or other focal cortical lesions and who are also mentally retarded. Refractory epilepsy may start or become severe at any age and may continue for years. In these already handicapped children, there is reluctance to consider the possibility of epilepsy surgery, for understandable reasons, including the idea that a positive outcome is much less likely than in children with normal intellect. However, this does not appear to be the case. With improved diagnostic techniques, surgical facilities, and experience, surgery is justifiably more often considered. Recent studies show that surgical management is possible and may improve the quality of life and the care of some of these children (Gleissner et al., 2006).

References

Battaglia, A. & Guerrini, R. (2005): Chromosomal disorders and epilepsy. *Epilept. Disord.* **7**, 181–192.

Besag, F.M.C. (1987): Cognitive deterioration in children with epilepsy. In: *Epilepsy, behavior and cognitive function*, eds. M. Trimble & E.H. Reynolds, pp. 113–127. New York: John Wiley & Sons.

Chaudhry, M.R. & Pond, D.A. (1961): Mental deterioration in epileptic children. *J. Neurol. Neurosurg. Psychiatry* **24**, 213–219.

DeLong, G.R. & Heinz, E.R. (1997): The clinical syndrome of early life bilateral hippocampal sclerosis. *Ann. Neurol.* **42**, 11–17.

Deonna, T. & Roulet-Perez, E. (2005): *Cognitive and behavioural disorders of epileptic origin in children*. London: MacKeith Press.

Deonna, T., Fohlen, M., Jalin, C., Delalande, O. & Ziegler, A.L. (2002): Epileptic stereotypies in children. In: *Epilepsy and movement disorders*, eds. R. Guerrini, J. Aicardi, F. Andermann & M. Hallett, pp. 319–332. Cambridge: Cambridge University Press.

Dulac, O. (2001): Epileptic encephalopathy. *Epilepsia* **42** (Suppl. 3), 23–26.

Gastaut, H., Broughton, R. & de Leo, G. (1982): Syncopal attacks compulsively self-induced by the Valsalva maneuver in children with mental retardation. *Electroencephalograph. Clin. Neurophysiol.* **35**, 323–329.

Gleissner, U., Clusmann, H., Sassen, R., Elger, C.E. & Helmstaedter, C. (2006): Postsurgical outcome in pediatric patients with epilepsy: a comparison of patients with intellectual disabilities, subaverage intelligence, and average-range intelligence. *Epilepsia* **47**, 406–414.

Goldsmith, I., Zupanc, M.L. & Buchhalter, J.R. (2000): Long-term seizure outcome in 74 patients with Lennox-Gastaut syndrome: effects of incorporating MRI head imaging in defining the cryptogenic subgroup. *Epilepsia* **41**, 395–399.

Harbord, M.G., Kyrkou, N.E., Kay, D. & Coulthard, K.P. (2004): Use of intranasal midazolam to treat seizures in paediatric community settings. *J. Paediatr. Child Health* **40**, 556–558.

Macleod, S., Mallik, A., Tolmie, J.L., Stephenson, J.B.P., O'Reagan, M. & Zuberi, S.M. (2005): Electro-clinical phenotypes of chromosome disorders associated with epilepsy in the absence of dysmorphism. *Brain Dev.* **27**, 118–124.

Pellock, J.M. & Hunt, P.A. (1995): A decade of modern epilepsy therapy in institutionalized mentally retarded patients. *Epilepsy Res.* **25**, 263–268.

Roubertie, A., Petit, J. & Genton, P. (2000): Ring chromosome 20: an identifiable epileptic syndrome. *Rev. Neurol.* (Paris) **156**, 149–153.

Roulet-Perez, E. & Deonna, T. (2006): Autism, epilepsy and EEG epileptiform activity. In: *Autism: a neurological disorder of early brain development*, eds. R. Tuchman & I. Rapin, pp. 174–188. London: MacKeith Press.

Roulet-Perez, E., Davidoff, V., Despland, P.A. & Deonna, T. (1993): Mental and behavioural deterioration of children with epilepsy and CSWS: acquired epileptic frontal syndrome. *Dev. Med. Child Neurol.* **35**, 661–674.

Roulet-Perez, E., Ballhousen, D., Bonafé, L., Cronel-Okayon, S. & Marder-Ingrar, M. (2007): Glucose-transporter deficiency (GLUT-1) presenting as idiopathic generalized seizures [abstract]. Pavia: Société de Neurologie Infantile, 18–21 April. Submitted July 2007.

Sillanpää, M. (2004): Epilepsy in people with intellectual disability. In: *Epilepsy in children*, 2nd ed., eds. S.J. Wallace & K. Farrell, pp. 281–286. London: Arnold

Uemura, N., Matsumoto, A., Nakamura, M., Watanabe, K., Negoro, T., Kumagai, T., Miura, K., Ohki, T., Mizuno, S., Okumura, A., Aso, K., Hayakawa, F. & Kondo, Y. (2005): Evolution of seizures and electroencephalographic findings in 23 cases of deletion type Angelman syndrome. *Brain Dev.* **27**, 383–388.

Vallenga, D., Grypdonck, M.H., Tan, F.I., Lendemeijer, B.H. & Boon, P.A. (2006): Decision-making about risk in people with epilepsy and intellectual disability. *J. Adv. Nurs.* **54**, 602–611.

Wang, D., Pascual, J.M., Yang, H., Engelstad, K., Jhung, S., Sun, R.P. & De Vivo, D.C. (2005): Glut-1 deficiency syndrome: clinical, genetic, and therapeutic aspects. *Ann. Neurol.* **57**, 111–118.

Yagi, K. (1996): Evolution of Lennox-Gastaut syndrome: a long-term longitudinal study. *Epilepsia* **37** (Suppl. 3), 48–51.

Chapter 4

Mental retardation in patients with neuromuscular disorders

Eugenio Mercuri, Marika Pane, Sonia Messina and Angela Beradinelli*

Paediatric Neurology Unit, Catholic University, Rome, Italy;
* Department of Child Neurology, Mondino Institute, Pavia, Italy
mercuri@rm.unicatt.it

Summary

Over the past few years advances in neuroimaging techniques and a better understanding of the genetic basis of neuromuscular disorders have resulted in a dramatic increase in the identification of the forms of neuromuscular disorders associated with mental retardation. It has become increasingly obvious that congenital myotonic dystrophy and Duchenne muscular dystrophy are not the only forms of neuromuscular disorder associated with mental retardation and that there are various newly identified forms with structural brain changes and severe mental retardation. In this chapter we review the state of the art on this topic, providing a practical approach to the classification that may help the clinician, subdividing the forms according to the presence and type of associated brain lesions.

Introduction

Until recently, with very few exceptions, the presence of mental retardation – or more generally of central nervous system (CNS) involvement – was considered one of the key elements for excluding a neuromuscular disorder in patients with hypotonia or contractures. In recent years, however, the advances in neuroimaging and in genetic diagnosis have completely changed our approach to these conditions. With neuroimaging techniques such as cranial ultrasound and brain magnetic resonance imaging (MRI) becoming more routinely used in infants and in children with hypotonia, there has been a dramatic increase in the detection of CNS pathology in neuromuscular disorders. This has resulted not only in a better understanding of the association between the peripheral and CNS involvement, but also of the relation between mental retardation and brain lesions, and of the mechanisms underlying these diseases.

Concomitant advances in the identification of genes responsible for different forms of neuromuscular disorders have been essential to achieve an improved classification of the various phenotypes. More specifically, it has become increasingly obvious that mental retardation is a feature of several forms of neuromuscular disorders and is not always related to the presence of lesions on brain MRI. Relatively minor lesions such as mild ventricular dilatation or non-specific periventricular white matter changes are frequent in infants with various neuromuscular disorders and they are often not associated with any clinical sign of mental retardation.

Structural brain changes, such as cerebellar hypoplasia or dysplasia or cortical migration disorders can be present in different forms of neuromuscular diseases, and although they are usually associated with mental retardation and epilepsy, this does not always hold true in individual cases.

Structural brain changes and neuromuscular disorders are both features of genetically distinct disease entities for which the gene defects have recently been identified. Most of these findings are, however, very recent and there are still many questions to be addressed. In this chapter we will discuss the prevalence, severity, and range of mental retardation and brain lesions in patients with primary neuromuscular disorders.

Association of muscle disorders with mental retardation

The incidence of mental retardation associated with neuromuscular disorders is not known, as in the forms of muscle with severe mental retardation – where there is often a predominance of clinical CNS signs – muscle involvement may not be identified diseases (see paragraph on congenital muscular dystrophies below). Another confounding factor is that very often infants and children with neuromuscular disorders are not formally assessed using age-specific cognitive assessments. It is not rare for children with prominent facial weakness to be misdiagnosed as having mental retardation because of their facial appearance or because of records of poor performance at school (often caused by poor attendance due to recurrent illness).

It is therefore very important that infants in whom there is a clinical suspicion of mental retardation should be formally assessed using age-appropriate tests assessing various aspects of cognitive function. When assessing these children one should also take into account that poor performance in timed items may reflect muscle weakness and the difficulty in performing motor actions with the same speed as the children's peers.

Types of muscle disorder associated with mental retardation

The forms of neuromuscular disorders that are classically associated with mental retardation are congenital myotonic dystrophies and Duchenne muscular dystrophy. More recently it has become evident that there are other forms of congenital muscular dystrophy that are also associated with mental retardation, some with and some without associated brain lesions.

From a practical point of view, it is important not only to establish the presence and severity of the mental retardation but also the presence, type, and severity of brain lesions on MRI.

An easy way to classify the forms of muscle disorders associated with mental retardation occurring in childhood is as follows:

- Mental retardation and muscle disorders without lesions on brain MRI.
- Mental retardation and muscle disorders with non-specific lesions on brain MRI.
- Mental retardation and muscle disorders with structural lesions on brain MRI.

We will also discuss separately one specific form of muscular dystrophy that is always associated with extensive changes in the white matter but not with mental retardation.

Mental retardation and muscle disorders without lesions on brain MRI

Duchenne muscular dystrophy is the most common form of neuromuscular disorder associated with mental retardation without any significant associated change detectable on brain MRI.

Duchenne muscular dystrophy (DMD) is an X-linked disorder caused by lack of a subsarcolemmal protein called dystrophin. The disease affects 1 in 3500 live male infants and is characterized by progressive weakness and wasting of skeletal muscles and lower limb contractures. Skeletal muscle weakness results in loss of walking ability and complete wheelchair dependence by the age of 13 years (mean age 9.5) followed by development of scoliosis in 90 per cent of the patients (Emery, 1993; 2001).

Although most attention is devoted to muscle weakness and to respiratory and cardiac failure, there are other features such as involvement of the CNS that should be considered because of their effect on everyday life. Several studies have reported that a significant proportion of boys with DMD have cognitive difficulties and specific verbal disabilities. This is hardly surprising as the proteins found to be deficient in muscle – the full-length dystrophin and its shorter isoforms – are normally present in specific areas of brain and cerebellum and are affected in patients with this disease. We will summarize the published data on mental retardation in DMD, both in humans and in animal models.

Signs of mental retardation were noted by Duchenne in a 7-year-old boy in his original paper on DMD: 'The intellect was dull and speech was difficult. The temporal regions were extremely projecting, as in certain hydrocephalics' (Duchenne, 1868). The association between DMD and intellectual impairment was confirmed in some of the early cases reported subsequently (Duchenne, 1872; Gowers, 1879; Erb, 1891). However, although a decrease in IQ in DMD boys compared with their peers has been reported in various papers since 1950, not all studies confirmed these data. It is now accepted that as a group DMD children do have a lower IQ than average for their peers but that this may not apply to individual cases. The reported mean IQ scores of children with DMD are approximately 1.0 to 1.5 standard deviations below the mean for age-matched controls (Allen & Rodgin, 1960; Worden & Vignos, 1962; Dubowitz, 1965; Cohen et al., 1968; Leibowitz & Dubowitz 1981), one-third of the patients presenting with non-progressive cognitive impairment when compared to patients with other neuromuscular disorders (Yoshioka et al., 1980; Emery, 1987).

The onset and progression of cognitive impairment do not follow the course and severity of the muscle weakness. It is not rare for medical advice to be sought for speech delay in a child with as yet undiagnosed DMD, at the time when there is no overt clinical sign of muscle weakness.

Over the years several studies have provided details of the profile of cognitive ability in these patients. In contrast with what has often been assumed, cognitive impairment is not related to the difficulties in performing non-verbal items because of weakness, but there is a general decrease in IQ, with a major deficit in verbal IQ. There are reports of a higher degree of impairment in verbal vs. non-verbal performance both in older (Bresolin et al., 1994) and younger patients (Dorman et al., 1988). Although in an extensive recent meta-analysis, Cotton et al. (2001) demonstrated there was no significant difference between verbal IQ and performance IQ scores among boys with DMD, many other studies have reported numerous deficits in verbal skills, such as limited expressive vocabulary, reading disability, impaired auditory selective attention, and verbal short-term working memory. Poor performance in digit span, story recall, and verbal comprehension are most common and can also occur in DMD patients who have a normal global IQ (Hinton et al., 2000).

Over the last two decades various papers have highlighted specific aspects of cognitive impairment in DMD but the results have not always been in agreement. Language delay and, in older children, language difficulties have been reported in several studies (Dorman *et al.*, 1988; Billard *et al.*, 1998; Hendriksen & Vles, 2006) and it has been hypothesized that the profile in DMD boys is similar to that observed in dysphonetic, dyseidetic dyslexia, though others have suggested that some of the cognitive difficulties may be related to attentional and memory impairment rather than directly to language difficulties.

Learning ability and long-term memory seem to be relatively normal among boys with DMD, as compared to short-term memory, which is significantly below normal. (Wicksell *et al.*, 2004).

A recent paper by Hendriksen & Vles (2006) provides new insight in the mechanisms underlying reading difficulties. The mean reading quotient in DMD patients in this study was significantly lower than the 85 per cent reported by Billard *et al.* (1998). DMD children were also found to have a low level of information processing, but this showed considerable variability and a weak correlation with reading disabilities, as the latter were also found in children with normal information processing capacities (Hendriksen & Vles, 2006).

Mental retardation in DMD boys: stable or progressive over the years?

The natural history of DMD is characterized by progressive weakness leading to loss of ambulation, and progressive impairment in cardiac and respiratory function. Cognitive impairment, in contrast, appears to be grossly stable, even though a few studies have suggested that some changes may take place over the years.

Cotton *et al.* (2005), reviewing a large amount of data from the previous studies, found that neither full scale IQ (FIQ) nor performance IQ (PIQ) changed with age in DMD boys. Other studies, in contrast, suggested possible changes such as a decrease in performance abilities, presumably reflecting progressive motor impairment. Moreover some investigators found different trends in the verbal IQ (VIQ) and PIQ over the years: some papers reported a decrease in PIQ; other studies reported either no change or even an improvement in PIQ with age; yet others reported an improvement in mean VIQ with better scores on verbal subtests such as information, similarities, arithmetic, comprehension, and digit span. Children assessed before the age of 11 years showed deficits in logical verbal abstract reasoning, language development, and mathematical/computational ability. They also had limited vocabulary and general knowledge. These deficits appeared to be less evident in the older age groups.

Why so much controversy? Mechanisms underlying mental retardation

Genetic background

The controversy regarding the incidence, profile, and evolution of cognitive difficulties in DMD probably reflects the populations studied. Several variables often not considered in many of the published studies could account for some of the variability or the controversy reported. Some of the problems arise from early days when cognitive impairment was thought to be secondary to the psychological consequences of the physical handicap or to other reasons, such as poor school attendance or difficulties in passing performance items because of the motor defect. Billard and coworkers (Billard *et al.*, 1998) were the first to discuss whether the reading difficulties found among boys with DMD resulted from the psychological and social consequences of the disorder. Based on studies in children with spinal muscular atrophy, these investigators concluded that the lower ability in reading skills found among children with DMD was due to the basic disorder rather than to the psychosocial consequences.

Following the possibility of identifying the specific gene defect in DMD and of achieving phenotype-genotype correlations, it has become obvious that cognitive impairment in DMD is often related to specific gene mutations and not to the psychological consequence of the physical handicap (Moizard et al., 1998). The mutations most often associated with cognitive impairment are preferentially located in the second part of the gene (including exons 45 to 54) (Lindlof et al., 1989; Covone et al., 1991; Hodgson et al., 1992; Nicholson et al., 1993; Bresolin et al., 1994; Bushby et al., 1995), with some investigators suggesting a specific association between deletion of exon 52 and low IQ (Rapaport et al., 1991). Most recently, increasing attention has been devoted to the localization of dystrophin in the brain and to the study of different mutations affecting shorter isoforms of dystrophin.

Brain dystrophin has been localized to the synapse, specifically to the postsynaptic density, and is absent in the *mdx* mouse, an animal model of human DMD. Kim et al. (1995) examined the protein in human DMD and found that the dystrophin was absent in the postsynaptic density from DMD brain but was normally expressed in the brain from an age-matched control subject. Dystrophin is deficient in human DMD cortical synapses and this provides a potential pathogenic mechanism for cognitive impairment. As dystrophin is expressed in neurons (Hoffmann et al., 1987; Hoffmann et al., 1988), it may play an important role in normal neuronal function, but is not clear why mental retardation does not occur in all cases of DMD. More recently, increased attention has been devoted to isoforms of dystrophin consisting of shorter C-terminal forms. These isoforms are encoded by distinct promoters in the DMD gene. It is believed that while the absence of full-length dystrophin affects cognitive function in various degrees, mutations affecting the shorter isoforms cause more severe cognitive impairment, as Moizard showed in 1998 for Dp 71 and Dp 120 (Lidov et al., 1995; Morris et al., 1995; Moizard et al., 1998; Bardoni et al., 2000; Felisari et al., 2000). Dp140 is brain-specific and is expressed mainly in foetal tissue and in very low quantity in adult brain, while Dp71 is expressed in glial and gyrus dentatus cells (den Dunnen et al., 1991; Rapaport et al., 1992). The Dp 140 translation start site is located in exon 51 but its promoter and the first exon lie in intron 44.

Mental retardation in the animal model (mdx mouse)

The *mdx* mouse is a murine model of DMD that lacks the full length dystrophin but retains all the shorter C-terminal isoforms, including the Dp71, while the mdx^{3cv} mouse also lacks the shorter isoforms. In 1991, Muntoni reported a cognitive deficit in *mdx* mice from 16 to 22 weeks, consisting of impairment in passive avoidance learning (Muntoni et al., 1991). Vaillend demonstrated later that *mdx* mice had specific problems in retaining information, though acquisition was normal (Vaillend et al., 1995). The loss of functional dystrophin did not affect behavioural exploration of novel objects, encoding of a new experience, or short-term memory for objects, but impaired the consolidation or expression of long-term recognition memory.

The available data suggest that the memory impairments cannot be attributed simply to muscle pathology, and that the memory deficits in *mdx* mice do not progress with age, at least within the first 6 months (Vaillend & Billard, 2002).

From pathological studies, it appears that a deficiency in brain full-length dystrophin leads to an impairment in both spatial and recognition memory. Neurophysiological analyses revealed a marked enhancement in the maintenance phase of long-term potentiation of synaptic efficacy, and of neuronal excitability in area CA1 of the hippocampus. As brain dystrophin is enriched in postsynaptic densities in the CA1 hippocampal area, there could be a direct relation between long-term memory deficits, altered synaptic plasticity, and dystrophin deficiency in the *mdx* mouse. The hippocampus is known to be implicated in spatial memory. Object recognition memory, at least after long delays, is also sensitive to hippocampal lesioning in rodents (Clark *et al.*, 2000) and to certain hippocampal-specific gene mutations (Rampon & Tsien, 2000; Genoux *et al.*, 2002; Pittenger *et al.*, 2002), although other parahippocampal cortices may also be implicated (Mumby *et al.*, 2002).

Mental retardation and muscle disorders with non-specific lesions on brain MRI

This group is composed of various forms of muscle disorders in which non-specific brain changes – though not a constant feature of the disease – are frequently observed. In most cases brain changes are minimal and consist of mild ventricular dilatation or focal periventricular white matter changes which are thought to be secondary to neonatal respiratory distress (which is not uncommon in infants with weak respiratory muscles). Non-specific changes have been reported in many muscle conditions with neonatal onset, including those in which mental retardation is not a feature, such as the severe form of spinal muscular atrophy. Although in this disease there is usually no associated CNS involvement, non-specific features such as cerebral atrophy or other ischaemic changes have been observed, mainly associated with prematurity or birth asphyxia (International Myotonic Dystrophy Consortium, 2000). The muscle disease most often associated with non-specific brain changes and mental retardation is congenital myotonic dystrophy.

Congenital myotonic dystrophy

Myotonic dystrophy (DM1) is the most frequently inherited neuromuscular disorder in the human population, with an incidence of 1 in 8000 and a prevalence of between 69 and 90 cases per million (Mostacciuolo *et al.*, 1987; Emery, 1991). The genetic basis is the amplification of a CTG trinucleotide repeat within the 3' untranslated region of the DM1 gene on chromosome 19, but the mechanism underlying the variable expressivity of the disease is still unclear (International Myotonic Dystrophy Consortium, 2000; Lieberman & Fischbeck, 2000). Recent studies have shown that in myotonic dystrophy the repeat number correlates with relevant clinical features such as disease severity and age of onset (Novelli *et al.*, 1993; Jaspert *et al.*, 1995).

The main presenting features in the neonate are general hypotonia and marked difficulty in sucking and swallowing, usually requiring tube feeding and generating contractures. Respiratory difficulties are also frequent and may be responsible for neonatal death (Rutherford *et al.*, 1989). Affected infants have a triangular shaped open mouth and are unable to close their eyes completely. Skeletal deformities such as talipes are very common.

In the children who survive, the severe neonatal weakness involving the respiratory and swallowing muscles gradually improves after the first months of life. Very severely affected neonates can, however, require ventilatory support for weeks, and some may never be weaned off the ventilator.

Several neuropsychological studies have shown the presence of mental retardation on neuropsychological tests (Woodward *et al.*, 1982; Bird *et al.*, 1983; Portwood *et al.*, 1986; Brumback, 1987; Perini *et al.*, 1989; Rubinsztein *et al.*, 1997). The estimates of mental retardation in DM1 vary from 20–80 per cent (Rubinsztein *et al.*, 1997; Broughton *et al.*, 1990) to 10–24 per cent (Portwood *et al.*, 1986), and have been reported to be associated with an abnormally large CTG repeat size (> 1000). Abnormal scores on measures of visual or verbal memory have been reported by some investigators (Rubinsztein *et al.*, 1997; Chang *et al.*, 1993). Meola and colleagues (Meola *et al.*, 1999; Meola *et al.*, 2003) have suggested that patients with DM1 present impairment of visuospatial recall, less significant impairment in visuospatial construction, and have deficits of verbal short-term and long-term memory. This impairment is more severe in the congenital form than in juvenile/adult onset (Tuikka *et al.*, 1993). Modoni *et al.* (2004) documented two distinct patterns of cognitive impairment in DM1: in particular, they confirmed the presence of a cognitive pattern characteristic of mental retardation in congenital cases, whereas in adult forms they documented an aging-related decline in frontal and temporal cognitive functions.

Cognitive impairment does not progress with time and it is considered a reflection of a developmental rather than a degenerative process in the central nervous system (Malloy *et al.*, 1990; Tuikka *et al.*, 1993). Perini *et al.* (1999) suggested that the cognitive impairment was a direct expression of the genetic involvement of the central nervous system and not a consequence of motor impairment. Previously Woodward *et al.* (1982) had suggested that there was no relation between general neuropsychological impairment and the degree of weakness, myotonia, or muscle atrophy in patients with myotonic dystrophy.

Psychiatric symptoms such as apathy, depression, and anxiety have also been described in DM1 patients (Brumback *et al.*, 1987; Colombo *et al.*, 1992).

Although the brain is structurally normal in these children, non-specific abnormalities are often observed. The incidence of ventricular dilatation in these infants has been reported at between 70 and 80 per cent. Other abnormalities such as intraventricular haemorrhage and periventricular leukomalacia have also been reported (Tanabe *et al.*, 1992; Hashimoto *et al.*, 1995).

Hashimoto *et al.* have reviewed MRI findings in seven cases of congenital myotonic dystrophy and showed ventricular dilatation in all, associated with periventricular or deep white matter changes (6/7), cortical atrophy (3/7), small corpus callosum (4/7), and a small brain stem (2/7) (Hashimoto *et al.*, 1995).

Mental retardation and muscle disorders with structural lesions on brain MRI

In the last decade there has been increasing evidence of the association between neuromuscular disorders and structural brain changes. Structural abnormalities are observed in patients with both motor neuron diseases, such as those with pontocerebellar hypoplasia, and primary muscle involvement. The congenital muscular dystrophies are the forms of muscle disorders that are most frequently associated with structural brain changes.

The congenital muscular dystrophies

The congenital muscular dystrophies (CMD) are a heterogeneous group of inherited neuromuscular disorders that occur at birth, or within the first few months of life, with hypotonia, muscle weakness, contractures, and motor developmental delay.

The most recent classification of CMD reflects the exciting advances in our understanding of their genetic basis and of the protein defects underlying the various CMD forms (Muntoni & Voit, 2004). This classification recognizes three main groups:

- CMD caused by mutations in genes encoding structural proteins of the basement membrane or extracellular matrix of skeletal muscle fibres. This group includes forms with mutations in the genes encoding collagen VI, laminin-$\alpha 2$ (merosin), and integrin-$\alpha 7$.
- CMD caused by mutations in genes encoding putative or proven glycosyltransferase enzymes. This group includes Fukuyama CMD, muscle-eye-brain disease, Walker-Warburg syndrome, MDC1C and MDC1D, with mutations in the *FCMD*, *POMGnT1*, *POMT1*, *POMT2*, *FKRP*, and *LARGE* genes.
- A form of CMD with rigid spine syndrome secondary to mutations in SEPN1, which encodes selenoprotein N, an endoplasmic reticulum protein of unknown function.

To date, 12 CMD forms have been mapped, and the genes responsible for 10 of these have been identified (Table 1).

Table 1. Genes responsible for congenital muscular dystrophies

Form	Distinctive clinical Features	MRI findings	Molecular data
FCMD	Severe MR, epilepsy, eye involvement	Micropolygyria, pachygyria, cerebellar involvement, abnormal signal in white matter	Fukutin/9q31
WWS	Severe MR, epilepsy, eye involvement	Type II lissencephaly, hydrocephalus, brain stem and cerebellar hypoplasia	Fukutin/9q31; POMT1/9q34.1; POMT2/14q24.3; FKRP/19q13.3
MEB	Severe MR, epilepsy, eye involvement	Pachygyria and polymicrogyria, brain stem and cerebellar hypoplasia, periventricular WM changes	POMGnT1/1q32-34 FKRP/19q13.3
MDC1B	Generalized muscle hypertrophy, rigidity of the spine, contractions	Normal	Gene unknown/ 1q42
MDC1C	Leg hypertrophy, wasting of upper limbs, variable CNS involvement or 'limb girdle phenotype'	Mostly normal or cerebellar cysts, cerebellar atrophy, WM changes	FKRP/19q13.3
MDC1D	1 case	Diffuse WM changes	LARGE/22q12.3-13.1
MDC1A	• Typical form: no severe MR, epilepsy 20%	Diffuse WM changes	LAMA2/6q22-23
	• Form with cortical dysplasia	WM changes and cortical dysplasia	LAMA2/6q22-23
	• Form with cerebellar hypoplasia: severe MR, epilepsy	WM changes and cerebellar hypoplasia	LAMA2/6q22-23
Ulrich syndrome	Contractures of proximal joints, distal laxity	Normal	Col6A1,A2/21q22.3 Col6 A3/2q37
CMD with rigid spine (RSMD1)	Rigidity of the spine, contractions, respiratory failure	Normal	SEPN1/1p35-36
Integrin $\alpha 7$-related CMD	3 cases, mild proximal muscle weakness	Normal	ITGA7/12q13

CMD, congenital muscular dystrophy; FCMD, Fukuyama CMD; MEB: muscle-eye-brain disease; MR, mental retardation; WWS, Walker-Warburg syndrome; WM, white matter.

From a practical point of view, however, it is useful to distinguish forms with CNS involvement from those in which this is absent or rare. With very few exceptions, the forms of CMD associated with mental retardation are usually also associated with structural brain changes on MRI and with abnormalities in the glycosylation of the α-dystroglycan, an important component of the dystrophin-glycoprotein complex. The glycosylation of this protein appears to be crucial in determining its ligand binding properties to components of the extracellular matrix and therefore to maintain the critical linkage between the extracellular matrix and the intracellular cytoskeleton (Michele & Campbell, 2003). These forms are collectively called dystroglycanopathies and the individual forms will be briefly discussed.

Dystroglycanopathies

The group includes all the forms of CMD associated with structural brain changes and ocular abnormalities, such as the Walker-Warburg syndrome, muscle-eye-brain disease, Fukuyama CMD, and other newly described forms with variable brain involvement such as MDC1C caused by mutations in the *FKRP* gene. Muscle pathology is similar in all these forms, with a dystrophic picture, severe depletion of α-dystroglycan, and a reduction in merosin expression on immunohistochemistry. Most of these patients have high creatine kinase (CK) levels.

Walker-Warburg syndrome

This is the most severe of the conditions with CNS involvement and is typically associated with death of affected individuals by the age of 3 years. However, 5–10 per cent of the patients survive beyond 5 years of age and they show profound mental and motor retardation. The diagnostic hallmark of the condition is the combination of severe brain malformations, muscular dystrophy, and structural eye abnormalities (Dobyns et al., 1989). There is neonatal onset with a combination of weakness and severe hypotonia suggestive of muscle involvement, and signs of CNS involvement, such as poor visual attention and decreased alertness, associated with ocular abnormalities including retinal dysgenesis, microphthalmia, or anterior chamber malformations (Dobyns et al., 1989).

Brain changes include type II lissencephaly with a micropolygyric cobblestone cortex often associated with absent or hypoplastic corpus callosum and septum pellucidum. The white matter is extensively involved, with diffuse changes throughout the cortex (Dobyns et al., 1985; Dobyns et al., 1989). Cerebellar malformation is seen in all patients with hypoplasia, particularly of the posterior vermis (Dobyns et al., 1989).

Muscle-eye-brain disease

This form was initially recognized in Finland but it has now been recognized worldwide. Clinical signs are usually present at birth or in the first months of life, with hypotonia and weakness. Ocular abnormalities may become evident only after the first few years, most commonly consisting of myopia and retinal hypoplasia (Santavuori et al., 1989; Dubowitz, 1994). These children invariably develop severe mental retardation and often epilepsy. The disease is progressive with the patients gradually losing their few acquired skills. Survival is variable and some patients reach adulthood (Dubowitz, 1994; Saito et al., 1999).

Brain MRI shows extensive abnormalities of neuronal migration, such as pachygyria and polymicrogyria, often with brain stem and cerebellar hypoplasia and periventricular white matter changes (Dubowitz & Fardeau, 1995).

Fukuyama congenital muscular dystrophy

This form was originally reported in Japan. The clinical features of Fukuyama CMD are mild to moderate hypotonia at birth and a progressive course with increasing weakness, joint contractures, high CK levels, moderate to severe mental retardation, and a frequent association with epilepsy. Ocular abnormalities occur in approximately 70 per cent of these children but are rarely severe, myopia being the most frequent abnormality (Honda & Yoshioka, 1978).

On brain MRI there is abnormal neuronal migration during development, with distorted cerebral gyral patterns. White matter changes are also frequent but are caused by delayed myelination rather than by demyelination, as they improve with age.

Congenital muscular dystrophy type 1C

The typical phenotype is characterized by wasting and severe weakness, most pronounced in the upper limbs, leg hypertrophy, and often macroglossia. These patients usually achieve the ability to sit but not to walk. They may experience feeding difficulties requiring gastrostomy, respiratory failure, and cardiac abnormalities with left ventricular dilatation.

MDC1C was originally described in people with normal intelligence and normal brain MRI, and these represent the vast majority of patients identified to date (Mercuri *et al.*, 2003). Nevertheless some patients with muscle and brain involvement have been reported (Topaloglu *et al.*, 2003; Louhichi *et al.*, 2004). These had mild mental retardation and cerebellar cysts, with or without cerebellar atrophy and white matter abnormalities.

Molecular genetics of the dystroglycanopathies

While until recently it was suggested that each of these forms was caused by mutations in a different gene (*fukutin* for Fukuyama CMD, *POMT1* for Walker-Warburg syndrome, *POMGnT1* for muscle-eye-brain disease, *FKRP* for MDC1C), in recent years it has become obvious that Walker-Warburg and muscle-eye-brain disease can be associated with mutations in all the genes involved in the glycosylation of the α-dystroglycan, namely *FKRP*, *fukutin*, *POMT1*, *POMT2*, for *POMGnT1* and *LARGE* (Table 1). Therefore, when confronted with a patient with clinical and imaging signs suggestive of a 'dystroglycanopathy' all these genes should be screened in order to reach a diagnosis.

Merosin-deficient congenital muscular dystrophy

Merosin (laminin α-2) is a subunit of laminin, an extracellular matrix protein that links with dystrophin on the inner side of the muscle membrane. This form is associated with mutations in the *LAMA2* gene and has autosomal recessive inheritance (Zhang *et al.*, 1996) (Table 1).

The reported incidence of this form ranges between 30 and 40 per cent of all the forms of CMD. Children with merosin deficiency are usually symptomatic at birth or in the first few weeks of life, with hypotonia and muscle weakness, weak cry, and, in 10 to 30 per cent of cases, contractures. Maximum motor ability is generally confined to sitting unsupported or standing with support; less commonly walking with support is achieved.

Children with merosin-negative CMD generally do not show structural brain changes but diffuse white matter changes on MRI are a constant feature in these children. These changes are not obvious on the conventional scans carried out in the first months of life, and become more evident around 6 months (Mercuri *et al.*, 1996; 2001). Despite their dramatic appearance on imaging, the changes are not usually associated with clinical signs of CNS involvement, the only sign of which is epilepsy. This has been observed in 10 to 30 per cent of affected children

(Voit et al., 1998). Mental retardation is rare and generally associated with the concomitant presence of other patterns of brain lesion, such as cerebellar hypoplasia or cortical dysplasia, which can be seen in a small proportion of these patients (Pini et al., 1996; Tan et al., 1997; Brett et al., 1998; Philpot et al., 1999).

Conclusions

On the basis of our experience and of a review of the literature, it appears that mental retardation is a frequent feature in patients with neuromuscular disorders. From a practical point of view there are a few general guidelines that may help the clinician in the differential diagnosis of these forms: (1) a detailed assessment of cognitive abilities should be carried out in order to obtain a reliable measure of the presence and severity of mental retardation; (2) brain MRI should be performed, paying particular attention to features and patterns, such as cerebellar cysts and focal dysplasia, that are known to be associated with specific genetic disorders; (3) muscle biopsy will also be of help in identifying specific abnormalities on immunohistochemistry and will provide further help in suggesting appropriate genetic analyses.

Identifying the specific genetic disorder will not only aid genetic counselling but will also help when informing the families about the specific features of the condition and its prognosis.

References

Allen, J.E. & Rodgin, D.W. (1960): Mental retardation in association with progressive muscular dystrophy. *Am. J. Dis. Child.* **100,** 208–211.

Bardoni, A., Felisari, G., Sironi, M., Comi, G., Lai, M., Robotti, M. & Bresolin, N. (2000): Loss of Dp140 regulatory sequences is associated with cognitive impairment in dystrophinopathies. *Neuromuscul. Disord.* **10,** 194–199.

Billard, C., Gillet, P., Barthez, M., Hommet, C. & Bertrand, P. (1998): Reading ability and processing in Duchenne muscular dystrophy and spinal muscular atrophy. *Dev. Med. Child Neurol.* **40,** 12–20.

Bird, T.D., Follett, C. & Griep, E. (1983): Cognitive and personality function in myotonic muscular dystrophy. *J. Neurol. Neurosurg. Psychiatry* **46,** 971–980.

Bresolin, N., Castelli, E., Comi, G.P., Felisari, G., Bardoni, A., Perani, D., Grassi, F., Turconi, A., Mazzucchelli, F., Gallotti, D., et al. (1994): Cognitive impairment in Duchenne muscular dystrophy. *Neuromuscul. Disord.* **4,** 359–369.

Brett, F.M., Costigan, D., Farrell, M.A., Heaphy, P., Thornton, J. & King, M.D. (1998): Merosin-deficient congenital muscular dystrophy and cortical dysplasia. *Eur. J. Paediatr. Neurol.* **2,** 77–82.

Broughton, R., Stuss, D., Kates, M., Roberts, J. & Dunham, W. (1990): Neuropsychological deficits and sleep in myotonic dystrophy. *Can. J. Neurol. Sci.* **17,** 410–415.

Brumback, R.A. (1987): Disturbed personality and psychosocial adjustment in myotonic dystrophy: relationship to intellectual/cognitive function and underlying affective disorder (depression) *Psychol. Rep.* **60,** 783–796.

Bushby, K.M., Appleton, R., Anderson, L.V., Welch, J.L., Kelly, P. & Gardner-Medwin, D. (1995): Deletion status and intellectual impairment in Duchenne muscular dystrophy. *Dev. Med. Child Neurol.* **37,** 260–269.

Chang, L., Anderson, T., Migneco, O.A., Boone, K., Mehringer, C.M., Villanueva-Meyer, J., Berman, N. & Mena I. (1993): Cerebral abnormalities in myotonic dystrophy. Cerebral blood flow, magnetic resonance imaging, and neuropsychological tests. *Arch. Neurol.* **50,** 917–923.

Clark, S.E., Hori, A., Putnam, A & Martin, T.P. (2000): Group collaboration in recognition memory. *J. Exp. Psychol. Learn. Mem. Cogn.* **26,** 1578–1588.

Cohen, H.J., Molnar, G.E. & Taft, L.T. (1968): The genetic relationship of progressive muscular dystrophy (Duchenne type) and mental retardation. *Dev. Med. Child Neurol.* **10,** 754–765.

Colombo, G., Perini, G.I., Miotti, M.V., Armani, M. & Angelini, C. (1992): Cognitive and psychiatric evaluation of 40 patients with myotonic dystrophy. *Ital. J. Neurol. Sci.* **13,** 53–58.

Cotton, S., Voudouris, N.J. & Greenwood, K.M. (2001): Intelligence and Duchenne muscular dystrophy: full-scale, verbal, and performance intelligence quotients. *Dev. Med. Child Neurol.* **43,** 497–501.

Cotton, S., Voudouris, N.J. & Greenwood, K.M. (2005): Association between intellectual functioning and age in children and young adults with Duchenne muscular dystrophy: further results from a meta-analysis. *Dev. Med. Child Neurol.* **47**, 257–265.

Covone, A.E., Lerone, M. & Romeo, G. (1991): Genotype-phenotype correlation and germline mosaicism in DMD/BMD patients with deletions of the dystrophin gene. *Hum Genet.* **87**, 353–360.

den Dunnen, J.T., Casula, L., Makover, A., Bakker, B., Yaffe, D., Nudel, U. & van Ommen, G.J. (1991): Mapping of dystrophin brain promoter: a deletion of this region is compatible with normal intellect. *Neuromuscul. Disord.* **1**, 327–331.

Dobyns, W.B., Kirkpatrick, J.B., Hittner, H.M., Roberts, R.M. & Kretzer, F.L. (1985): Syndromes with lissencephaly. II: Walker-Warburg and cerebro-oculo-muscular syndromes and a new syndrome with type II lissencephaly. *Am. J. Med. Genet.* **22**, 157–195.

Dobyns, W.B., Pagon, R.A., Armstrong, D., Curry, C.J., Greenberg, F., Grix, A., Holmes, L.B., Laxova, R., Michels, W., Robinow, M., *et al.* (1989): Diagnostic criteria for Walker-Warburg syndrome. *Am. J. Med. Genet.* **32**, 195–210.

Dorman, C., Hurley, A.D. & D'Avignon, J. (1988): Language and learning disorders of older boys with Duchenne muscular dystrophy. *Dev. Med. Child Neurol.* **30**, 316–327.

Dubowitz, V. (1965): Intellectual impairment in muscular dystrophy. *Arch. Dis. Child.* **40**, 296–301.

Dubowitz, V. (1994): Proceedings of the 22nd ENMC Sponsored Workshop on Congenital Muscular Dystrophy, Netherlands, 14–16 May, 1993. *Neuromuscul. Disord.* **4**, 75–81.

Dubowitz, V. & Fardeau, M. (1995): Proceedings of the 27th ENMC Sponsored Workshop on Congenital Muscular Dystrophy, Netherlands, 22–24 April, 1994. *Neuromuscul. Disord.* **5**, 253–258.

Duchenne, G. (1868): Recherches sur la paralysie musculaire pseudo-hypertrophique, ou paralysie myosclérosique. *Arch. Gen. Med.* **11**, 5–25, 179–209, 305–321, 421–443, 552–588.

Duchenne, G.B. (1872): *De l'électrisation localisée et de son application à la pathologie et à la thérapeutique*, 3rd ed. Paris: Baillière.

Emery, A.E.H. (1987): The European Neuromuscular Centre (ENMC): importance of collaborative research. *Neuromuscul. Disord.* **7**, 135–137.

Emery, A.E.H. (1991): Population frequencies of inherited neuromuscular diseases: a world survey. *Neuromuscul. Disord.* **1**, 19–29.

Emery, A.E.H. (1993): *Duchenne muscular dystrophy*, 2nd ed., pp. 115–120. Oxford: Oxford University Press.

Emery, A.E.H. (2001): Duchenne muscular dystrophy or Meryon's disease. In: *The muscular dystrophies*, ed. A.E.H. Emery, pp. 55–71. Oxford: Oxford Medical Publications.

Erb, W.H. (1891): Dystrophia muscolaris progressive. Klinische und pathologisch-anatomische Studien. *Deutsche Zeitschrift fur Nervenheilkunde* **1**, 13–84, 173–261.

Felisari, G., Martinelli Boneschi, F., Bardoni, A., Sironi, M., Comi, G.P., Robotti, M., Turconi, A.C., Lai, M., Corrao, G. & Bresolin, N. (2000): Loss of Dp140 dystrophin isoform and intellectual impairment in Duchenne dystrophy. *Neurology* **55**, 559–564.

Genoux, D., Haditsch, U., Knobloch, M., Michalon, A., Storm D, & Mansuy, I.M. (2002): Protein phosphatase 1 is a molecular constraint on learning and memory. *Nature* **29**, 970–975.

Gowers, W.R. (1879): Clinical lecture on pseudohypertrophic muscular paralysis. *Lancet ii*, 73–75, 113–116.

Hashimoto, T., Tayama, M., Yoshimoto, T., Miyazaki, M., Harada, M., Miyoshi, H., Tanouchi, M. & Kuroda, Y. (1995): Proton magnetic resonance spectroscopy of brain in congenital myotonic dystrophy. *Pediatr. Neurol.* **12**, 335–340.

Hendriksen, J.G.M. & Vles, J.S.H. (2006): Are males with Duchenne muscular dystrophy at risk for reading disabilities? *Pediatr. Neurol.* **34**, 296–300.

Hinton, V.J., De Vivo, D.C., Nereo, N.E., Goldstein, E. & Stern, Y. (2000): Poor verbal working memory across intellectual level in boys with Duchenne dystrophy. *Neurology* **54**, 2127–2132.

Hodgson, S.V., Abbs, S., Clark, S., Manzur, A., Heckmatt, J.Z., Dubowitz, V. & Bobrow, M. (1992): Correlation of clinical and deletion data in Duchenne and Becker muscular dystrophy, with special reference to mental ability. *Neuromuscul. Disord.* **2**, 269–276.

Hoffman, E.P., Brown, R.H. & Kunkel, L.M. (1987): Dystrophin: the protein product of the Duchenne muscular dystrophy locus. *Cell* **51**, 919–928.

Hoffman, E.P., Hudecki, M.S., Rosemberg, P.A., Pollina, C.M. & Kunkel, L.M. (1988): Cell and fiber-type distribution of dystrophin. *Neuron* **1**, 411–420.

Honda, Y. & Yoshioka, M. (1978): Ophthalmological findings of muscular dystrophies: a survey of 53 cases. *J. Pediatr. Ophthalmol. Strabismus* **15**, 236–238.

International Myotonic Dystrophy Consortium (IDMC) (2000): New nomenclature and DNA testing guidelines for myotonic dystrophy type 1 (DM1). *Neurology* **54**, 1218–1221.

Kim, T.W., Wu, K. & Black, I.B. (1995) Deficiency of brain synaptic dystrophin in human Duchenne muscular dystrophy. *Ann. Neurol.* **38**, 446–449.

Jaspert, A., Fahsold, R., Grehl, H. & Claus, D. (1995): Myotonic dystrophy: correlation of clinical symptoms with the size of the CTG trinucleotide repeat. *J. Neurol.* **242**, 99–104.

Leibowitz, D. & Dubowitz, V. (1981): Intellect and behaviour in Duchenne muscular dystrophy. *Dev. Med. Child Neurol.* **23**, 577–590.

Lidov, H.G., Selig, S. & Kunkel, L.M. (1995): Dp140: a novel 140 kDa CNS transcript from the dystrophin locus. *Hum. Mol. Genet.* **4**, 329–335.

Lieberman, A.P. & Fischbeck, K.H. (2000): Triplet repeat expansion in neuromuscular disease. *Muscle Nerve* **23**, 843–850.

Lindlof, M., Kiuru, A., Kaariainen, H., Kalimo, H., Lang, H., Pihko, H., Rapola, J., Somer, H., Somer, M. & Savontaus, M.L. (1989): Gene deletions in X-linked muscular dystrophy. *Am. J. Hum. Genet.* **44**, 496–503.

Louhichi, N., Triki, C., Quijano-Roy, S., Richard, P., Makri, S., Meziou, M., Estournet, B., Mrad, S., Romero, N.B., Ayadi, H., Guicheney, P. & Fakhfakh, F. (2004): New FKRP mutations causing congenital muscular dystrophy associated with mental retardation and central nervous system abnormalities. Identification of a founder mutation in Tunisian families. *Neurogenetics* **5**, 27–34.

Malloy, P., Mishra, S.K. & Adler, S.H. (1990): Neuropsychological deficits in myotonic muscular dystrophy. *J. Neurol. Neurosurg. Psychiatry* **53**, 1011–1013.

Meola, G., Sansone, V., Perani, D., Colleluori, A., Cappa, S., Cotelli, M., Fazio, F., Thornton, C.A. & Moxley, R.T. (1999): Reduced cerebral blood flow and impaired visual-spatial function in proximal myotonic myopathy. *Neurology* **53**, 1042–1050.

Meola, G., Sansone, V., Perani, D., Scarone, S., Cappa, S., Dragoni, C., Cattaneo, E., Cotelli, M., Gobbo, C., Fazio, F., Siciliano, G., Mancuso, M., Vitelli, E., Zhang, S., Krahe, R. & Moxley, R.T. (2003): Executive dysfunction and avoidant personality trait in myotonic dystrophy type 1 (DM-1) and in proximal myotonic myopathy (PROMM/DM-2). *Neuromuscul. Disord.* **13**, 813–821.

Mercuri, E., Pennock, J., Goodwin, F., Sewry, C., Cowan, F., Dubowitz, V. & Muntoni, F. (1996): Sequential study of central and peripheral nervous system involvement in an infant with merosin-deficient congenital muscular dystrophy. *Neuromuscul. Disord.* **6**, 425–429.

Mercuri, E., Rutherford, M., De Vile, C., Counsell, S., Sewry, C., Brown, S. Bydder, G., Dubowitz, V. & Muntoni, F. (2001): Early white matter changes on brain magnetic resonance imaging in a newborn affected by merosin-deficient congenital muscular dystrophy. *Neuromuscul. Disord.* **11**, 297–299.

Mercuri, E., Brockington, M., Straub, V., Quijano-Roy, S., Yuva, Y., Herrmann, R., Brown, S.C., Torelli, S., Dubowitz, V., Blake, D.J., Romero, N.B., Estournet, B., Sewry, C.A., Guicheney, P., Voit, T. & Muntoni, F. (2003): Phenotypic spectrum associated with mutations in the fukutin-related protein gene. *Ann. Neurol.* **53**, 537–542.

Michele, D.E. & Campbell, K.P. (2003): Dystrophin-glycoprotein complex: post-translational processing and dystroglycan function. *J. Biol. Chem.* **278**, 15457–15460.

Modoni, A., Silvestri, G., Pomponi, M.G., Mangiola, F., Tonali, P.A. & Marra, C. (2004): Characterization of the pattern of cognitive impairment in myotonic dystrophy type 1. *Arch. Neurol.* **61**, 1943–1947.

Moizard, M.P., Billard, C., Toutain, A., Berret, F., Marmin, N. & Moraine, C. (1998): Are Dp71 and Dp140 brain dystrophin isoforms related to cognitive impairment in Duchenne muscular dystrophy? *Am. J. Med. Genet.* **80**, 32–41.

Morris, G.E., Simmons, C. & Nguyen, T.M. (1995): Apo-dystrophins (Dp140 and Dp71) and dystrophin splicing isoforms in developing brain. *Biochem. Biophys. Res. Commun.* **215**, 361–367.

Mostacciuolo, M.L., Barbujani, G., Armani, M., Danieli, G.A. & Angelini, C. (1987): Genetic epidemiology of myotonic dystrophy. *Genet. Epidemiol.* **4**, 289–298.

Mumby, D.G., Glenn, M.J., Nesbitt, C. & Kyriazis, D.A. (2002): Dissociation in retrograde memory for object discriminations and object recognition in rats with perirhinal cortex damage. *Behav. Brain Res.* **132**, 215–226.

Muntoni, F. & Voit, T. (2004): The congenital muscular dystrophies in 2004 a century of exciting progress. *Neuromuscul. Disord.* **14**, 635–649.

Muntoni, F., Mateddu, A. & Serra, G. (1991): Passive avoidance behaviour deficit in the mdx mouse. *Neuromuscul. Disord.* **1**, 121–123.

Nicholson, L.V., Johson, M.A., Bushby, K.M. & Gardner-Medwin, D. (1993): Functional significance of dystrophin positive fibres in Duchenne muscular dystrophy. *Arch. Dis. Child.* **68**, 632–636.

Novelli, G., Gennarelli, M., Menegazzo, E., Mostacciuolo, M.L., Pizzuti, A., Fattorini, C., Tessarolo, D., Tomelleri, G., Giacanelli, M., Danieli, G.A., et al. (1993): (CTG)n triplet mutation and phenotype manifestations in myotonic dystrophy patients. *Biochem. Med. Metab. Biol.* **50**, 85–92.

Perini, G.I., Colombo, G., Armani, M., Pellegrini, A., Ermani, M., Miotti, M. & Angelini, C. (1989): Intellectual impairment and cognitive evoked potentials in myotonic dystrophy. *J. Nerv. Ment. Dis.* **177**, 750–754.

Perini, G.I., Menegazzo, E., Ermani, M., Zara, M., Gemma, A., Ferruzza, E., Gennarelli, M. & Angelini, C. (1999): Cognitive impairment and (CTG)n expansion in myotonic dystrophy patients. *Biol. Psychiatry* **46**, 425–431.

Philpot, J., Bagnall, A., King, C., Dubowitz, V. & Muntoni, F. (1999): Feeding problems in merosin deficient congenital muscular dystrophy. *Arch. Dis. Child.* **80**, 542–547.

Pini, A., Merlini, L., Tome, F.M., Chevallay, M. & Gobbi, G. (1996): Merosin-negative congenital muscular dystrophy, occipital epilepsy with periodic spasms and focal cortical dysplasia. Report of three Italian cases in two families. *Brain Dev.* **18**, 316–322.

Pittenger, C., Huang, Y.Y., Paletzki, R.F., Bourtchouladze, R., Scanlin, H., Vronskaya, S. & Kandel, E.R. (2002): Reversible inhibition of CREB/ATF transcription factors in region CA1 of the dorsal hippocampus disrupts hippocampus-dependent spatial memory. *Neuron* **34**, 447–462.

Portwood, M.M., Wicks, J.J., Lieberman, J.S. & Duveneck, M.J. (1986): Intellectual and cognitive function in adults with myotonic muscular dystrophy. *Arch. Phys. Med. Rehabil.* **67**, 299-303.

Rampon, C. & Tsien, J.Z. (2000): Genetic analysis of learning behaviour-induced structural plasticity. *Hippocampus* **10**, 605–609.

Rapaport, D., Passos-Bueno, M.R., Brandao, L., Love D., Vainzof, M. & Zatz, M. (1991): Apparent association of mental retardation and specific patterns of deletions screened with probes cf56a and cf23a in Duchenne muscular dystrophy. *Am. J. Med. Genet.* **39**, 437–441.

Rapaport, D., Passos-Bueno, M.R., Takata, R.I., Campiotto, S., Eggers, S., Vainzof, M., Makover, A., Nudel, U., Yaffe, D. & Zatz, M. (1992): A deletion including the brain promoter of the Duchenne muscular dystrophy gene is not associated with mental retardation. *Neuromuscul. Disord.* **2**, 117–120.

Rubinsztein, J.S., Rubinsztein, D.C., McKenna, P.J., Goodburn, S. & Holland, A.J. (1997): Mild myotonic dystrophy is associated with memory impairment in the context of normal general intelligence. *J. Med. Genet.* **34**, 229–233.

Rutherford, M.A., Heckmatt, J.Z. & Dubowitz, V. (1989): Congenital myotonic dystrophy: respiratory function at birth determines survival. *Arch. Dis. Child.* **64**, 191–195.

Saito, Y., Murayama, S., Kawai, M. & Nakano, I. (1999): Breached cerebral glia limitans-basal lamina complex in Fukuyama-type congenital muscular dystrophy. *Acta Neuropathol. (Berl.)* **98**, 330–336.

Santavuori, P., Somer, H., Sainio, K., Rapola, J., Kruus, S., Nikitin, T., Ketonen, L. & Leisti, J. (1989): Muscle-eye-brain disease (MEB). *Brain Dev.* **11**, 147–153.

Tan, E., Topaloglu, H., Sewry, C., Zorlu, Y., Naom, I., Erdem, S., D'Alessandro, M., Muntoni, F. & Dubowitz, V. (1997): Late onset muscular dystrophy with cerebral white matter changes due to partial merosin deficiency. *Neuromuscul. Disord.* **7**, 85–89.

Tanabe, Y., Iai, M., Tamai, K., Fujimoto, N. & Sugita, K. (1992): Neuroradiological findings in children with congenital myotonic dystrophy. *Acta Paediatr.* **81**, 613–717.

Topaloglu, H., Brockington, M., Yuva, Y., Talim, B., Haliloglu, G., Blake, D., Torelli, S., Brown, S.C. & Muntoni, F. (2003): FKRP gene mutations cause congenital muscular dystrophy, mental retardation, and cerebellar cysts. *Neurology* **60**, 988–992.

Tuikka, R.A., Laaksonen, R.K. & Somer, H.V. (1993): Cognitive function in myotonic dystrophy: a follow-up study. *Eur. Neurol.* **33**, 436–441.

Vaillend, C., Rendon, A., Misslin, R. & Ungerer, A. (1995): Influence of dystrophin-gene mutation on mdx mouse behaviour. I. Retention deficits at long delays in spontaneous alternation and bar-pressing tasks. *Behav. Genet.* **25**, 569–579.

Vaillend, C. & Billard, J.M. (2002): Facilitated CA1 hippocampal synaptic plasticity in dystrophin-deficient mice: role for GABAA receptors? *Hippocampus* **12**, 713–717.

Voit, T. (1998) : Congenital muscular dystrophies: 1997 update. *Brain Dev.* **20**, 65–74.

Wicksell, R.K., Kihlgren, M., Melin, L. & Eeg-Olofsson, O. (2004): Specific cognitive deficits are common in children with Duchenne muscular dystrophy. *Dev. Med. Child Neurol.* **46**, 154–159.

Woodward, J.B., Heaton, R.K., Simon, D.B. & Ringel, S.P. (1982): Neuropsychological findings in myotonic dystrophy. *J. Clin. Neuropsychol.* **4**, 335–342.

Worden, D.K. & Vignos, P.J. (1962): Intellectual function in childhood progressive muscular dystrophy. *Pediatrics* **29**, 968–977.

Yoshioka, M., Okuno, T., Honda, Y. & Nakano, Y. (1980): Central nervous system involvement in progressive muscular dystrophy. *Arch. Dis. Child.* **55,** 589–594.

Zhang, X., Vuolteenaho, R. & Tryggvason, K. (1996): Structure of the human laminin alpha2-chain gene (LAMA2), which is affected in congenital muscular dystrophy. *J. Biol. Chem.* **271,** 27664–27669.

Chapter 5

Mental retardation in paediatric disease

Angelo Selicorni, Marta Cerutti, Cecilia Vellani, Melissa Bellini and Donatella Milani

Clinical Genetics, I Paediatric Clinic, University of Milan, Fondazione IRCCS Ospedale Maggiore Policlinico, via Commenda 9, 20122 Milan, Italy
ambulatorio@gencli.it

Summary

Mental retardation is a common problem in the paediatric age range. The incidence appears to be between 1 and 10 per cent of the general population. The aetiology is heterogeneous. Current evidence suggests that a genetic defect is the basic disorder in most cases. However, a large proportion of patients (30 to 40 per cent) remain undiagnosed, despite advances in cytogenetics and molecular medicine.
In this chapter we describe the diagnostic work-up in the paediatric age range to diagnose or exclude a malformation syndrome. We outline the difficulties faced by clinicians. The most common are related to the wide variability of clinical expression, to genetic heterogeneity, and to the lack of defined and specific diagnostic criteria in some of the commonest diseases. We emphasize that the aetiological diagnosis is not the clinician's final goal but merely the starting point in the long-term care of the patient and their family. Finally, we discuss the problems of assessing the patient's prognosis.

Introduction

The prevalence of mental retardation among paediatric patients is quite variable. It can be estimated from various different studies to be between 1 and 10 per cent of the general population, with a sex ratio (male to female) of 1.5. The higher proportion of affected males certainly reflects the significant contribution of X-linked diseases associated with mental retardation – that is, genetic conditions (syndromic or isolated mental retardation) caused by mutation of genes localized on the X chromosome.

Fig. 1 shows the distribution of causes of mental retardation (Stevenson *et al.*, 2003). Two facts are clear: first, there is still a very high percentage of patients who suffer from mental deficits of unknown cause; and second, the great majority of known causes of mental retardation are in various ways related to genetic anomalies at chromosomal or single gene level. Moreover, it is also clear that when a new cause is identified, it often falls within the genetic aetiology group thanks to the discovery of new biological techniques, new genes, and new phenotypes. Thus one of the main points in the clinical approach to the mentally retarded patient is to define whether mental retardation is an isolated and unique impairment or whether it is one of the manifestations of a more complex disease such as a malformation syndrome.

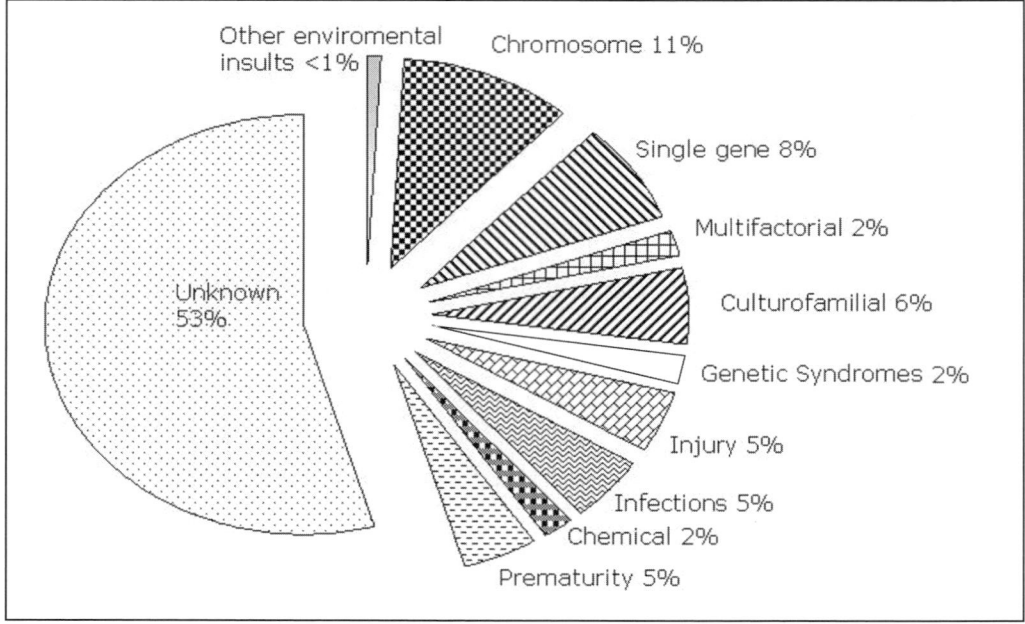

Fig. 1. *Causes of mental retardation* (Stevenson *et al.*, 2003, *Am. J. Med. Genet.*)

Nature of malformation syndromes and tools for diagnosis

From a practical point of view a malformation syndrome is the most logical reason for the coexistence of various different and sometimes rare medical problems in the same child. Every medical practitioner should always remember this possibility when examining a child, abandoning any strictly specialist viewpoint.

A malformation syndrome may also be defined in a more scientific way as a complex disease which combines in variable ways different categories of medical problems or features – abnormalities of physical growth (both growth deficiency and overgrowth), the presence of major-malformations of different organs or appendages, abnormalities of psychomotor and mental development, and the presence of minor anomalies or dysmorphisms. The peculiarity of this combination of problems is that it has a common unique constitutional cause: an anomaly in the genome of the affected child, which can be defined by a genetic test or hypothesized at a clinical level.

In a malformation syndrome we consider the presence of the following:

• Peculiar features that must be assessed very carefully at the clinical diagnostic level.

• Occasional anomalies. These refer to medical problems that are more frequent in that particular group of patients in comparison with the general population, but where their presence or absence is not decisive for a clinical diagnosis.

• Medical complications or clinical paediatric problems which are more common in the affected patients than in the general population. A knowledge of the natural history of each syndrome is the basis for protocols of medical follow-up.

Tables 1, 2, and 3 show examples of these various features in a fairly common malformation syndrome, Williams syndrome. Table 4 shows the follow-up protocol available as suggested by the American Academy of Pediatrics and the Italian Society of Medical Genetics.

Among the diagnostic tools available, clinical evaluation remains the most important, though recent years have witnessed rapid advances in molecular biology and cytogenetics.

Clinical evaluation of a suspected malformation syndrome associated with mental retardation

The starting point of every clinical evaluation is a detailed history, as normally obtained in any paediatric case. It is important to collect information on family history, pregnancy, the neonatal period, growth, psychomotor milestones, and pathological data with particular reference to major malformations or neurological diseases. It should be remembered that even apparently trivial information may be an important clue supporting a specific clinical suspicion.

Genetic tests and any specialist evaluations or examinations carried out on the patient should also be considered.

After performing a complete paediatric examination and collecting the basic auxological data (weight, length/height, head circumference), the most specific part of the clinical evaluation is the evaluation of any dysmorphological features. This consists of a thorough examination, from head to foot, looking for and recording every possible minor anomaly that can be found. We

Table 1. Main features in Williams' syndrome

Peculiar facies
Psychomotor retardation
Congenital heart disease
Short stature

Table 2. Occasional features in Williams' syndrome

Urinary tract malformations
Thyroid malformations
Inguinal and/or umbilical hernia

Table 3. Complications in Williams' syndrome

Orthopaedic
Ocular
Vascular
Dental
Otic
Gastrointestinal
Renal

define a minor anomaly as a congenital abnormality with no clinical significance but with an aesthetic impact. Most of these affect the face but they may also be found in other parts of the body (Aase, 1990; Bankier, 1988). Anthropometric defects can be estimated using growth charts specific for different parts of the body (inner and outer canthal distances, philtrum length, ear length, hand length, middle finger length, and so on). Fig. 2 shows an example of these growth charts.

It should be noted that anyone can have one or two minor anomalies without any specific pathologic meaning, and family resemblances should be considered. The observer should start the examination by studying the appearance of the face from top to bottom, both frontally and laterally, and then continue with the neck, trunk, and extremities following a standard scheme. Figs. 3 and 4 show some referral diagrams available on the computerized system POSSUM.

The importance of an accurate description of the patient's features is well described by Stevenson *et al.* (2003), in which it is considered that 'the physical phenotype appears to be more helpful than the severity of mental retardation, presence of seizures or other neurobehavioural attributes in identification of causation of mental retardation itself'.

After the history has been obtained and the physical evaluation made, there are various possible pathways to follow in order to formulate a diagnosis:

• In a patient with mental retardation and dysmorphic features, basic genetic testing (standard karyotype, molecular analysis of the *FMR1* gene for fragile-X syndrome) may be an easy and quick way to obtain a final diagnosis.

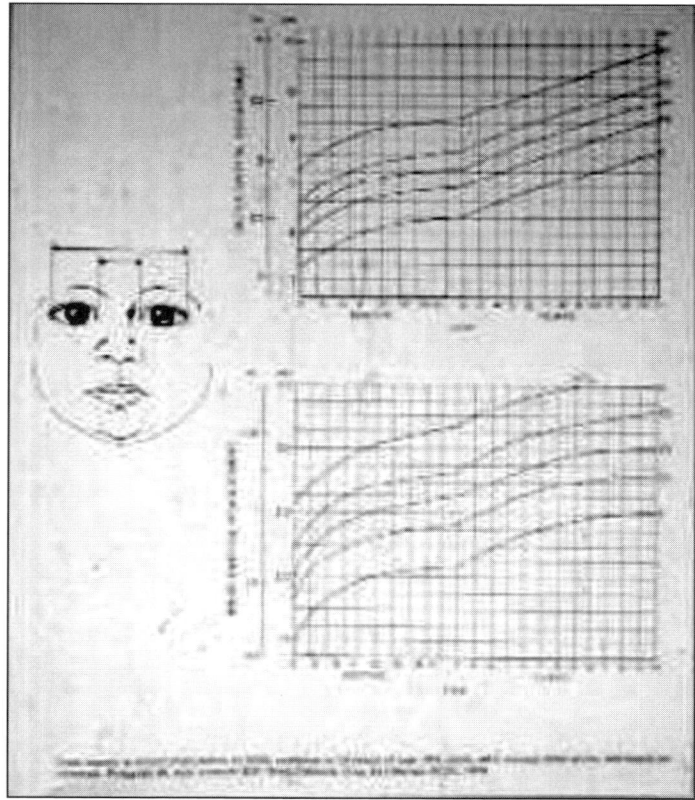

Fig. 2. Growth charts.

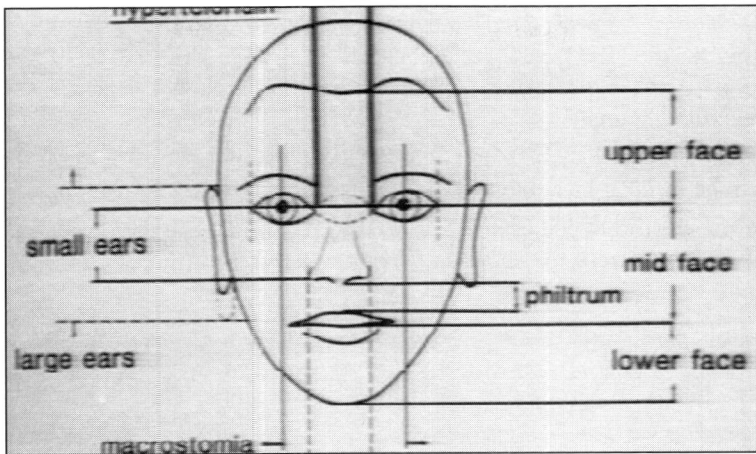

Fig. 3. Face traits, comparative drawings (frontal view).

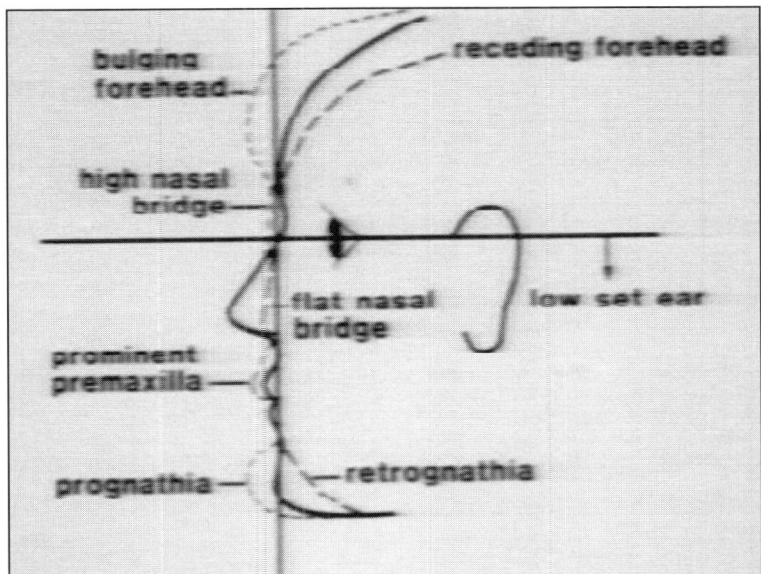

Fig. 4. Face traits, comparative drawings (lateral view).

- If the combination of clinical problems and dysmorphic features is so typical that the disease can be recognized by the clinician, we have what is defined as a 'gestalt diagnosis'. The gestaltic hypothesis can then be supported or refuted by specific genetic tests. Table 5 shows a list of relatively common syndromes that can be recognized by gestalt diagnosis.
- In the great majority of cases there is no help from basic genetic tests and no gestalt diagnosis is possible. In these situations the task of the clinician is particularly hard and involves compiling a list of possible differential diagnoses based on any particularly abnormal features in the patient.

In this latter case, computerized dysmorphology systems such as POSSUM and OMD (Oxford Medical Database) are very helpful. On submission of the specific features present in the patient (termed 'handles'), the databases offer a list of possible conditions compatible with the signs and symptoms supplied. These databases are not 'expert systems' but 'systems for experts'; only the experience of a clinician will lead to the correct diagnosis. By the end of the evaluation, three situations are possible:

(1) We have a specific hypothesis which is confirmable through a genetic test. The specific genetic test can then be made.

(2) We have a specific hypothesis with no available laboratory test to confirm it. In this case we need to search the medical literature and discuss the case with other experts in dysmorphology.

(3) We have no specific hypothesis so we need to reconsider the data, or we may decide to follow up the patient in case the situation becomes clearer with time.

Table 4. Follow-up protocols in Williams' syndrome

	Age 0–1 years		2–5 years		6–12 years		13–18 years	
Assessments	A.P.	I.P.	A.P.	I.P.	A.P	I.P.	A.P.	I.P.
Complete clinical examination	+	+	+(#)	+(#)	+(#)	+(#)	+(#)	+(#)
Eye examination	+	+	+(#)	+(**)	+(#)	+(#)	+	+(#)
Ear examination	+	+	+(#)	+(**)	+(#)	+(#)	+	+(#)
Dental examination	–	–	+	+	–	–	–	–
Orthopaedic examination	–	–	+	+	+	+	+	+
Neurocognitive examination	+	+	+	+(**)	+	+	+	
Arterial pressure measure	+	+	+(#)	+(#)	+(#)	+(#)	+(#)	+(#)
Heart examination	+	+	+(#)	+(**)	+(§)	+(§)	+(§)	+(§)
Abdominal ultrasound	+	+	–	–	–	–	+(§§)	–
Thyroid ultrasound	–	–	–	–	–	–	–	–
Thyroid biochemistry	+	+	+(***)	+(°)	+(***)	+(°)	+(***)	+(°)
Serum calcium	+	+	+(*)	+(*)	+(°°)	+(°°)	+(°°)	+(°°)
Azotaemia	–	–	–	+(***)	–	+(***)	–	+(***)
Urinary calcium/creatinine ratio	+	+	+(°)	+(°)	+(°)	+(°)	+(°°)	+(°)
Plasma creatinine	+	+	+(***)	–	+(°)	–	+(***)	–
Complete urine examination	+	+	+(#)	+	+(#)	+(#)	+(#)	+(#)
Coeliac disease	–	–	–	+(°)	–	+(°)	–	+(°)

(#) Yearly examinations.
(*) Check once a year if symptomatic, check every 2 or 3 years if basal value is normal.
(**) Check once a year under 3 years of age.
(***) Check every 4 years.
(°) Check every 2 years.
(§) If previous examinations are negative, repeat the evaluation for aortic stenosis and hypertension at puberty.
(°°) Check once a year if basal value was high on previous examination or if the child is symptomatic, every 4 years if basal value was normal.
(°°°) Yearly evaluation of plasmatic calcium if the teenager becomes symptomatic, otherwise check every 4 years.
(§§) Check at puberty onset and then every 5 years.
A.P., American protocol; I.P., Italian protocol.

Mental retardation and paediatric disease

In everyday life, mental retardation is often the main problem that brings a patient to medical attention and triggers a diagnostic pathway, while in other situations it is discovered after a syndromic diagnosis has been made. Consider, for example, a newborn baby with bilateral cryptorchidism, defective suckling and severe hypotonia. If we apply accepted suspicion criteria for Prader-Willi syndrome there is a clear indication for performing a methylation test which will give us a pathological result with this condition. Once we have obtained a clinical diagnosis of Prader-Willi syndrome we will communicate the results to the family. Communication of a diagnosis means a full explanation of the disorder and its prognosis, based on knowledge of the natural history of the disease. In our example, this implies a discussion about mental retardation, which is one of the main features of Prader-Willi syndrome, though we also need to discuss the wide variability in expression of this feature. The parents should also be prepared to cope with behavioural problems, particularly those related to the search for food (a striking feature of Prader-Willi syndrome).

Table 5. Frequent gestaltic diagnoses

Disease	Caused by:
Down syndrome	Chromosome 21 trisomy
Turner syndrome	X monosomy
Cri du chat syndrome	Deletion/microdeletion 5p
Edwards syndrome	Chromosome 18 trisomy
Patau syndrome	Chromosome 13 trisomy
Wolf-Hirschhorn syndrome	Deletion/microdeletion 4p
Williams syndrome	Microdeletion 7q11.23
Microdeletion 22q syndrome (Di George)	Microdeletion 22q11.2
Noonan syndrome	Mutation in *PTPN11*, *KRAS*, *SOS1* gene
Cornelia de Lange syndrome	*NIPBL*, *SMC1*
Rubinstein-Taybi syndrome	Microdeletion 16p13.3, mutation of gene *CBP*
Treacher-Collins syndrome	Mutation of *Treacle* gene
Silver-Russell syndrome	Maternal uniparental disomy of chromosome 7 in 10% of patients
Sotos syndrome	Deletion 5q35, mutation in gene *NSD1* in about 70% of patients
Ocular-auricular-vertebral spectrum	Unknown genetic test. Clinical diagnosis
Achondroplasia	Mutation in gene *FGFR3* in 98% of patients
Apert syndrome	Mutation in gene *FGFR2*

Occasionally the clinician's work is relatively simple, but there are specific issues that must be considered which may complicate the task of making a diagnosis and determining the prognosis in a very young patient. Some examples of these are the variability of clinical expression, lack of clarity in defining diagnostic criteria, the genetic heterogeneity of various syndromes, and the difficulty in determining the prognosis for future development in very young children.

Variability of clinical expression

It is well known that the dysmorphic phenotype typical of a particular condition can be very mild in some patients and fully expressed in others. An example is the Cornelia de Lange syndrome. In 1993 it was accepted that there were both a classical phenotype and a mild phenotype. In the classical phenotype the patients have particular facial dysmorphisms which are often recognizable at birth or soon after, while in the mild form it may be difficult to recognize the phenotypical appearance even in the young adult. The same variability is evident in other malformation syndromes – the phenotype related to microdeletion 22q11.2 is another example.

The variability of the phenotype is also evident in the evolution of the facial features in some patients affected by specific conditions. In many situations the phenotype becomes more evident as the child gets older. Before the discovery of the genetic defect that causes Williams syndrome (microdeletion 7q11.2), the mean age of the diagnosis was internationally reported to be at around 6 years, when the typical elf face becomes fully recognizable. In mild cases of Cornelia de Lange syndrome there are examples of an evolving facial phenotype where the features are atypical in the first years of life but become clearly evident by 4–5 years. It is also important to remember that in many syndromes it may not be easy to recognize the dysmorphology in the adult patient because of the natural evolution of somatic traits.

A practical consequence of these various problems is that it is important to follow up those patients who do not yet have a specific diagnosis, especially if the initial evaluation was done at a young age. It can also be useful to ask adult patients in whom the phenotype is not diagnostic to provide photographs of their appearance at a younger age, if available.

Variability of expression is also shown in the presence or absence of major malformations and other medical problems. Once again microdeletion 22q11.2 is a good example. It is well known that patients with this complex disease can have important cardiac malformations (mostly conotruncal defects), structural or functional anomalies at the palate, defects of cell-mediated immunity because of hypoplasia or agenesis of the thymus, and hypocalcaemia secondary to parathyroid hypoplasia or aplasia. Looking at large groups of affected subjects we can see how variable the combination of these principal congenital defects may be in individual patients. About 10 per cent of cases of microdeletion 22q11.2 are familial, which means that one of the parents has the same genetic deletion as the child. Careful examination may show that the disease phenotype is very mildly expressed in one of the parents, so the diagnosis is made in the parent only as a result of the correct diagnosis in the offspring.

Another important concept to consider is that medical problems which can be particularly important as diagnostic criteria for a specific disease can have an age-dependent onset. In obesity/mental retardation syndromes such as Cohen or Bardet-Biedl syndrome, it is known that retinitis pigmentosa – which is a feature of these syndromes – is not congenital but becomes evident only after some years. Another example is Costello syndrome. Before the definition of the phenotype and the discovery of gene defect (in *H-RAS* gene) in this disorder, the diagnosis was strongly dependent on the presence of perioral/perianal papillomata, but these benign tumours may not make their first appearance for several years after birth.

Unclear definition of clinical diagnostic criteria

The evolution of molecular genetics in recent years has allowed us to use molecular tests for many of the most common malformation syndromes. The detection rate of these tests rarely approaches 100 per cent, and the more we know the more it becomes clear that genetic heterogeneity is the rule rather than the exception. If we take into account the practical difficulties in finding fully equipped laboratories capable of carrying out complex and multiple genetic analyses, we can understand why clinical diagnostic criteria are still so important.

Unfortunately the more we know about natural history and clinical phenotypes of these syndromes, the more difficult it becomes to define the clinical criteria. The story of the Kabuki Make-up syndrome is a good example. The Japanese investigators Niikawa and Kuroki wrote about this syndrome for the first time in 1981, when no accepted genetic defect had been discovered. After the first study of about 60 affected patients, the Japanese authors suggested quite rigid and defined diagnostic criteria (Table 6), writing that 'the core of phenotypic spectrum of Kabuki Make-up syndrome is quite narrow.' In the following years, more patients were observed in non-Asiatic populations, and multiple reports appeared in the medical literature, leading to a better defined phenotype and a list of reported medical complications of the syndrome. A couple of European investigators suggested new possible diagnostic algorithms slightly different from the original one (Tables 7 and 8). After these new proposals, the problem seemed no easier to solve, as outlined by Amstrong et al. (2005) in a review of Kabuki syndrome, writing '... the diagnosis of Kabuki syndrome is a clinical one for which no validated diagnostic criteria have been published.' Obviously this kind of problem increases the difficulties of making a definitive diagnosis in many situations in which molecular tests are not conclusive or are not available. The only possible way forward for these patients is to establish a process of validation of the clinical diagnosis accepted by experts in the field of clinical genetics and dysmorphology.

Genetic heterogeneity of various syndromes

In recent years molecular cytogenetics and molecular biology have greatly improved the genetic basis for defining various syndromes. New genes have been discovered and new microdeletion syndromes delineated. The following questions remain: What if we have a clinical suspicion of a specific syndrome and genetic testing gives us a negative result? Did we suggest the wrong diagnosis or does the genetic test have a low detection rate, not close to 100 per cent? These questions may be easy to resolve in situations such as Noonan syndrome or Cornelia de Lange syndrome, in which the first genes identified (*PTPN11* and *NIPBL*) show a mutation in fewer than 50 per cent of classically affected children. The solution may be more complex in other situations. An interesting recent example is the Smith-Magenis syndrome. This condition is clinically characterized by the presence of peculiar facial dysmorphisms, short stature, mental retardation, brachydactyly, and very typical behavioural problems. At a genetic level, affected patients show a deletion of the short arm of chromosome 17 at the p11.2 band of about 3.5–4.0 Mb. Some patients with larger deletions can be diagnosed directly with a standard karyotype with more than 550 bands; in the great majority, however, the deletion can be highlighted only through fluorescence *in situ* hybridization (FISH) analysis with specific probes. Recent studies have shown that the critical region for the development of Smith-Magenis phenotype is not investigated with the available commercial probes which do not include *RAI1* gene. More recently, a truncating mutation of *RAI1* gene itself has been diagnosed in some rare patients with Smith-Magenis phenotype and negative FISH studies. This is clear evidence that the Smith-Magenis phenotype can have different genetic defects which should be always considered in planning the laboratory confirmation of a clinical diagnosis such as this. At the moment it is very difficult to say whether mutated patients are more common than microdeleted patients, and it is also unknown whether patients with negative results in all the available

Table 6. Diagnostic criteria for Kabuki syndrome (Nikawa et al., 1988)

Peculiar facial dysmorphism
Psychomotor retardation
Postnatal growth failure
Skeletal anomalies
Dermatoglyphic anomalies

Table 7. Diagnostic criteria for Kabuki syndrome, updated (Schrander-Stumpel et al., 1994)

Peculiar facies and mild to moderate mental retardation
Short stature
Skeletal anomalies
Major malformations (not compulsory)
Fetal pads (useful but not pathognomonic)

Table 8. Diagnostic criteria for Kabuki syndrome (Digilio et al., 2001)

Peculiar facies and at least three of the following:
Mental retardation
Congenital heart disease
Short stature
Skeletal anomalies
Fetal pads

laboratory investigations (at a cytogenetic, molecular cytogenetic, and molecular level) should be considered unaffected or whether new genes may be discovered in the future to be related to this phenotype.

The meaning of all this is that if we have a convincing clinical diagnosis of a specific disease which is not confirmed by any available genetic tests we should first reconsider our conclusions. If our suspicions remain, we cannot exclude the possibility that other genetic defects will be discovered in the future.

Difficulties in forecasting outcome in very young patients

At the time when the diagnosis is made, in the neonatal period or slightly later, there are two very common and important questions asked by parents of children with a malformation syndrome associated with mental retardation: What degree of retardation will our child have? If the disease is known to have variability of expression, will the phenotype of our child be mild or severe?

We need to consider the following two possibilities:
- the existence of a correlation between genotype and phenotype;
- if the genetic defect of the syndrome is unknown or no genotype-phenotype correlation exists, the presence of a relation between phenotypic features and functional severity.

Unfortunately in the great majority of well known conditions, these correlations are not direct or evident. We will discuss some examples of common genetic syndromes.

In Wolf-Hirschhorn syndrome, Zollino et al. (2000) identified three classes of deletion based on the width of the deletion (Table 9). A comparison between the amount of missing DNA and the clinical phenotype showed some level of correlation with the presence or absence of major malformations, but a weaker correlation with the severity of mental retardation.

Table 9. Genotype-phenotype correlations in Wolf-Hirschhorn syndrome (Zollino et al., 2000)

Class 1: Large deletion
Class 2: Large molecular deletion (4.4–3.2 Mb)
Class 3: Small molecular or no deletion (< 2.8 Mb) • Positive correlation with presence/absence of major malformations • Minor correlation with severity of mental retardation

Williams syndrome is another microdeletion syndrome in which 98 per cent of patients have a loss of DNA on the long arm of chromosome 7 (7q11.2). Recent studies have shown that the great majority of Williams syndrome patients lose the same amount of genetic material because of the presence of two very similar sequences of DNA at the beginning and end of the commonly deleted region of about 1.8 Mb. In spite of the similarity of genetic deficiency, we know that Williams syndrome patients show wide variability in severity at both a clinical and a functional level, and the reasons for this remain unknown. Accurate clinical studies have failed to demonstrate any correlation between the presence or absence of a specific feature and the level of severity of the mental retardation.

In Angelman syndrome we are now aware of the existence of at least four genetic classes of patients – related to different possible anomalies of the 15q11.2 region – as summarized in Fig. 5. Various studies on the existence of possible correlations between a specific genetic class and certain clinical features have been carried out. The results show a gradient of severity, starting from deleted patients (who are the most severely affected) and proceeding to UBE3A-mutated patients, IC-mutated patients, and UPD-mutated patients, who are the least affected.

On the other hand, Rubinstein-Taybi syndrome – a dysmorphic syndrome characterized by facial dysmorphisms, short stature, mental retardation, and large/adducted/duplicated halluces and toes – does not show any evident difference between patients with microdeletion of 16p13 and those with *CBP* gene mutations.

The final example is related to Cornelia de Lange syndrome, a genetic syndrome characterized by a characteristic dysmorphic face, hirsutism, prenatal and postnatal growth retardation, mental retardation, and smallness of the hands and feet or the presence of a severe limb reduction defect of the upper limbs. From 1993 the existence of a classical and a mild phenotype has been accepted (Van Allen et al., 1993). In subsequent years it has become evident that the phenotype of this patients can be greatly variable and that a specific separation into two different classes is not easy. At a genetic level it is now clear that about 50 per cent of patients show a mutation in the *NIPBL* gene (Musio et al., 2006). Available data regarding correlations between genotype and phenotype seem to suggest more severe involvement in mutated patients, affecting prenatal and postnatal growth, language delay, and the prevalence of limb reduction defects. The main problem is that, though this may be true in general terms, there are examples of very mildly affected people with truncating mutations in the same gene. A second gene was recently associated with Cornelia de Lange syndrome *(SMC1L1)* but data are too scarce to properly discuss a possible phenotype related to mutations of this gene (Gillis *et al.*, 2004).

At a clinical level two variables seems to correlate with the severity of functional involvement: low birth weight and limb reduction defects.

The prevalence of severe mental retardation increases as the birth weight diminishes, though this is not an absolute correlation – some affected children with low birth weight (under 2500 g) have substantially better mental development than others of the same low birth weight.

The other powerful clinical feature is the presence of a limb reduction defect. In this case the correlation is more direct: all patients with this kind of malformation have severely impaired mental development. Thus the presence of this type of malformation can be considered a sign of a poor prognosis. Unfortunately we know that the absence of this sign cannot be considered

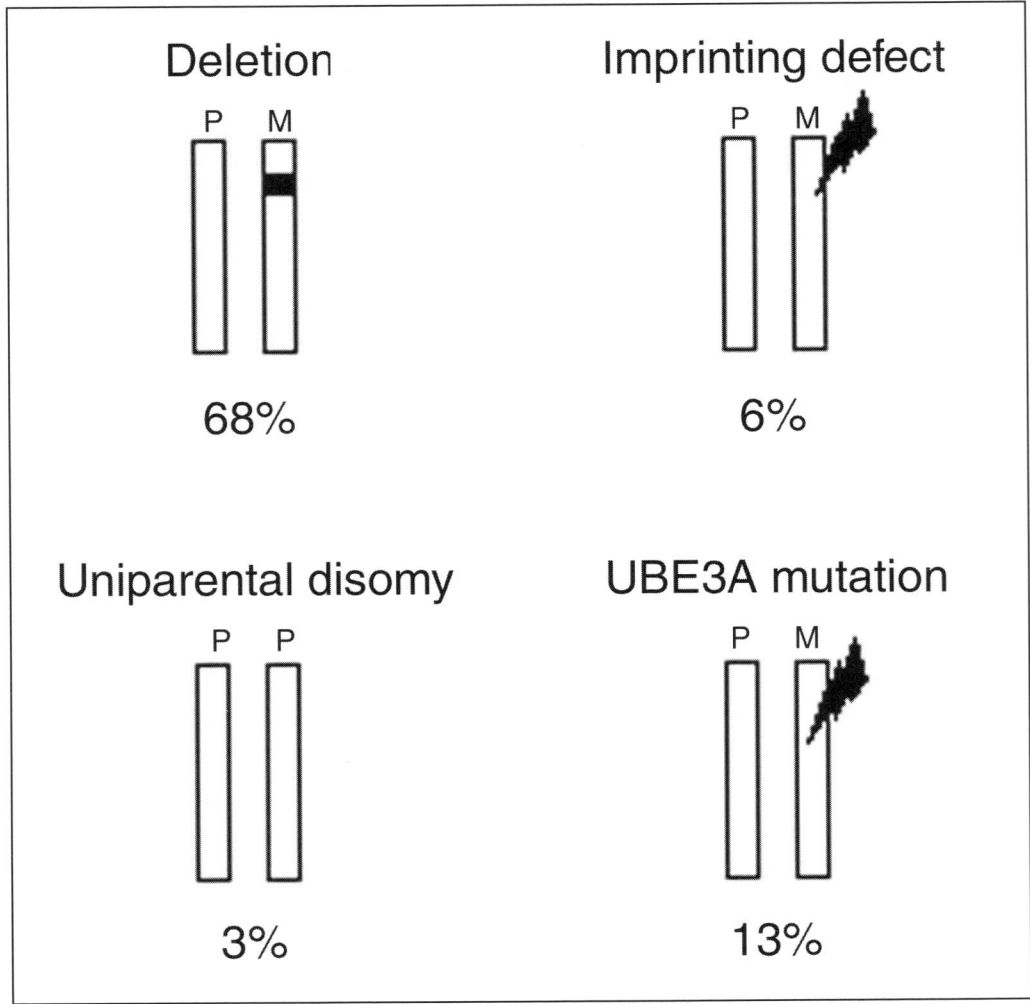

Fig. 5. *Different possible genetic mechanisms of Angelman syndrome* (Williams, 2005, *Brain Dev.*). M, maternal; P, paternal.

predictive of a good prognosis because severe mental retardation may occur in patients with Cornelia de Lange syndrome who have normal birth weight and no limb malformations.

These examples are useful in showing how difficult the interpretation of the correlation between genotype and phenotype can be at a clinical level. From a biological point of view they demonstrate the complex way in which the expression of the genetic material is regulated, and how far we are from understanding all the mechanisms.

What is the diagnostic end point of the process?

The final point of our discussion is the significance of the diagnosis. We are convinced that making the correct diagnosis will have important practical consequences for the assistance we can offer to our patients. By making a specific diagnosis, we can provide the family with genetic counselling and anticipate possible medical complications associated with the condition, which may be generic or specific. Generic medical complications are common to all children with mental retardation and result from their reduced mobility and their neurological involvement. Table 10 lists these possible medical problems. None of them is specific for a particular syndrome but all are relatively common in many conditions and have a direct correlation with the severity of mental and neurological involvement. The ability to suspect, accurately diagnose, and properly treat these complications is very important because their clinical presentation in a malformed, mentally retarded child may be quite atypical.

Table 10. Clinical problems found in patients with mental retardation

Alimentary disturbance
Gastro-oesophageal reflux/oesophagitis
Recurrent infections at the upper and lower airways/chronic obstructive bronchopneumonopathy
Odontostomatological problems
Sleep disturbance
Constipation
Scoliosis/kyphosis
Predisposition to obesity in young-adult age

Another important chapter of this long story is related to the prevalence of behavioural problems which are very common in children with genetic syndromes. Neurobehavioural studies are being undertaken to describe the symptoms, to classify them, and to relate them to the different syndromes. It is important not to forget that these manifestations can also be an expression of the interaction between underdiagnosed medical problems causing discomfort or pain and the very poor ability of such children to describe their symptoms. The practical significance of this at both a diagnostic and a therapeutic level is obvious.

Conclusions

The examples given show how the medical approach to these special patients needs to create strong multidisciplinary alliances between paediatrics, genetics, neurology, and neuropsychiatry, which can offer global assistance to the children and their families, not forgetting the educational, social, emotional, and psychological issues. This task is both essential and urgent and can be summarized by the reminder that these patients and their families 'are not a separate world but a part of our world'.

References

Aase, J. (1990): *Diagnostic Dismorphology*. Amsterdam: Kluwer Academic Publishers.

American Academy of Pediatrics (2001): Health care supervision for children with Williams Syndrome. *Pediatrics* **107**, 1192-1204.

Armstrong, L., Abd El Moneim, A., Aleck, K., Aughton, D.J., Baumann, C., Braddock, S.R., Gillesen-Kaesbach, G., Graham, J.M., Grebe, T.A., Gripp, K.W., Hall, B.D., Hennekam, R., Hunter, A., Keppler-Noreuil, K., Lacombe, D., Lin, A.E., Ming, J.E., Kokitsu-Nakata, N.M., Nikkel, S.M., Philip, N., Raas-Rothschild, A., Sommer, A., Verloes, A., Walter, C., Wieczorek, D., Williams, M.S., Zackai, E. & Allanson, J.E. (2005): Further delineation of Kabuki syndrome in 48 well-defined new individuals. *Am. J. Med. Genet. A.* **132**, 265-272.

Bankier, A. (1998): Dismorphology: problems in nomenclature. *Dysmorphol. Clin. Genet.* **2**, 24-50.

Battaglia, A. & Carey, J. (2003): Diagnostic evaluation of developmental delay/mental retardation. *Am. J. Med. Genet. Part C*, **117C**, 3-14.

Digilio, M.C., Marino, B., Toscano, A., Giannotti, A. & Dallapiccola, B. (2001): Congenital heart defects in Kabuki syndrome. *Am. J. Med. Genet.* **100**, 269-274.

Gillis, L.A., McCallum, J., Kaur, M., DeScipio, C., Yaeger, D., Mariani, A., Kline, A.D., Li, H.H., Devoto, M., Jackson, L.G. & Krantz, I.D. (2004): NIPBL mutational analysis in 120 individuals with Cornelia de Lange syndrome and evaluation of genotype-phenotype correlations. *Am. J. Hum. Genet.* **75**, 610-623.

Musio, A., Selicorni, A., Focarelli, M.L., Gervasini, C., Milani, D., Russo, S., Vezzosi, P. & Larizza, L. (2006): X-linked Cornelia de Lange syndrome owing to SMC1L1 mutations. *Nat. Genet.* **38**, 528-530.

Niikawa, N., Kuroki, Y., Kajii, T., *et al.* (1988): Kabuki make-up (Niikawa-Kuroki) syndrome: a study of 62 patients. *Am. J. Med. Genet.* **31**, 565-590.

Schrander-Stumpel, C., Meinecker, P., Wilson, G., Gillessen-Kaesbach, G., Tinschert, S., Konig, R., Philip, N., Rizzo, R., Schrander, J., Pfeiffer, L., *et al.* (1994): The Kabuki (Niikawa-Kuroki) syndrome: further delineation of the phenotype in 29 non-Japanese patients. *Eur. J. Pediatr.* **153**, 438-445.

SIGU (2000): Linee guida per la Sindrome di Williams. *Riv. It. Pediatr.* **26**, 244-253.

Stevenson, R.E., Procopio-Allen, A.M., Schroer, R.J. & Collins, J.S. (2003): Genetic syndromes among individuals with mental retardation. *Am. J. Med. Genet.* **123**, 29-32.

Van Allen, M.I., Filippi, G., Siegel-Bartelt, J., *et al.* (1993): Clinical variability within Brachmann-de Lange syndrome: a proposed classification system. *Am. J. Med. Genet.* **47**, 947-958.

Williams, C.A. (2005): Neurological aspects of the Angelman syndrome. *Brain Dev.* **27**, 88-94.

Zollino, M., Di Stefano, C., Zampino, G., Mastroiacovo, P., Wright, T. J., Sorge, G., Selicorni, A., Tenconi, R., Zappala, A., Battaglia, A., Di Rocco, M., Palka, G., Pallotta, R., Altherr, M.R. & Neri, G. (2000): Genotype-phenotype correlations and clinical diagnostic criteria in Wolf-Hirschorn syndrome. *Am. J. Med. Genet.* **94**, 254-261.

Chapter 6

Laboratory: instructions for proper use of genetic tests

Angelo Selicorni, Cecilia Vellani, Marta Cerutti, Melissa Bellini and Donatella Milani

Clinical Genetics, I Paediatric Clinic, University of Milan, Fondazione IRCCS Ospedale Maggiore Policlinico, via Commenda 9, 20122 Milan, Italy
ambulatorio@gencli.it

Summary

In recent years, biological research has increased the possibilities for detailed study of the organization of the human genome. The result is that we are presented with various possibilities for using new and more sophisticated tests to confirm specific diagnoses.
Some of the genetic tests available can be used at all levels of resolution (standard karyotype, FRM1 gene molecular tests, subtelomeric studies, array-CGH analysis) without needing to confirm a specific hypothesis. On the other hand, with other types of analysis – for example fluorescence *in situ* hybridization (FISH) studies looking for specific microdeletions, and molecular tests of known genes to identify causal mutations – it is mandatory to have a well defined clinical hypothesis.
The more we know, the more it emerges that an important feature of many genetic syndromes is represented by genetic heterogeneity. This means that in some syndromes more than one genetic defect can be identified in the same but variable disease. In certain cases the different types of genetic mutation cover the entire spectrum of disease variability; in others the clinical diagnosis may still be valid even when all the available genetic studies have given normal results. The genetic heterogeneity of an increasing number of the different conditions sometimes makes the confirmation of a clinical diagnosis a multistep pathway. For this reason, clinicians involved in the diagnostic work-up should be informed about the quality, numbers, and detection rates of the genetic tests available, in order to establish an accurate diagnostic work-up and to interpret the results of the analyses correctly.

A genetic test is an analysis of DNA, RNA, chromosomes, proteins, metabolites, or other products carried out to define a genotype, phenotype, or karyotype, whether related or not to a human heritable disease. There are several different types of genetic test: diagnostic tests, presymptomatic tests, susceptibility tests, genetic tests to identify carriers of a mutation, and tests used for legal purposes.

In everyday practice, it is very important that the physician who plans to perform a genetic test is aware of all the possible results of the test (its possibilities and limitations) and of the possible consequences of the test for the patient and the whole family in terms of genetic counselling. The test should be strictly related to the clinical problem under investigation and should be

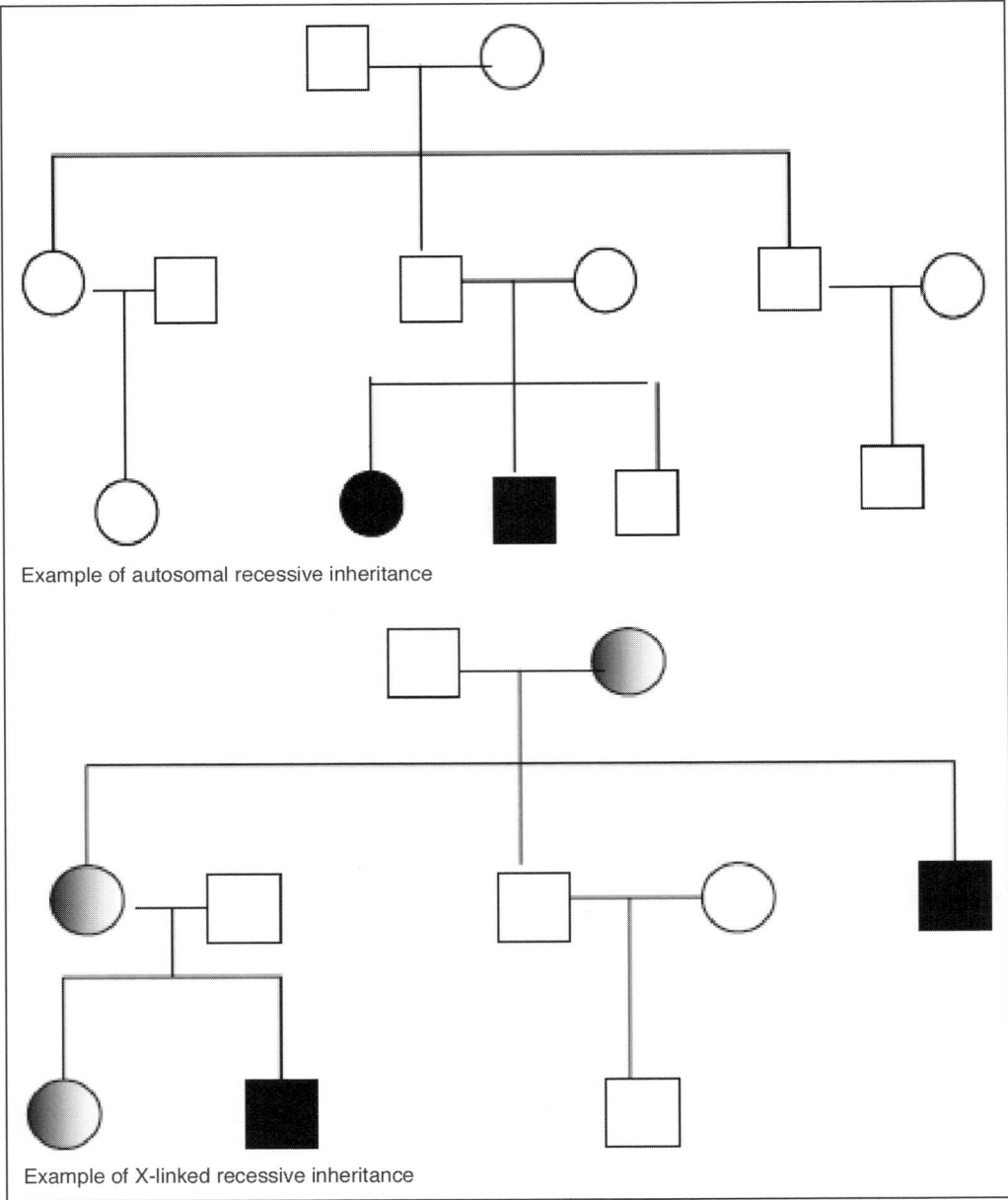

Fig. 1. Top: Example of autosomal recessive inheritance. Bottom: Example of X-linked recessive inheritance.

consistent with the pattern of inheritance identified in the patient's family. Fig. 1 shows two examples which suggest an autosomal recessive and an X-linked recessive disease, respectively.

The physician who suggests the test should be aware whether the test will be totally or only partially informative with respect to diagnosis, and should also consider which healthy members of the family should be tested to define their genetic risks or to make a further evaluation of the results on the patient. In particular, the diagnosis of a specific mutation will guide the clinician towards a study of other healthy members of the family – the relatives could be carriers of the same mutation and could therefore have affected children. The further situation relates to the interpretation of a new mutation in a specific gene. Before classifying this as a pathogenic mutation, both parents should be screened to rule out the possibility of a polymorphism.

Table 1 shows the classification of genetic diseases according to the underlying genetic anomaly. Obviously we have different types of genetic test which may confirm or disclose various types of abnormality. Genetic tests have different levels of resolution, ranging from the common type of cytogenetic testing to the most accurate mutation analysis.

Table 1. Classification of genetic diseases according to genetic anomaly

• Chromosomal	Number of aberrations Structural defects
• Monogenic	Autosomal dominant Autosomal recessive X-linked dominant X-linked recessive
• Multifactorial	
• Mitochondrial	

Cytogenetic analysis

The oldest and easiest way to analyse our genome is by standard cytogenetic analysis. This test is carried out on a blood sample and detects the presence or absence of abnormalities in chromosome numbers or structure. Fig. 2 shows an example of a chromosomal analysis. Whole chromosomes are characterized by a well defined sequence of black, grey, and white bands that depend on the type of stain used. Various types of banding are able to define specific regions of different chromosomes. Communication and interaction with the laboratory guarantee the most effective approach. It should be remembered that recent standard cytogenetic analyses have a higher resolution than 10 or more years ago, so that the possibility of detecting a structural anomaly has greatly improved. A direct consequence of this evolution in technology is that it is advisable to repeat a standard karyotype analysis if it was first done more than 10 years earlier. Table 2 defines the guidelines for standard karyotypes in children. The main question is whether in this molecular age a simple standard karyotype should be carried out to define the diagnosis in a child with mental retardation. Recently published reports apparently give us different answers. Rauch et al. (2006) studied a large unselected group of patients with mental retardation and found that 16 per cent of them were affected by a chromosomal anomaly evident in a standard karyotype. On the other hand, Macayran et al. (2006) found no cytogenetic anomaly in 113 patients affected by isolated mental retardation. The results of these two reports seem discordant, but those of the latter were affected by a different choice of reference population which might be considered a source of bias. However, both studies emphasized that the presence of associated dysmorphic features and medical problems (major malformations, growth anomalies) increase the likelihood of there being a chromosomal anomaly as a cause of the mental problem.

Table 3 lists some of the most common chromosomal aneuploidy syndromes. It is important to bear in mind that chromosomal mosaicisms are very common types of chromosomal defect.

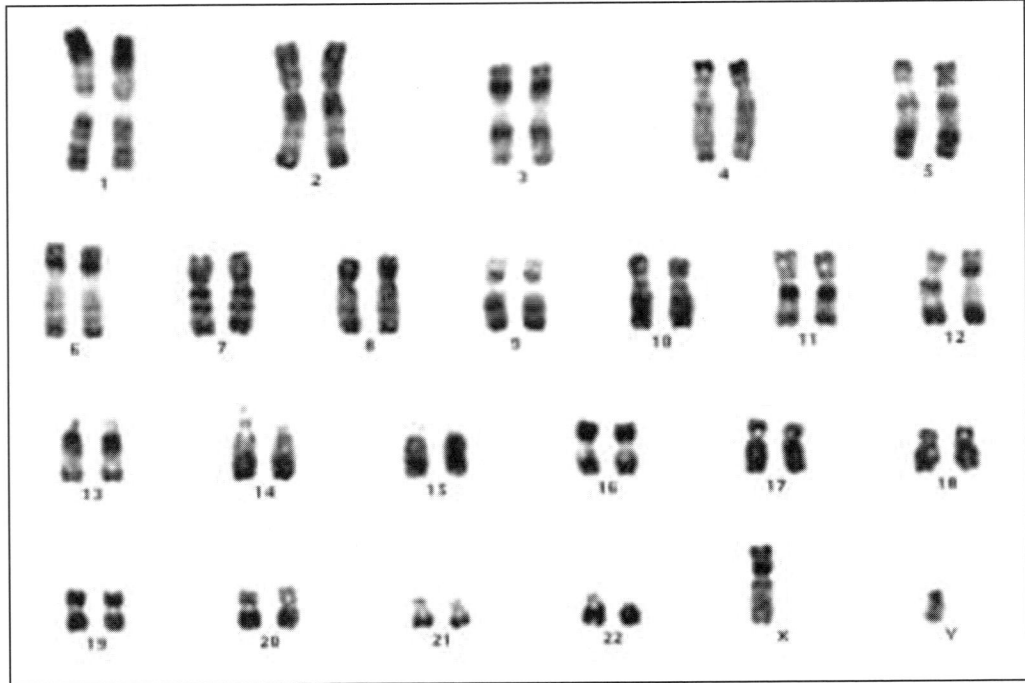

Fig. 2. Example of a chromosomal analysis.

We define mosaicism as a condition in which the patient has at least two different cell lines: one with a normal and the other with an abnormal karyotype. Common classical examples are Down syndrome and Turner syndrome, in which mosaicism is relatively common. If the physician suspects a mosaicism or wishes to rule out this possibility, the following should be done:

- The hypothesis of a mosaicism should be explained very clearly to the laboratory scientist, who will then analyse a larger number of metaphases.
- If a standard karyotype done earlier was reported as normal on the basis of only a small number of metaphases, it should be repeated.
- The type of tissue analysed must be the correct one to detect the suspected mosaicism.

Table 2. Guidelines for undertaking standard karyotyping in children

• Mental retardation of unknown origin
• Multiple major malformations/dysmorphic features associated with one malformation
• Ambiguous genitalia
• Short stature in females
• Relatives of individuals with chromosomal aberrations

This last recommendation refers to the rare situation in which a properly conducted analysis of a blood sample fails to demonstrate the pathological cell line. An example is the Pallister-Killian syndrome, a condition caused by the presence of a pathological cell line with an extra chromosome characterized by two copies of the short arm of chromosome 12 (isochromosome 12p). For unknown reasons, this chromosomal abnormality cannot be found in the blood but only in certain other types of tissue, for example skin fibroblasts. Affected individuals show peculiar facial dysmorphic features with a typical fronto-temporal hairline, severe to profound mental retardation, epilepsy, absent or nearly absent speech, and various associated anomalies.

As previously stated, a standard karyotype can also show the presence of various structural chromosomal abnormalities which may cause a disease when they are associated with loss (deletion) or gain (duplication) of a piece of DNA. Table 4 lists possible structural chromosomal anomalies, describing them very simply. It is important to discuss those situations in which the karyotype shows the presence of an abnormal structure without loss or duplication of DNA which could be associated with a pathological phenotype. Obviously, the first hypothesis is that the chromosomal abnormality is not responsible for the pathological phenotype. The medical literature provides examples, in which a patient affected by a specific syndrome has a mutation of the specific disease-related gene and, for example, an apparently balanced reciprocal *de novo* translocation between two chromosomes. Apart from this very rare situation, it is important to consider how deeply to explore these issues. The apparently balanced structural anomaly in our patient must be *'de novo'* – that is to say, not present as a result of segregation from one of the healthy parents. At the end of this chapter, we review how to demonstrate more precisely whether there is neither an excess nor a deficit of DNA. Nevertheless a relation between karyotype and pathological phenotype should always be considered, for the following reasons: first, the structural chromosomal anomaly breaks a gene at one of the breakpoints and is responsible for the phenotype; second, in the region in which the structural abnormalities take place there could be a sequence of genes functionally related to each another: the new structure of the chromosomes disrupts this functional sequence, even when no gene is damaged.

Table 3. Some of the most common chromosomal aneuploidy syndromes

• Trisomy 21
• Trisomy 18
• Trisomy 13
• Trisomy 8
• Trisomy 9
• Klinefelter syndrome (47,XXY)
• Turner syndrome (45,X)

It is important to discuss the clinical application of prometaphase studies. This approach allows to obtain more despiralized chromosomes with an increased number of bands. In the past, these studies were widely used to detect a few chromosomal anomalies or to study in detail an apparently balanced chromosomal translocation. These techniques are still useful even though new approaches are now available and seem to be more powerful. Indeed, the use of a prometaphase study without a specific diagnostic question is not advisable.

Table 4. Structural chromosomal anomalies

- Translocation
- Insertion
- Duplication
- Deletion
- Inversion
- Ring chromosome
- Isochromosome

Molecular cytogenetics

FISH analysis

An important and relatively new technique applied in the last 10 years to confirm clinical diagnoses is fluorescent *in situ* hybridization (FISH). With this technique we can verify the absence (or duplication) of very short sequences of DNA using a complementary molecular probe labelled with a fluorescent pigment. The probe used can be complementary to a centromeric, subtelomeric, interstitial chromosomal region or can paint the whole chromosome. Fig. 3 shows an example of this type of analysis, while Table 5 lists the practical applications of FISH.

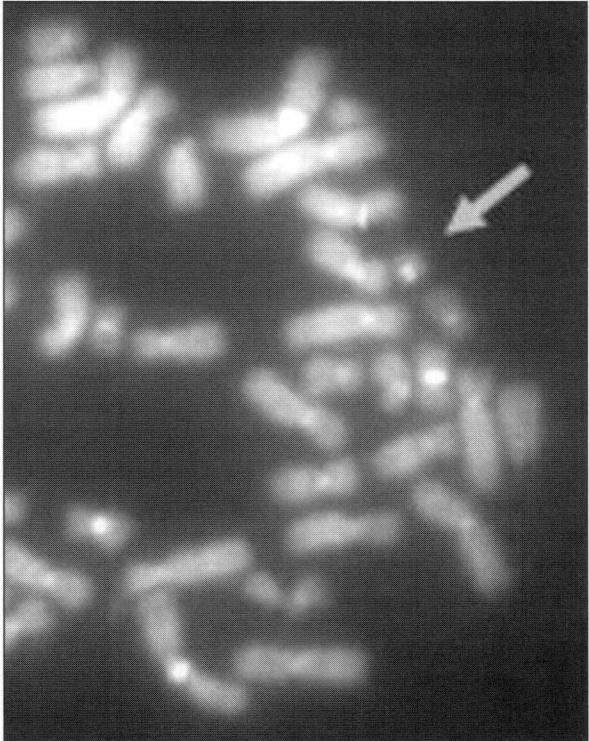

Fig. 3. An example of fluorescent in situ *hybridization (FISH).*

Table 5. Indications for fluorescent *in situ* hybridization (FISH)

• Translocations study and their breakage points
• Identification/characterization of supernumerary markers/ring chromosomes
• Identification of cryptic rearrangement (microdeletion, microduplication)

FISH analysis is very useful for confirming the clinical suspicion of a microdeletion syndrome which cannot be revealed by standard or high-resolution cytogenetic techniques. Table 6 lists the most commonly investigated microdeletion syndromes with their main clinical features and their chromosomal localization. It is important to emphasize that in different situations the detection rate of FISH analyses may be relatively variable. In Williams syndrome, for example, we know now that 97 to 98 per cent of patients will have a typical microdeletion; thus a negative result from FISH analysis should force the clinician to reconsider the clinical diagnosis. Wolf-Hirschhorn syndrome shows a very wide variety of chromosomal defects – some patients carry a deletion that is detectable by standard cytogenetics because it is very large or because it is related to the presence of an unbalanced chromosomal translocation. However, many Wolf-Hirschhorn patients show a deletion only when FISH is applied. In the past, knowledge about the minimal critical region lacked precision, so FISH analysis with initially normal results might not be confirmed by a study done later, using different and more appropriate probes. Angelman and Prader-Willi syndromes are examples of clinical conditions caused by various different genetic defects, so a negative FISH result is only one step in the diagnostic pathway; other molecular tests must be used in order to complete the diagnostic process. Recent evidence shows that this may also be the case in Smith-Magenis and Alagille syndromes, in which both chromosomal microdeletions and point mutations of a specific gene localized in the critical region (RAI 1 and JAG 1, respectively) can be responsible for the clinical phenotype. In the majority of the patients with neurofibromatosis type 1 the molecular defect is a mutation of the neurofibromin gene. A relatively small percentage of subjects show a true microdeletion of the 17q region surrounding the *NF1* gene. Furthermore, microdeletion 22q11.2 is very variable in its extension, even though there is no linear correlation between the width of the deletion and the severity of phenotype, which is well known to be extremely variable.

Table 6. The most investigated microdeletion syndromes

Syndrome	Microdeletion
Wolf-Hirschhorn	4p16.3
Williams	7q11.23
Langer-Giedion	8q24.1
WAGR	11p13
Miller-Diecker	17p13.3
Smith-Magenis	17q11.2
Angelman/Prader-Willi	15q11-q13
Di George	22q11.2

WAGR, Wilms tumour-aniridia-genitourinary anomalies-mental retardation syndrome.

It is therefore easy to understand how necessary it is to make a provisional clinical diagnosis when asking the laboratory to carry out the appropriate analysis, and how essential it is to have a thorough knowledge of the application of the FISH technique to specific diseases when evaluating negative results and planning new diagnostic strategies.

What is the role of microdeletion syndromes in clinical practice in relation to individuals with mental retardation? Rauch *et al.* (2006) reported that up to 5.3 per cent of mentally retarded patients were affected by a microdeletion syndrome.

Subtelometric analysis

As previously stated, the probe that we use can be complementary to sequences of DNA located in the terminal parts of chromosomes (that is, the subtelomeric regions). This is the biological and technical basis for another molecular cytogenetic approach, *subtelomeric analysis*, which has become an essential part of the diagnostic work-up in patients with a suspected complex constitutional disease.

From a biological point of view, the subtelomeric regions of every chromosome are hybridized with specific probes which show whether subtle, cryptic rearrangements are present even when they cannot be detected by standard cytogenetic banding. The importance of this assessment lies in the fact that we now know that the subtelomeric regions are extremely rich in genes, which is why even small rearrangements may be responsible for complex diseases. It is important to emphasize that familial mental retardation, even in cases with strong phenotypic differences, constitutes a major indication. Mentally retarded patients with different phenotypes could in fact be the result of an unbalanced segregation of familial balanced cryptic chromosomal translocation, as in the family shown in Fig. 4.

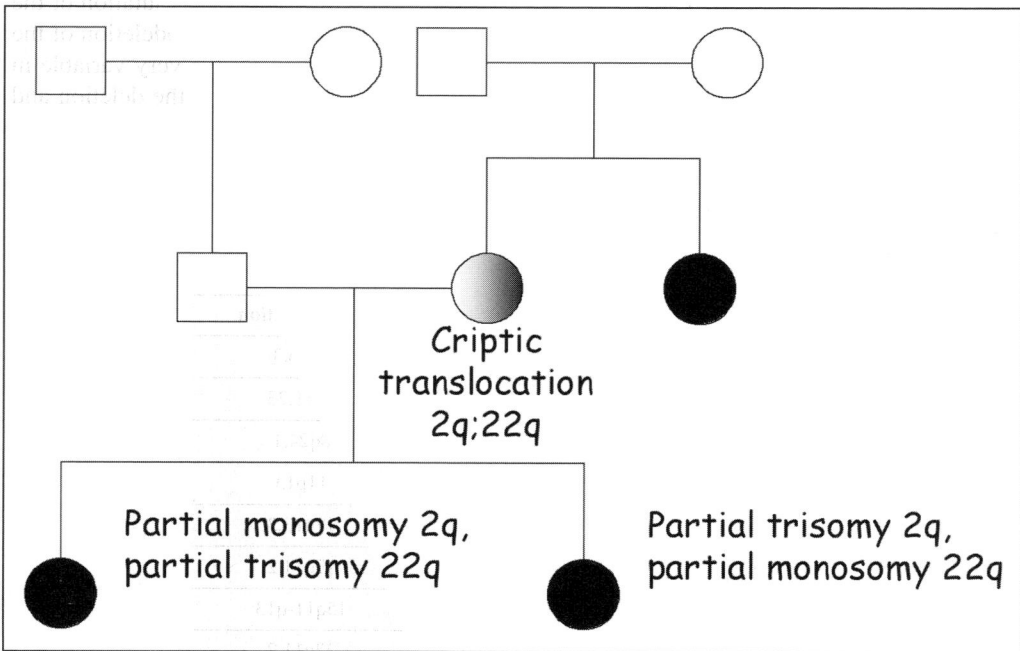

Fig. 4. An example of familiar balanced cryptic chromosomal translocation.

This new approach proved the existence of clinical syndromes that are clinically well characterized and relatively frequent (for example, the famous microdeletion syndromes that we have previously discussed).

It is evident that, apart from these examples and possibly a few others, the use of subtelomeric studies depends on the methodological application of a sequence of examinations instead of a search for confirmation of a clinical diagnosis, as happens with most other microdeletion conditions. It is therefore very important to define the detection rate that can be expected from these kinds of test procedures. Published reports are obviously quite variable and depend strongly on the types of patients considered. The great majority of studies, however, suggest that around 3 to 5 per cent of mentally retarded patients can be diagnosed as having a specific disorder thanks to subtelomeric analysis. This is very important because 50 per cent of cases are caused by a balanced cryptic anomaly evident in one of the two parents and, possibly, in their part of the family. The highest detection rates are found when the clinical selection is more accurate; therefore, when the patient has a so-called 'chromosomal phenotype', there is a strong possibility of finding a cryptic subtelomeric anomaly. Table 7 shows a practical algorithm suggested by de Vries et al. in 2001 to select the patients for subtelomeric analysis. According to this study, with a score below 3 it is very unlikely that the diagnosis will be missed by not doing the test, even if the numbers of patients analysed were greatly reduced. For higher scores, the detection rate is greater but the false negative results also increase.

Molecular biology

Although we do not propose to go deeply into this subject, we will discuss the general approach and the most common problems and considerations related to this kind of genetic test.

First, we have to differentiate between indirect and direct molecular tests. An indirect molecular test – also known as a linkage study – refers to situations in which we do not know exactly the gene of interest but we do know the chromosomal site. A similar situation is where a known gene is too large to be analysed directly. In both situations, we need to study many members of the family, as well as affected and healthy relatives. A molecular study aims to analyse the segregation of genetic polymorphisms which are very close to the possible locus of the gene (or within the gene itself in the case of a well known large gene) in the family members, to determine which of the family have or have not received pathological genetic information. This kind of study is not always effective. It depends on the numbers of family members and type of genetic polymorphism analysed.

Table 7. Medical indications for subtelomeric study

Feature	Score
Family history of mental retardation	1
Compatible with mendelian inheritance	2
Incompatible with mendelian inheritance	2
Postnatal growth retardation or excessive growth	2
Microcephaly, macrocephaly, short/tall stature	1 point for each anomaly (maximum 2 points)
More than two facial dysmorphic features	2
Non-facial minor anomalies and/or major malformations	2

A score of 3 or more is an indication for subtelomeric study.

In direct analysis, we study the whole gene, searching for the presence of a mutation – that is to say, a variation in the sequence causing a disease (Strachan & Read, 2003). We can be confronted with various different situations. If we are studying the *FGFR2* gene for Apert syndrome or the *FGFR3* gene for achondroplasia, we know that there are a few possible mutations that are responsible for more than 98 per cent of affected patients. By searching for these directly we will quickly have a specific answer. A negative result can rule out our clinical diagnosis. For the *PTPN11* gene (Fig. 5) the situation is different. We know that there are no specific mutational hotspots, and the laboratory must analyse the whole gene in order to find a mutation. It is therefore a longer and more difficult task.

A similar situation is encountered in the study of another new gene, *NIPBL*, which is related to Cornelia de Lange syndrome. The gene maps on the short arm of chromosome 5, it is very large (47 exons), and no mutation hot spots have been characterized so far. Studying this gene implies the analysis of all its exons, the promoter regions, and the intron/exon regions. After the first reports, it was clear that this gene is very rich in benign genetic polymorphisms, so that finding a variation in the DNA sequence does not necessarily mean a genuine pathological mutation of the gene. If this kind of DNA sequence variation has not been described previously, we need to consider the possibility of a familial polymorphism, and both healthy parents should be studied before attributing a pathological result to the genetic test. For the *NIPBL* gene and Cornelia de Lange syndrome, and also for the *PTPN11* gene and Noonan syndrome, it is well known that the detection rate is very far from 100 per cent. This is because of the genetic heterogeneity of these diseases which characterizes a large number of monogenic syndromes in which the pathological phenotype may be caused by mutations of different but sometimes functionally related genes. From a practical point of view, the clinician needs to know the detection rate for each single test and must explain to the family the possibilities and limitations of the tests. The clinician's task is also to plan a strategy if there is a negative result in patients where there is strong clinical suspicion. In many cases, a negative genetic result does not rule out the clinical diagnosis, even when there are no new methods available to define the problem in molecular terms. In Cornelia de Lange syndrome, for example, the detection rate of a mutational analysis of the *NIPBL* gene is about 50 per cent; if the first test is negative, two other genes, *SMC1A* and *SMC3*, should be considered. The detection rate for these genes is very low and it is poorly characterized, but it is estimated to account for no more than 10 per cent of affected patients. After extensive and accurate molecular studies, the diagnosis remains a clinical one in about 40 per cent of possible Cornelia de Lange syndrome patients. In this molecular era, it is mandatory to store DNA from affected patients for future analysis and to keep in touch with the family because of possible advances in diagnostic procedures. Molecular defects related to the well known mechanism of 'genomic imprinting' are very specific. Genomic imprinting is a mechanism for regulating the expression of the genome. It is the differential expression (activation/inactivation) of specific genes or regions of specific chromosomes which is related to the parental origin of that gene or region. This means that during gametogenesis, specific portions of our genome undergo a modification through methylation/demethylation which inactivates some genes and activates others. This phenomenon is reversible in the sense that a gene activated because of its paternal origin can be transmitted to the following generation in an inactive form through a maternal chromosome. The normal functioning of the whole genome depends on a balance between active and inactive genes; every mutation which modifies this balance can cause a disease. Among human diseases, some examples are the 15q11.2 region (Angelman and Prader-Willi syndrome) (Valera *et al.*, 2004), the 11p15.5 region (Beckwith-Wiedemann and Silver-Russell syndrome) and the 7q region (Silver-Russell syndrome).

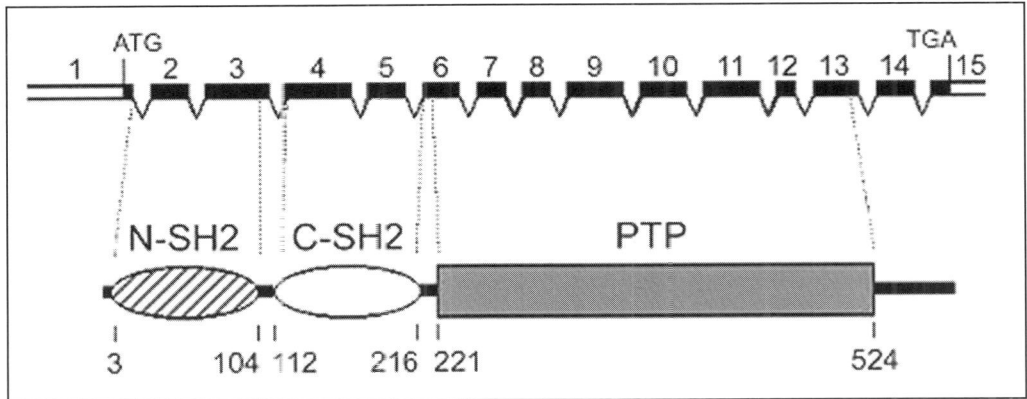

Fig. 5. The PTPN11 gene.

Another important issue is related to the so-called dynamic mutations. This term refers to a specific new mechanism of gene mutation caused by abnormal amplification of the number of repeated triplets of nucleotidic bases. In some of our genes there are regions in which we can observe a variable number of repetitions of a triplet (for example CGG = cytosine-guanine-guanine, as in the promoter of *FMR1* gene). There is a specific range for normal variation; if the number of repetitions increases above the normal limit, the gene can become unstable during both meiosis and mitosis, leading to an abnormal gene. This mechanism is typical of diseases such as fragile-X syndrome, a common cause of mental retardation in the paediatric age range. The phenotype of this syndrome is not very striking as the patients are young, so the suspicion index must be very high. The test should be considered as a screening test for mentally retarded patients with no specific diagnosis. There are a few exclusion criteria (for example, the presence of microcephaly). The gene is located on the long arm of the X chromosome, in the Xq27.3 band, and it shows the presence of a repetition of the CGG triplet within the promoter region. If the number of triplets exceeds the normal value of 55, there is a premutation – that is, the gene is still normal but is unstable and prone to a further increase in the number of triplets (when there are more than 200 triplets the gene is considered to be fully mutated). The increase in triplet number from premutation to full mutation is typical of female gametogenesis, so that a female with a premutation stage can generate males with a full mutation who are therefore affected by fragile-X syndrome. Table 8 shows a practical algorithm for selecting the patients on whom this genetic test should be carried out. De Vries *et al.* (1999) stated that using their scoring system in a wide population of mentally retarded patients and testing all the patients with a score equal to or above 5, they did not miss any affected subjects and avoided carrying out the test in a large proportion of cases. Fragile-X is an example of a large class of diseases referred to as X-linked mental retardation (XLMR). In a recent issue of the *Journal of Medical Genetics*, Raymond offered a useful way of approaching this problem, while another paper published in the *American Journal of Human Genetics* (Plenge *et al.*, 2002) outlined an important genetic feature which can be sometimes observed in the mothers of children with possible XLMR, known as 'skewed X inactivation'. In practical terms, the normal random inactivation of one of the two X chromosomes typical of every female is altered in some mothers of children with XLMR, with preferential inactivation of the X chromosome which carries the mutated gene. The study of X inactivation in these mothers can show whether the XLMR mutated gene is present in that family or not.

Table 8. Algorithm for fragile-X syndrome molecular testing

Feature	Score
Familial history of mental retardation	
• Affected brother, maternal uncle, nephew or cousin	2
• Every affected relative (compatible with XL)	1
Face	
• Elongated mandible/prominent and high forehead	2
• One of the two previous signs	1
Ears	
• Large and prominent	2
• Only large	1
Joints	
• Metacarpophalangeal laxity	2
• 5th finger laxity	1
Skin	
• Soft and redundant palmar skin	2
• Soft palmar skin	1
Testes	
• Both > 30 ml	2
• One > 30 ml	1
Behaviour	
• Shyness, poor visual contact, then friendly and hyperverbal	2
• Some of these features	1

Comparative genomic hybridization

The most recent and very promising technique for analysing DNA is comparative genomic hybridization (CGH). The aim of this new approach is to detect very small chromosomal rearrangements (microdeletions or microduplications) that may be present in the whole chromosome. Thus CGH allows very detailed examination not only of the terminal part of the chromosome, as in subtelomeric studies, but also of the interstitial regions. The importance of being able to study the interstitial regions of chromosomes in detail lies in the fact that small rearrangements quite often affect these sites (about two to three times more often than the terminal parts of the chromosome). The indications for the use of this technique are clearly the same as for subtelomeric studies, although a positive family history of mental retardation is not a strong indication for CGH because interstitial microrearrangements are usually *de novo* and less often familial. The name itself gives us an idea of the type of analysis that is performed. In practical terms, the entire DNA of the patient is compared with a control sample of DNA by using a large number of small consecutive segments of DNA. This comparison can determine whether the patient has the same amount of DNA in every sequence analysed or – when considering a specific trait – has less or more DNA than the control sample. When the latter situation occurs, it means that the patient has a microdeletion (less DNA than the control DNA) or a microduplication (more DNA than the control DNA). The detection rate of array-CGH is clearly influenced by how accurately we select the patients (a 'chromosomal phenotype' leads to a higher prevalence of anomalies) and by the level of resolution that is used. The level of resolution has improved as a very detailed panel of control DNA samples has become available and permits the identification of very small rearrangements.

The detection rate of array-CGH is described in four reports published between 2004 and 2006. These are: Kirchhoff *et al.* (2004), 8.6 per cent; Miyake *et al.* (2006), 10 per cent; Rosenberg *et al.* (2006), 16 per cent; and Poss *et al.* (2006), 8.8 per cent. It is evident that in a variable but consistent proportion of undiagnosed patients (between 8 and 16 per cent) a specific disorder can be identified. Analysis of the types of anomaly showed that about one-third of the interstitial anomalies detected were large enough to be identified by standard karyotyping, even though this was not diagnosed previously. CGH in these cases can enable the laboratory to repeat classical cytogenetic studies more accurately.

A large number of patients with multiple anomalies and mental retardation with a *de novo* 'apparently balanced chromosomal translocation' in fact have an unbalanced condition, and their medical problems are closely correlated with the chromosomal abnormality.

The first results of array-CGH have revealed the existence of atypical presentations of known deletion/microdeletion syndromes, and have shown that the human genome has a greater variability than previously suspected. Before classifying a particular feature found in a patient's genome as pathological, a study of the parents' genome should be undertaken to determine whether the same

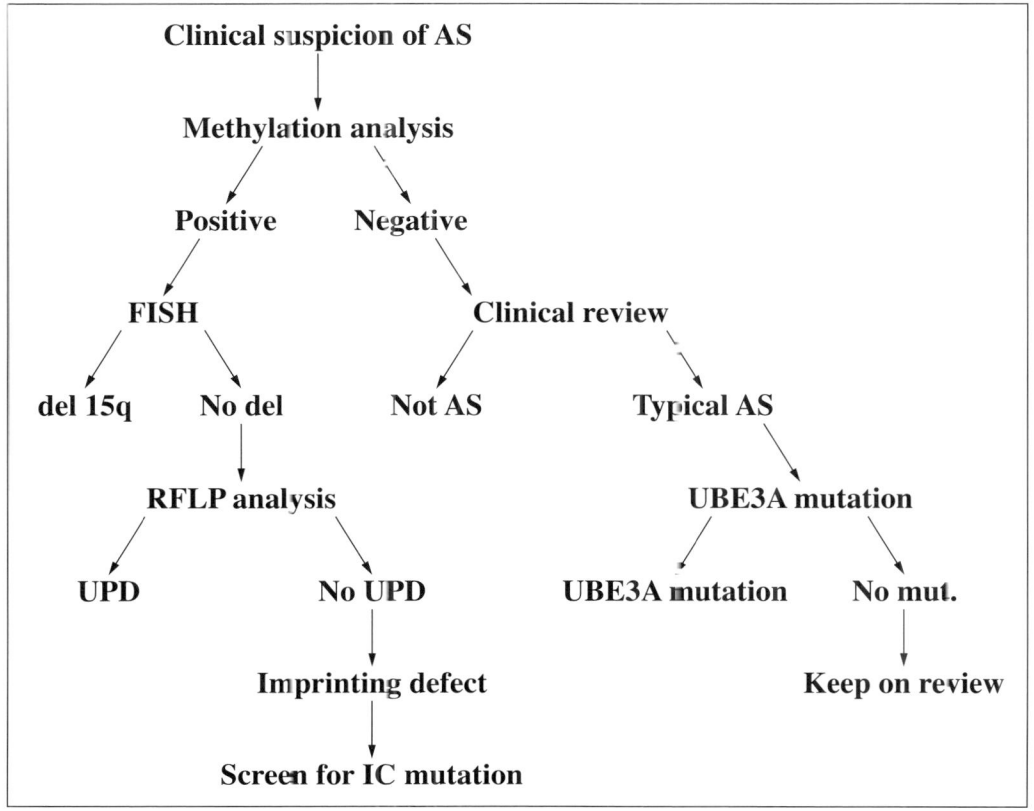

Fig. 6. An algorithm for genetic testing for Angelman syndrome.

characteristic is present, especially if the type of 'anomaly' has not previously been described and characterized as pathological. Many normal variants in different chromosomal regions have been discovered in this way (small duplications or deletions not related to a pathological phenotype).

We are just beginning to gain insight into interstitial chromosomal microrearrangements. In apparently familial non-pathological variants, further research will be necessary to determine whether the patient's phenotype results from varied expression of DNA caused by genomic imprinting, or from a difference in the width of the variant from parent to child.

The more we know about the genetic basis of different syndromes, the more aware we become that the same phenotype can have different genetic causes – for example, chromosomal deletions *versus* microdeletions (as in Wolf-Hirshhorn syndrome), chromosomal microdeletions *versus* mutation of a single gene (such as in Prader-Willi, Angelman, or Smith-Magenis syndromes), or mutation of different single genes producing genetic heterogeneity (Noonan syndrome, Cornelia de Lange syndrome).

The practical consequence of this heterogeneity is that a well defined clinical suspicion will rarely be supported by a single genetic test – the road to a definite diagnosis can be long, and parents need to be aware of this. Fig. 6 shows the complex algorithm for genetic confirmation of a clinical diagnosis of Angelman syndrome.

Current knowledge about the genetic basis of many syndromes suggests that in some patients a genetic confirmation is not possible because the detection rate of genetic tests is not 100 per cent. This means there is a need for continuous clinical assessment so that patients can be tested with new techniques or for new genes, and so that any new clinical features that develop can be assessed. This is very important as new information may greatly modify our knowledge of the recurrence risks of a specific condition. When the correlation between a mutation of the *UBE3A* gene and Angelman syndrome was discovered, we learned that in a some families with this disease the risk of recurrence could be as high as 50 per cent. Recently, it has been stated that five per cent of patients with Cornelia de Lange syndrome have a mutation in the *SMC1* gene, an X-linked gene, and this altered the basis of genetic counselling, especially in isolated male patients.

Though we are in the molecular and cytogenetic molecular era, the role of the clinician is no less important than in the past. Accurate evaluation of the clinical phenotype and a definite clinical diagnosis are the only possible ways to interpret the results of various genetic tests and to plan the most precise and cost-effective genetic analyses.

It is also extremely important that clinicians improve their biological knowledge and obtain information about the different available techniques and about the implications of genetic heterogeneity. They also need to establish close relations with their local laboratory to ensure that each patient is studied by the best and most specific pathway.

References

de Vries, B.B., Mohkamsing, S., van den Ouweland, A.M., Mol, E., Gelsema, K., van Rijn, M., Tibben, A., Halley, D.J., Duivenvoorden, H.J., Oostra, B.A. & Niermeijer, M.F. (1999): Screening for the fragile X syndrome among the mentally retarded: a clinical study. The collaborative fragile X study group. *J. Med. Genet.* **36**, 467–470.

de Vries, B.B., White, S.M., Knight, S.J., Regan, R., Homfray, T., Young, I.D., Super, M., McKeown, C., Splitt, M., Quarrell, O.W., Trainer, A.H., Niermeijer, M.F., Malcolm, S., Flint, J., Hurst, J.A. & Winter, R.M. (2001): Clinical studies on submicroscopic subtelomeric rearrangements: a checklist. *J. Med. Genet.* **38**, 145–150.

Kirchhoff, M., Pedersen, S., Kjeldsen, E., Rose, H., Duno, M., Kolvraa, S. & Lundsteen, C. (2004): Prospective study comparing HR-CGH and subtelomeric FISH for investigation of individuals with mental retardation and dysmorphic features and an update of a study using only HR-CGH. *Am. J. Med. Genet. A* **127**, 111–117.

Macayran, J.F., Cederbaum, S.D. & Fox, M.A. (2006): Diagnostic yield of chromosome analysis in patients with developmental delay or mental retardation who are otherwise nondysmorphic. *Am. J. Med. Genet.* **140**, 2320–2323.

Miyake, N., Shimokawa, O., Harada, N., Sosonkina, N., Okubo, A., Kawara, H., Okamoto, N., Kurosawa, K., Kawame, H., Iwakoshi, M., Kosho, T., Fukushima, Y., Makita, Y., Yokoyama, Y., Yamagata, T., Kato, M., Hiraki, Y., Nomura, M., Yoshiura, K., Kishino, T., Ohta, T., Mizuguchi, T., Niikawa, N. & Matsumoto, N. (2006): BAC array CGH reveals genomic aberrations in idiopathic mental retardation. *Am. J. Med. Genet. A* **140**, 205–211.

Plenge, R.M., Stevenson, R.A., Lubs, H.A., Schwartz, C.E. & Willard, H.F. (2002): Skewed X-chromosome inactivation is a common feature of X-linked mental retardation disorders. *Am. J. Hum. Genet.* **71** (Suppl. 1), 168-173.

Poss, A.F., Goldenberg, P.C., Fehder, C.W., Kearney, H.M., Koeberl, D.D. & McDonald, M.T. (2006): Clinical experience with array CGH: case presentations from nine months of practice. *Am. J. Med. Genet. A* **140**, 2050–2056.

Rauch, A., Hoyer, J., Guth, S., Zweier, C., Kraus, C., Becker, C., Zenker, M. Huffmeier, U., Thiel, C., Ruschendorf, F., Nurnberg, P., Reis, A., Trautmann, U., et al. (2006): Diagnostic yield of various genetic approaches in patients with unexplained developmental delay or mental retardation. *Am. J. Med. Genet.* **140**, 2063–2074.

Raymond, F.L. (2006): X-linked mental retardation: a clinical guide. *J. Med. Genet.* **43** (Suppl. 3), 193-200

Rosenberg, C., Knijnenburg, J., Bakker, E., Vianna-Morgante, A.M., Sloos, W., Otto, P.A., Kriek, M., Hansson, K., Krepischi-Santos, A.C., Fiegler, H., Carter, N.P., Bijlsma, E.K., van Haeringen, A., Szuhai, K. & Tanke, H.J. (2006): Array-CGH detection of micro rearrangements in mentally retarded individuals: clinical significance of imbalances present both in affected children and normal parents. *J. Med. Genet.* **43**, 180–186.

Chapter 7

X-linked mental retardation: a diagnostic, clinical and molecular update

Rossella Caselli, Filomena T. Papa, Francesca Ariani, Ilaria Meloni and Alessandra Renieri

Medical Genetics, Department of Molecular Biology, University of Siena, Policlinico 'Le Scotte', viale Bracci 2, 53100 Siena, Italy
renieri@unisi.it

Summary

X-linked mental retardation (XLMR) is a heterogeneous condition subdivided into two main clinical categories: syndromic XLMR (MRXS) and non-syndromic XLMR (MRX). The number of genes involved has grown rapidly in recent years. This review focuses on the 27 identified genes involved in MRX, wherever possible pointing out the signalling pathways involved and the emerging common mechanisms. Most of the proteins are involved in three distinct mechanisms: (1) modulation of neuronal differentiation and synaptic plasticity; (2) regulation of synaptic vesicle cycling; (3) gene expression regulation. From a clinical perspective, this review emphasizes that mutations in several of these mental retardation genes can result in non-syndromic as well as syndromic forms of XLMR. Reported findings suggest that an accurate current and retrospective clinical evaluation of the patient and of the family history is still fundamental for the initial phenotypic classification of the family before undertaking molecular analysis. In this review, the Italian XLMR Network and its role in the diagnostic and research fields of mental retardation are briefly discussed. One of the major aims of the Network is to increase significantly the proportion of patients with mental retardation who will receive a molecular diagnosis and consequently the appropriate clinical management.

Definition and prevalence of X-linked mental retardation

Mental retardation is defined as a disability characterized by significant limitations in intellectual functioning and in adaptive behaviour, with onset before the age of 18 years (Chelly & Mandel, 2001). Intellectual functioning is defined by the intelligence quotient (IQ), and adaptive behaviour refers to how an individual responds to the demands of everyday life. On the basis of the IQ value, mental retardation may be classified in four categories of severity: mild (IQ 50–70), moderate (IQ 35–50), severe (IQ 20–35), and profound (IQ < 20). In developed countries, mental retardation represents the most frequent cause of severe handicap in children and one of the main reasons for referral in clinical genetic practice. Reported estimates are of about two to three per cent of the general population, and the genetic causes may account for 25–50 per cent of cases of severe mental retardation (Gecz, 2004). Mental retardation is significantly more common in males than in females. The excess of about 30 per cent reflects the presence of several causative genes on the X chromosome, responsible for so called X-linked mental retardation (XLMR) (Baird & Sadovnick, 1985; McLaren & Bryson, 1987; Neri & Chiurazzi, 1999). Based on clinical studies, Turner & Partington (1991) estimated that 20 to 25 per cent of mental retardation in men is caused by X-linked gene defects. Traditionally, XLMR conditions are distinguished into 'syndromic' (MRXS) and 'non-syndromic' or 'non-specific' (MRX), depending on their clinical presentation, although the distinction is gradually becoming less clear (Kerr *et al.*, 1991; Frints *et al.*, 2002; Renieri *et al.*, 2005).

Non-syndromic mental retardation (MRX) and causative genes

The term non-syndromic X-linked mental retardation (MRX) was introduced by Kerr *et al.* in 1991 to indicate a condition segregating in an X-linked manner in which male patients have no consistent phenotypic manifestations other than mental retardation (Kerr *et al.*, 1991; Mulley *et al.*, 1992). To date, 27 genes responsible for MRX have been identified (Table 1; Fig. 1) (Ropers, 2006). Most are responsible for a very small percentage of XLMR cases (0.1 to 1 per cent). For all MRX genes identified up to now, knowledge of the pathogenesis is limited. The corresponding proteins apparently have very different functions. In recent years, as new genes are found considerable effort has been made to identify common pathways. At present, 24 genes seem to be involved in four distinct signalling pathways. For the remaining three genes, no linkage has been possible.

The first genes identified were frequently signalling molecules involved in the Rho GTPase pathway (*FMR1, OPHN1, GDI1, PAK3, ARHGEF6, TM4SF2,* and *FGD1*). Proteins belonging to the Rho GTPases cycle play a key role in regulating dendritic outgrowth and dendritic spine formation and dynamics (Luo, 2000). Rho GTPases are signalling proteins that transduce extra-cellular signals inside the cell, thus orchestrating changes in the actin cytoskeleton. These changes are essential for a number of processes including morphological differentiation, neurite outgrowth and pathfinding, establishment of cell polarity, dendritic spine formation and remodelling, synapse formation, and synaptic plasticity (Hall, 1998; Ramakers, 2002; Chechlacz & Gleeson, 2003). It has long been known that in MRX children these spines are reduced in number and abnormally shaped, with a predominance of very long and thin spines at the expense of stubby and mushroom-like spines (Purpura, 1974). Thus a disruption of the Rho GTPases pathway by mutations in upstream (*OPHN1, ARHGEF6,* and *GDI1*) or downstream *(PAK3)* effectors may lead to a deregulation of neurite sprouting and dendritic spine formation. On the other hand, *TM4SF2*, encoding Tetraspanin 2, and *FMR1*, encoding FMRP, seem to be involved in signalling cascades indirectly linked to the Rho GTPases pathway. In any case, mutations of these genes should have an effect on the regulation of actin cytoskeleton dynamics and neurite outgrowth (Renieri *et al.*, 2005). In addition to the cycle of the small GTPases of Rho, another important cellular process that is altered in patients with mental retardation is the regulation of gene expression. Selective expression or inhibition of different genes is necessary for the correct differentiation and functioning of all cell types, including neurons. Gene expression can be regulated either by the modulation of chromatin structure or by the regulation of activity of the molecules involved in the multistage process leading from the gene to the mature functional protein. In particular, four MRX genes codify for proteins involved in chromatin remodelling (*RPS6KA3, ATRX, MECP2,* and *JARID1C*) and other three for closely related transcription factors (*ZNF41, ZNF81,* and *ZNF674*) (Renieri *et al.*, 2005) (http://www.ggc.org/xlmr.htm). In addition, other MRX genes are involved at various levels in these processes:

Table 1. Known MRX genes

Gene symbol	Protein name	Potential protein function	Reference
Rho GTPases cycle and dendritic outgrowth regulation			
OPHN1	OPHN1	Rho-GTPase-activating protein for RhoA, Rac1 and cdc42	Billuart P., 1998
PAK3	PAK3	Serine-threonine protein kinase downstream of Rac1 and cdc42	Allen K., 1998
ARHGEF6	α-Pix	Guanine-nucleotide exchange factor protein for Rac and cdc42	Kutsche H., 2000
TM4SF2	TM4SF2	Membrane protein interacting with integrins	Zemni R., 2000
FMR1	FMRP	RNA-binding protein; regulator of gene expression at the post-transcriptional level	Rousseau F., 1994
FGD1	FGD1	RhoGEF: possible role in stimulation of neurite outgrowth	Lebel R.R., 2002
Gene expression regulation			
RPS6KA3	RSK2	Serine-threonine protein kinase	Merienne K., 1999
ATRX	XNP	ATP-dependent DNA-helicase	Yntema H., 2002
MECP2	MeCP2	Methyl CpG binding protein	Couvert P., 2001
JARID1C	JAD1C	Role in chromatin remodelling	Jensen L.R., 2005
ZNF41	ZNF41	Zinc-finger protein; transcriptional repressor?	Shoichet S., 2003
ZNF81	ZNF81	Zinc-finger protein; transcriptional repressor?	Kleefstra T., 2004
ZNF674	ZNF674	Zinc-finger protein; transcriptional repressor?	Lugtenberg D., 2006
ARX	ARX	Transcription factor?	Stromme P., 2002
FMR2	FMR2P	Transcription factor	Gecz J., 1996
PQBP1	PQBP-1	Poly-glutamine binding protein 1; interacts with components of the spliceosome; transcriptional repressor	Kalscheuer V.M., 2003
FTSJ1	FTSJ1	RNA methyltransferase	Freude K., 2004
CDKL5	CDKL5	Serine-threonine kinase	Kalscheuer V.M., 2003
Synaptic vesicle transport			
GDI1	α-GDI	GDP-dissociation inhibitor for Rab proteins	D'Adamo P., 1998
IL1RAPL1	ILRAPL	Unknown; involved in stimulated neurotransmitter exocytosis?	Carrie A., 1999
NLGN4	HNLX	Post-synaptic membrane protein; involved in induction of presynaptic structures; linked to NMDA-type-glutamatergic receptors	Laumonnier F., 2004
DLG3	SAP102	Post-synaptic scaffolding protein linked to NMDA-type-glutamatergic receptors	Tarpey P., 2004
AP1S2	AP1S2	Adaptin protein in the assembly of endocytic vesicles	Tarpey P., 2006
SLC6A8	SC6A8	Neurotransmitter transporter	Salomons G., 2001
Orphan mechanisms			
SLC16A2	MCT8	Creatine transporter	Friesema E.C., 2004
AGTR2	AT2	Receptor for angiotensin II	Vervoort V., 2002
ACSL4	ACSL4	Long-chain acyl-CoA synthetase	Meloni I., 2002

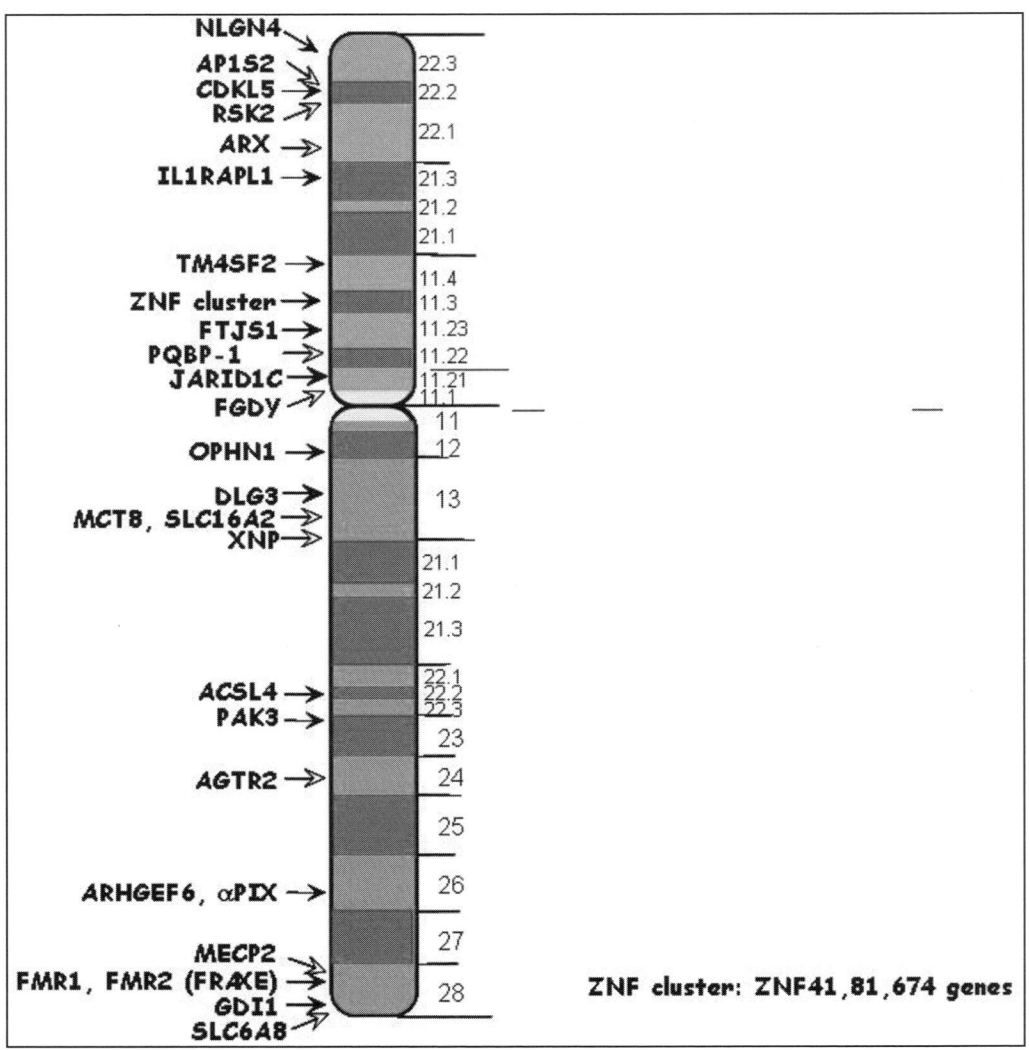

Fig. 1. *Non-syndromic XLMR genes. Modified from Greenwood Genetic Center XLMR Update (http://www.ggc.org/xlmr.htm).*

FMR2, which codifies for a strong transcriptional activator that might participate in the regulation of the Ras/MAPK (mitogen-activated protein kinase) signal transduction pathway; *ARX*, which has been hypothesized to participate in transcriptional complexes regulating genes required for cognitive development (Bienvenu et al., 2002); *PQBP1*, which interacts with components of the spliceosome; *FTSJ1*, which may be involved in the processing and modification of rRNA (Feder et al., 2003; Freude et al., 2004); and *CDKL5*, which encodes for a serine-threonine kinase that interacts with *MECP2* and thus might be indirectly involved in gene regulation (Mari et al., 2005).

More recently, proteins involved in synaptic vesicles cycling have been found to be defective. In particular, mutations have been found in four genes the products of which are located in synaptic vesicles or are necessary for their formation: *SLC6A8*, *NLGN4*, *DLG3*, and *GDI1* (also involved in the Rho GTPase pathway). In addition, *IL1RAPL1* may regulate calcium-dependent exocytosis and thereby play a role in neurotransmitter release (Bahi *et al.*, 2003). Very recently, *AP1S2* has been found to be mutated in three unrelated MRX families (Tarpey *et al.*, 2006). *AP1S2* is the first reported XLMR gene encoding a protein directly involved in the assembly of endocytic vesicles as it constitutes part of the complex that mediates the recruitment of clathrin to the vesicle membrane. Consequently, the pathway of synaptic vesicle transport and recycling regulating neurotransmitter release is potentially altered in MRX patients. Tight regulation of this process is essential for granting the correct temporal and quantitative control of neurotransmitter release and the maintenance of a neurotransmitter reservoir. This in turn is essential for correct synapse functionality and thus for normal brain functioning.

Little is known about the function of the other MRX genes, for which no common pathways have been identified so far (*SLC16A2*, *AGTR2*, and *FACL4*). *SLC16A2* encodes for a creatine transporter belonging to a protein superfamily of transporters responsible for neurotransmitter uptake (Salomons *et al.*, 2003). Thus, one hypothesis is that mutations in *SLC16A2* might result in an alteration in neurotransmitter release, as for *SLC6A8*. *AGTR2* encodes for AT2, a seven transmembrane domain G-protein-coupled type 2 receptor for angiotensin II (Gallinat *et al.*, 2000). Its exact function in brain is presently unknown. It seems to be involved in several functions in neurons, including ionic fluxes, cell differentiation, and axonal regeneration (Lucius *et al.*, 1998; Gendron *et al.*, 1999; Van Bohlen *et al.*, 2001; Rosenstiel *et al.*, 2002), suggesting that an alteration in one of these pathways following *AGTR2* absence might lead to mental retardation. *FACL4* (fatty acid-CoA ligase 4), renamed *ACSL4* (Mashek *et al.*, 2004), has been found mutated by our group in three different MRX families (Meloni *et al.*, 2002; Longo *et al.*, 2003). This gene encodes for a protein which adds coenzyme-A to long chain fatty acids and has a high substrate preference for arachidonic acid, which is abundant in lipids of the nervous system. It is difficult to establish how the reduced function of this acyl-CoA ligase could lead to mental retardation. It is possible that the absence of *ACSL4* function may lead to precocious apoptosis in neurons and to disruption of brain development (Meloni *et al.*, 2002).

Syndromic X-linked mental retardation (MRXS) and causative genes

MRXS conditions are clinically recognizable because mental retardation is present in association with a specific pattern of physical, neurological, or metabolic abnormalities. Presently, it is difficult to estimate the proportion of XLMR that accounts for the MRXS disorder. Until now, about 150 MRXS disorders have been described, for which 51 MRXS genes have been cloned (Fig. 2) (http://www.ggc.org/xlmr.htm). Despite the presence of distinctive features among MRXS patients, the definition of the correct diagnosis can be difficult. In particular, the diagnostic approach is often more difficult in adolescents and adults than in younger children because of the effects of age on physical features and changes in the family structure. A good example of these problems is the family with an *ATRX* mutation reported by Yntema (Yntema *et al.*, 2002). In this family, two patients had a phenotype suggestive of ATR-X (X-linked mental retardation accompanied by α-thalassaemia) while the other two displayed mental retardation only. Following the identification of the *ATRX* mutation, a retrospective evaluation of these two latter patients revealed the presence in childhood of some mild dysmorphic features reminiscent of the typical ATR-X facial appearance. As they were examined in adulthood, no molecular analysis of the *ATRX* gene would have been performed in these two patients in the absence of the two typical ATR-X brothers or of an accurate retrospective evaluation. On the other hand, there are syndrome-specific symptoms (for example, characteristic facial features and large testes in fragile X syndrome) that are not always recognizable in early childhood. Finally, if the facial features are very mild, as in the two ATR-X patients of the example, they may not be sufficient *per se* to direct molecular analysis toward a specific gene, complicating the definition of the correct diagnosis. However, it is clear that an accurate present and retrospective clinical evaluation of the patient and of their family history is still fundamental, even if it does not necessarily achieve a diagnosis.

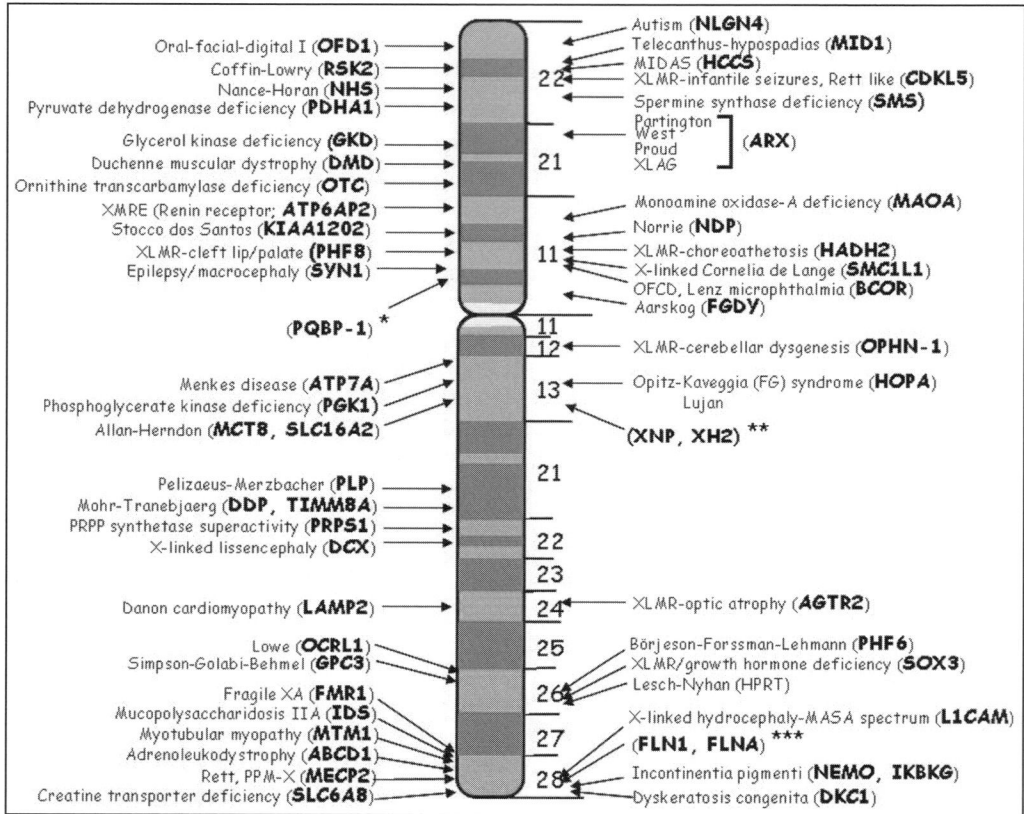

Fig. 2. *Syndromic XLMR genes and associated syndromes. The genes with asterisk (PQBP1, XNP, and FLN1) are associated with several syndromes. In particular, mutations in PQBP1 gene were found in Sutherland-Haan, Hamel cerebropalatocardiac, Golabi-Ito-Hall, Porteous, and Renpenning syndromes. The phenotype caused by mutation in the ATRX gene is indicated with the term XLMR-Hypotonic Facies and includes: Carpenter-Waziri, Holmes-Gang, Chudley-Lowry, Juberg-Marsidi, Smith-Fineman-Myers syndromes and α-thalassaemia/mental retardation sindrome with the addition of α-thalassaemia and HbH inclusion bodies in erythrocytes. FLN1 gene is associated with periventricular nodular heterotopia, otopalotodigital 1 and 2, and Melnick-Needles syndrome. Modified from Greenwood Genetic Center XLMR Update (http://www.ggc.org/xlmr.htm).*

It has long been speculated that the two XLMR conditions might have distinct genetic bases, with *MRXS* genes encoding for proteins with a broad range of molecular targets and *MRX* genes being involved in more specific tasks. However, this hypothesis has been questioned by the identification of mutations in the same genes in both MRX and MRXS patients (Fig. 1, 2). Several genes – such as *FMR1*, *RPS6KA3*, *MECP2*, and *ATRX*, which were initially identified as causative genes for MRXS – have been found mutated in patients with isolated mental retardation (Renieri *et al.*, 2005). In addition, mutations in the same gene can produce a wide variety of distinguishable syndromes. For example, mutations in *ARX*, considered to be the second most common cause of XLMR, have been found in several distinct syndromic conditions, including West syndrome, Partington syndrome, and X-linked lissencephaly with abnormal genitalia (XLAG) (Stromme *et al.*, 2002; Kato *et al.*, 2004). Although from these molecular data the distinction between MRX and MRXS is becoming less clear, it is still useful in clinical practice for a first phenotypic classification of the family, before undertaking molecular analysis.

The Italian XLMR bank

The large number of known XLMR genes, and the fact that no major genes seem to exist, make it difficult to offer a molecular diagnosis in patients with mental retardation. In particular, for those cases in which mental retardation is the only consistent feature, it is not possible to define the genes that are most likely to be altered. In these cases it is necessary to offer screening for mutations in all known MRX genes. Currently, systematic screening of the MRX genes in this mental retardation population in a clinical diagnostic setting is a difficult issue because of the high costs and the fact that it is very time consuming. For these reasons, in 2003 we proposed the creation of the Italian X-linked Mental Retardation Network to collect data on a vast number of patients with mental retardation, with detailed clinical information recorded according to common criteria, and to analyse known mental retardation genes (Pescucci *et al.*, 2007). The network includes 12 laboratories and 26 clinical centres spread all over Italy (the list of participants is available on the home page of the XLMR bank website at the address http://xlmr.unini.it/homepage.asp). The Network collects both syndromic (unknown syndromes) and non-specific mental retardation cases negative for FRAXA, chromosomal, and subtelomeric rearrangements. Collected samples and the clinical information are inserted in a web-based database available at the address http://xlmr.unisi.it. The overall design of the XLMR bank database includes three distinct parts with a password-restricted access. Each part is organized in several electronic schedules in order to collect detailed clinical and molecular data. Part I of the database includes forms filled by the clinical centre that has seen the patient and collected the biological samples (Fig. 3). Part II is filled by the biobank curators and includes information on the source and the type of stored biological samples. Currently, the following biological samples are stored: DNA, plasma, lymphocytes, and lymphoblastoid cell lines in DMSO medium. Part III is filled by the laboratories that join the Network and includes information about the laboratory tests carried out on each sample collected (Fig. 4). Using the 'Search' option the external users can visualize the complete list of patients collected in the database, the pedigree, and the provisional or definitive diagnosis (Fig. 5).

Each laboratory in the network can carry out analysis on one or two genes, and the molecular results are regularly inserted in the on-line database. Each newly identified mental retardation gene can be added to the list of the molecular tests performed as soon as a laboratory becomes available. New clinical centres and laboratories can join the Network at any time, only requiring an appropriate level password to the bank curator. At the same time, the members of the Network may decide to cease analysing genes which are of unproven value according to the latest scientific information.

The network represents a useful tool both for diagnostic purposes and research. Large scale analysis of the majority of known XLMR genes may allow many patients to receive a molecular diagnosis. In addition, given the low frequency of mutations in each MRX gene (at least for

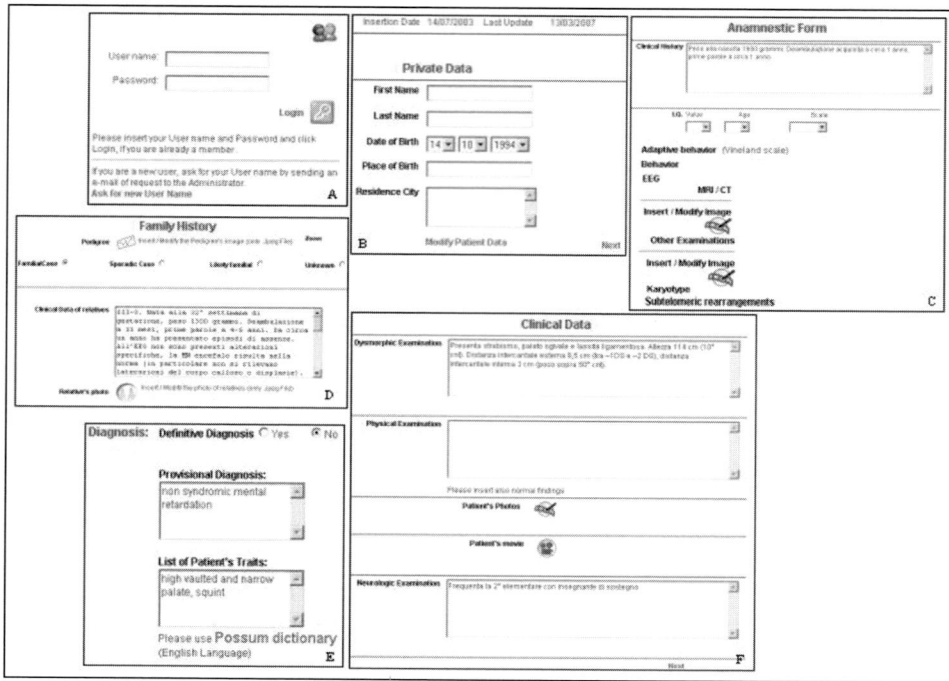

Fig. 3. Part I of the XLMR bank database. The access to this section is password restricted (panel A). Each panel indicates the different schedules included in this section and filled by the clinical centre that has examined the patient (panels from B to F).

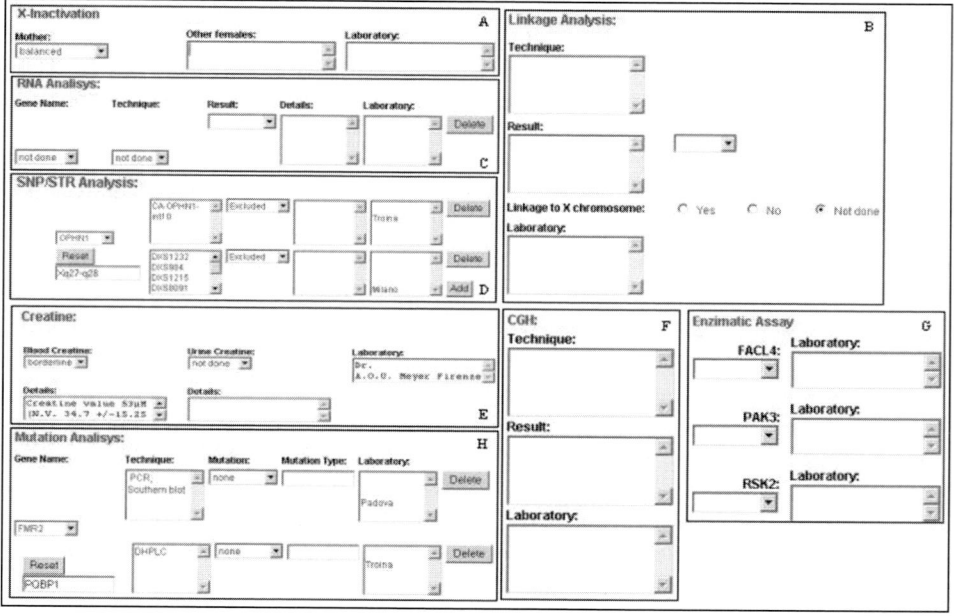

Fig. 4. Part III of the XLMR bank database. Each frame of this section includes information about the laboratory tests performed on each collected samples. Note that different tests may be added or deleted on the bases of the ongoing work.

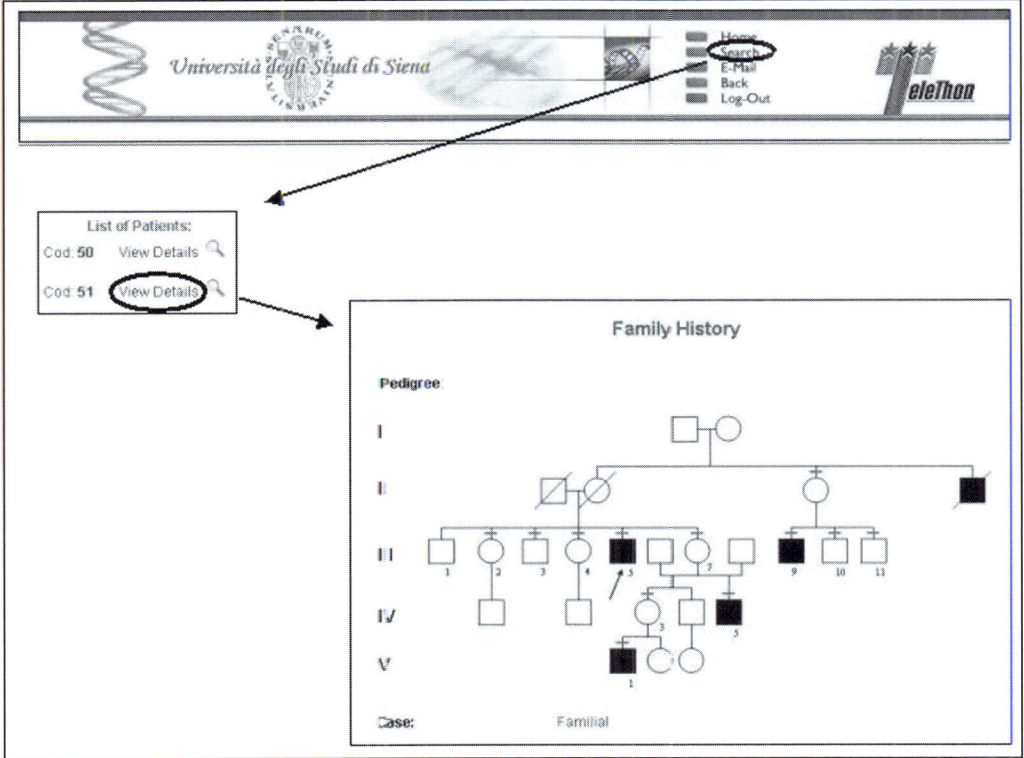

Fig. 5. Home page of the XLMR bank (http://xlmr.unisi.it). Using the 'Search' option available at the home page, users can visualize the complete list of patients recorded in the bank and consult their pedigree. This set of information is also available for 'external users' without password access.

those already identified), it is necessary to have a large panel of patients when searching for pathogenic mutations in any potential new MRX gene. The establishment of a network of laboratories sharing patients and molecular results can provide a large patient panel in which mutations in the known MRX genes have been excluded.

Future perspectives

During recent years, additional genes have been implicated in XLMR and several syndromic forms have been found to be caused by mutations in already known XLMR genes. However, much work remains to be done, as it is estimated that there might be as many as 100 MRX genes (Chelly & Mandel, 2001). In order to identify the remaining genes on the X chromosome which cause mental retardation, a systematic approach is needed. The Italian XLMR Network represents a useful tool to reach this final goal. The maintenance and improvement of the biobank will allow the scientific community to gain access to a large collection of biological samples and to detailed clinical information related to each patient, for research purposes. The Network is also fundamental to establish the percentage of Italian patients with mutations in the already known XLMR genes. An important ongoing effort to identify the causes of XLMR is represented by the medical sequencing proposal for X-linked mental retardation and related X-linked disorders which are under revision by the National Institutes of

Health. This is an international project aimed at determining the molecular basis of XLMR by sequencing all functionally important segments of the X chromosome in a large cohort of unrelated XLMR patients, using the platforms of the Human Genome Project (Wellcome Trust Sanger Center, NHGRI). The Italian XLMR Network participates to this project with 63 selected XLMR patients negative for mutations in the known genes. This collaboration may give impulse to the identification of new causative genes for mental retardation and to the delineation of new syndromes.

Establishing the genetic causes in patients with mental retardation is fundamental for improving clinical management, defining the prognosis, and facilitating genetic counselling of the families. In the future it will help develop therapeutic strategies for mental retardation.

Acknowledgments: The XLMR bank was funded by grants from Pierfranco and Luisa Mariani Foundation and Telethon Foundation (GTF02006; GTF05005 to A.R.). The work on FACL4 was funded by Telethon Foundation (GGP040102 to A.R.). Our special thanks to the families of our patients.

References

Allen, R.C., Zoghbi, H.Y., Moseley, A.B., Rosenblatt, H.M. & Belmont, J.W. (1992): Methylation of HpaII and HhaI sites near the polymorphic CAG repeat in the human adrogen-receptor gene correlates with X chromosome inactivation. *Am. J. Hum. Genet.* **51**, 1229-1239.

Bahi, N., Friocourt, G., Carrie, A., Graham, M.E., Weiss, J.L., Chafey, P., Fauchereau, F., Burgoyne, R.D. & Chelly, J. (2003): IL1 receptor accessory protein like, a protein involved in X-linked mental retardation, interacts with neuronal calcium sensor-1 and regulates exocytosis. *Hum. Mol. Genet.* **12**, 1415-1425.

Baird, P.A. & Sadovnick, A.D. (1985): Mental retardation in over half-a-million consecutive livebirths: an epidemiological study. *Am. J. Ment. Defic.* **89**, 323-30.

Bienvenu, T., Poirier, K., Friocourt, G., Bahi, N., Beaumont, D., Fauchereau, F., Ben Jeema, L., Zemni, R., Vinet, M., Francis, F., Couvert, P., Gomot, M., Moraine, C., van Bokhoven, H., Kalscheuer, V., Frints, S., Gecz, J., Ohzaki, K., Chaabouni, H., Fryns, J., Desportes, V., Beldjord, C. & Chelly, J. (2002): ARX, a novel Prd-class-homeobox gene highly expressed in the telencephalon, is mutated in X-linked mental retardation. *Hum. Mol. Genet.* **11**, 981-991.

Billuart, P., Vinet, M.C., des Portes, V., Llense, S., Richard, L., Moutard, M.L., Recan, D., Bruls, T., Bienvenu, T., Kahn, A., Beldjord, C. & Chelly, J. (1996): Identication of STS PCR screening of a microdeletion in Xp21.3-22.1 associated with non-specific mental retardation. *Hum. Molec. Genet.* **5**, 977-979.

Carrie, A., Jun, L., Bienvenu, T., Vinet, M., McDonell, N., Couvert, P., Zemni, R., Cardona, A., Van Buggenhout, G., Frints, S., Hamel, B., Moraine, C., Ropers, H., Strom, T., Howell, G., Whittaker, A., Ross, M., Kahn, A., Fryns, J., Beldjord, C., Marynen, P. & Chelly, J. (1999): A new member of the IL-1 receptor family highly expressed in hippocampus and involved in X-linked mental retardation. *Nat. Genet.* **23**, 25-31.

Chechlacz, M. & Gleeson, J.G. (2003): Is mental retardation a defect of synapse structure and function? *Pediatr. Neurol.* **29**, 11-17.

Chelly, J. & Mandel, J. (2001): Monogenic causes of X-linked mental retardation. *Nat. Rev. Genet.* **2**, 669-680.

Couvert, P., Bienvenu, T., Aquaviva, C., Poirier, K., Moraine, C., Gendrot, C., Verloes, A., Andres, C., Le Fevre, A.C., Souville, I., Steffann, J., des Portes, V., Ropers, H.H., Yntema, H.G., Fryns, J.P., Briault, S., Chelly, J. & Cherif, B. (2001): MECP2 is highly mutated in X-linked mental retardation. *Hum. Mol. Genet.* **10**, 941-946.

D'Adamo, P., Menegon, A., Lo Nigro, C., Grasso, M., Gulisano, M., Tamanini, F., Bienvenu, T., Gedeon, A., Oostra, B., Wu, S., Tandon, A., Valtorta, F., Balch, W., Chelly, J. & Toniolo, D. (1998): Mutations in GDI1 are responsible for X-linked non-specific mental retardation. *Nat. Genet.* **19**, 134-139.

Feder, M., Pas, J., Wyrwicz, L.S. & Bujnicki, J.M. (2003): Molecular phylogenetics of the RrmJ/fibrillarin superfamily of ribose 2'-O-methyltransferases. *Gene* **302** (Suppl. 1-2), 129-138.

Freude, K., Hoffmann, K., Jensen, L.R., Delatycki, M.B., des Portes, V., Moser, B., Hamel, B., van Bokhoven, H., Moraine, C., Fryns, J.P., Chelly, J., Gecz, J., Lenzner, S., Kalscheuer, V.M. & Ropers, H.H. (2004): Mutations in the FTSJ1 gene coding for a novel S-adenosylmethionine-binding protein cause nonsyndromic X-linked mental retardation. *Am. J. Hum. Genet.* **75**, 305-309.

Friesema, E.C., Grueters, A., Biebermann, H., Krude, H., von Moers, A., Reeser, M., Barrett, T.G., Mancilla, E.E., Svensson, J., Kester, M.H., Kuiper, G.G., Balkassmi, S., Uitterlinden, A.G., Koehrle, J., Rodien, P., Halestrap, A.P.

& Visser, T.J. (2004): Association between mutations in a thyroid hormone transporter and severe X-linked psychomotor retardation. *Lancet* **364**, 1435-1437.

Frints, S.G., Froyen, G., Marynen, P., Willekens, D., Legius, E. & Fryns, J.P. (2002): Re-evaluation of MRX36 family after discovery of an ARX gene mutation reveals mild neurological features of Partington syndrome. *Am. J. Med. Genet.* **112**, 427-428.

Gallinat, S., Busche, S., Raizada, M.K. & Sumners, C. (2000): The angiotensin II type 2 receptor: an enigma with multiple variations. *Am. J. Physiol. Endocrinol. Metab.* **278**, E357-74.

Gecz, J. (2004): The molecular basis of intellectual disability: novel genes with naturally occurring mutations causing altered gene expression in the brain. *Front. Biosci.* **9**, 1-7.

Gecz, J., Gedeon, A., Sutherland, G. & Mulley, J. (1996): Identification of the gene FMR2, associated with FRAXE mental retardation. *Nat. Genet.* **13**, 105-108.

Gendron, L., Laflamme, L., Rivard, N., Asselin, C., Payet, M. & Gallo-Payet, N. (1999): Signals from the AT2 (angiotensin type 2) receptor of angiotensin IIinhibit p21 ras and activate MAPK (mitogen activated protein kinase) to induce morphological neuronal differentiation in NG108-15 cells. *Mol. Endocrinol.* **13**, 1615-1626.

Hall, A. (1998): Rho GTPases and the actin cytoskeleton. *Science* **279**, 509-514.

Jensen, L.R., Amende, M., Gurok, U., Moser, B., Gimmel, V., Tzschach, A. Janecke, A.R., Tariverdian, G., Chelly, J., Fryns, J.P., Van Esch, H., Kleefstra, T., Hamel, B., Moraine, C., Gecz, J., Turner, G., Reinhardt, R., Kalscheuer, V.M., Ropers, H.H. & Lenzner, S. (2005): Mutations in the JARID1C gene, which is involved in transcriptional regulation and chromatin remodelling, cause X-linked mental retardation. *Am. J. Hum. Genet.* **76**, 227-236.

Kalscheuer, V.M., Freude, K., Musante, L., Jensen, L.R., Yntema, H.G., Gecz, J., Sefiani, A., Hoffmann, K., Moser, B., Haas, S., Gurok, U., Haesler, S., Aranda, B., Nshedjan, A., Tzschach, A., Hartmann, N., Roloff, T.C., Shoichet, S., Hagens, O., Tao, J., Van Bokhoven, H., Turner, G., Chelly, J., Moraine, C., Fryns, J.P., Nuber, U., Hoeltzenbein, M., Scharff, C., Scherthan, H., Lenzner, S., Hamel, B.C., Schweiger, S. & Ropers, H.H. (2003a): Mutations in the polyglutamine binding protein 1 gene cause X-linked mental retardation. *Nat. Genet.* **35**, 313-315.

Kalscheuer, V.M., Tao, J., Donnelly, A., Hollway, G., Schwinger, E., Kubart, S., Menzel, C., Hoeltzenbein, M., Tommerup, N., Eyre, H., Harbord, M., Haan, E., Sutherland, G.R., Ropers, H.H. & Gecz, J. (2003b): Disruption of the serine/threonine kinase 9 gene causes severe X-linked infantile spasms and mental retardation. *Am. J. Hum. Genet.* **72**, 1401-1411.

Kato, M., Das, S., Petras, K., Kitamura, K., Morohashi, K., Abuelo, D.N., Barr, M., Bonneau, D., Brady, A.F., Carpenter, N.J., Cipero, K.L., Frisone, F., Fukuda, T., Guerrini, R., Iida, E., Itoh, M., Lewanda, A.F., Nanba Y., Oka, A., Proud, V.K., Saugier-Veber, P., Schelley, S.L., Selicorni, A., Shaner, R., Silengo, M., Stewart, F., Sugiyama, N., Toyama, J., Toutain, A., Vargas, A.L., Yanazawa, M., Zackai, E.H. & Dobyns, W.B. (2004): Mutations of ARX are associated with striking pleiotropy and consistent genotype-phenotype correlation. *Hum. Mutat.* **23**, 147-159.

Kerr, B., Turner, G., Mulley, J., Gedeon, A. & Partington, M. (1991): Non-specific X-linked mental retardation. *J. Med. Genet.* **28**, 378-382.

Kleefstra, T., Yntema, H.G., Oudakker, A.R., Banning, M.J., Kalscheuer, V.M., Chelly, J., Moraine, C., Ropers, H.H., Fryns, J.P., Janssen, I.M., Sistermans, E.A., Nillesen, W.N., de Vries, L.B., Hamel, B.C. & van Bokhoven, H. (2004): Zinc finger 81 (ZNF81) mutations associated with X-linked mental retardation. *J. Med. Genet.* **41**, 394-399.

Kutsche, K., Yntema, H., Brandt, A., Jantke, I., Nothwang, H., Orth, U., Boavida, M., David, D., Chelly, J., Fryns, J., Moraine, C., Ropers, H., Hamel, B., van Bokhoven, H. & Gal, A. (2000): Mutations in ARHGEF6, encoding a guanine nucleotide exchange factor for Rho GTPases, in patients with X-linked mental retardation. *Nat. Genet.* **26**, 247-250.

Laumonnier, F., Bonnet-Brilhault, F., Gomot, M., Blanc, R., David, A., Moizard, M.P., Raynaud, M., Ronce, N., Lemonnier, E., Calvas, P., Laudier, B., Chelly, J., Fryns, J.P., Ropers, H.H., Hamel, B.C., Andres, C., Barthelemy, C., Moraine, C. & Briault, S. (2004): X-linked mental retardation and autism are associated with a mutation in the NLGN4 gene, a member of the neuroligin family. *Am. J. Hum. Genet.* **74**, 552-557.

Lebel, R.R., May, M., Pouls, S., Lubs, H.A., Stevenson, R.E. & Schwartz, C.E. (2002): Non-syndromic X-linked mental retardation associated with a missense mutation (P312L) in the FGD1 gene. *Clin. Genet.* **61**, 139-145.

Longo, I., Frints, S.G., Fryns, J.P., Meloni, I., Pescucci, C., Ariani, F., Borghgraef, M., Raynaud, M., Marynen, P., Schwartz, C., Renieri, A. & Froyen, G. (2003): A third MRX family (MRX68) is the result of mutation in the long-chain fatty acid-CoA ligase 4 (FACL4) gene: proposal of a rapid enzymatic assay for screening mentally retarded patients. *J. Med. Genet.* **40**, 11-17.

Lucius, R., Gallinat, S., Rosenstiel, P., Herdegen, T., Sievers, J. & Unger, T. (1998): The angiotensin II type 2 (AT2) receptor promotes axonal regeneration in the optic nerve of adult rats. *J. Exp. Med.* **188**, 661-670.

Lugtenberg, D., Yntema, H.G., Banning, M.J., Oudakker, A.R., Firth, H.V., Willatt, L., Raynaud, M., Kleefstra, T., Fryns, J.P., Ropers, H.H., Chelly, J., Moraine, C., Gecz, J., Reeuwijk, J., Nabuurs, S.B., de Vries, B.B., Hamel, B.C., de Brouwer, A.P. & Bokhoven, H. (2006): ZNF674: a New Kruppel-Associated Box-Containing Zinc-Finger Gene Involved in nonsyndromic X-linked mental retardation. *Am. J. Hum. Genet.* **78**, 265-278.

Luo, L. (2000): Rho GTPases in neuronal morphogenesis. *Nat. Rev. Neurosci.* **1**, 173-180.

Mari, F., Azimonti, S., Bertani, I., Bolognese, F., Colombo, E., Caselli, R., Scala, E., Longo, I., Grosso, S., Pescucci, C., Ariani, F., Hayek, G., Balestri, P., Bergo, A., Badaracco, G., Zappella, M., Broccoli, V., Renieri, A., Kilstrup-Nielsen, C. & Landsberger, N. (2005): CDKL5 belongs to the same molecular pathway of MeCP2 and it is responsible for the early-onset seizure variant of Rett syndrome. *Hum. Mol. Genet.* **14**, 1935-1946.

Mashek, D.G., Bornfeldt, K.E., Coleman, R.A., Berger, J., Bernlohr, D.A., Black, P., DiRusso, C.C., Farber, S.A., Guo, W., Hashimoto, N., Khodiyar, V., Kuypers, F.A., Maltais, L.J., Nebert, D.W., Renieri, A., Schaffer, J.E., Stahl, A., Watkins, P.A., Vasiliou, V. & Yamamoto, T.T. (2004): Revised nomenclature for the mammalian long-chain acyl-CoA synthetase gene family. *J. Lipid. Res.* **45**, 1958-1961.

McLaren, J. & Bryson, S.E. (1987): Review of recent epidemiological studies of mental retardation: prevalence, associated disorders, and aetiology. *Am. J. Ment. Retard.* **92**, 243-254.

Meloni, I., Muscettola, M., Raynaud, M., Longo, I., Bruttini, M., Moizard, M., Gomot, M., Chelly, J., das Portes, V., Fryns, J., Ropers, H., Magi, B., Bellan, C., Volpi, N., Yntema, H., Lewis, S., Schaffer, J. & Renieri, A. (2002): FACL4, ancoding fatty acid-CoA ligase 4, is mutated in nonspecific X-linked mental retardation. *Nat. Genet.* **30**, 436-440.

Merienne, K., Jacquot, S., Pannetier, S., Zeniou, M., Bankier, A., Gecz, J., Mandel, J.L., Mulley, J., Sassone-Corsi, P. & Hanauer, A. (1999): A missense mutation in RPS6KA3 (RSK2) responsible for non-specific mental retardation. *Nat. Genet.* **22**, 13-14.

Mulley, J.C., Kerr, B., Stevenson, R. & Lubs, H. (1992): Nomenclature guidelines for X-linked mental retardation. *Am. J. Med. Genet.* **43**, 383-391.

Neri, G. & Chiurazzi, P. (1999): X-linked mental retardation. *Adv. Genet.* **41**, 55-94.

Pescucci, C., Caselli, R., Mari, F., Speciale, C., Ariani, F., Bruttini, M., Sampieri, K., Mencarelli, M.A., Scala, E., Longo, I., Artuso, R., Renieri, A. & Meloni, I. (2007): The Italian XLMR bank: a clinical and molecular database. *Hum. Mutat.* **28**, 13-18.

Purpura, D.P. (1974): Dendritic spine 'dysgenesis' and mental retardation. *Science* **186**, 1126-1128.

Ramakers, G.J. (2002): Rho proteins, mental retardation and the cellular basis of cognition. *Trends Neurosci.* **25**, 191-199.

Renieri, A., Pescucci, C., Longo, I., Ariani, F., Mari, F. & Meloni, I. (2005): Non-syndromic X-linked mental retardation: from a molecular to a clinical point of view. *J. Cell. Physiol.* **204**, 8-20.

Ropers, H.H. (2006): X-linked mental retardation: many genes for a complex disorder. *Curr. Opin. Genet. Dev.* **16**, 260-269.

Rosenstiel, P., Gallinat, S., Arlt, A., Unger, T., Sievers, J. & Lucius, R. (2002): Angiotensin AT2 receptor ligands: do they have potential as future treatments for neurological disease? *CNS Drugs* **16**, 145-153.

Rousseau, F., Heitz, D., Tarleton, J., MacPherson, J., Malmgren, H., Dahl, N., Barnicoat, A., Mathew, C., Mornet, E., Tejada, I., Maddalena, A., Spiegel, R., Schinzel, A., Marcos, G., Schorderet, D., Schaap, T., Maccioni, L., Russo, S., Jacobs, A., Schwartz, C. & Mandel, J.L. (1994): A multicenter study on genotype-phenotype correlation in the fragile X syndrome, using direct diagnosis with probe StB12.3: the first 2253 cases. *Am. J. Hum. Genet.* **55**, 225-237.

Salomons, G.S., van Dooren, S.J., Verhoeven, N.M., Cecil, K.M., Ball, W.S., Degrauw, T.J. & Jakobs, C. (2001): X-linked creatine-transporter gene (SLC6A8) defect: a new creatine-deficiency syndrome. *Am. J. Hum. Genet.* **68**, 1497-1500.

Salomons, G.S., van Dooren, S.J., Verhoeven, N.M., Marsden, D., Schwartz, C., Cecil, K.M., DeGrauw, T.J. & Jakobs, C. (2003): X-linked creatine transporter defect: an overview. *J. Inherit. Metab. Dis.* **26**, 309-318.

Shoichet, S.A., Hoffmann, K., Menzel, C., Trautmann, U., Moser, B., Hoeltzenbein, M., Echenne, B., Partington, M., Van Bokhoven, H., Moraine, C., Fryns, J.P., Chelly, J., Rott, H.D., Ropers, H.H. & Kalscheuer, V.M. (2003): Mutations in the ZNF41 gene are associated with cognitive deficits: identification of a new candidate for X-linked mental retardation. *Am. J. Hum. Genet.* **73**, 1341-1354.

Stromme, P., Mangelsdorf, M., Shaw, M., Lower, K., Lewis, S., Bruyere, H., Lutcherath, V., Gedeon, A., Wallace, R., Scheffer, I., Turner, G., Partington, M., Frints, S., Fryns, J., Sutherland, G., Mulley, J. & Gecz, J. (2002): Mutations in the human ortholog of Aristaless cause X-linked mental retardation and epilepsy. *Nat. Genet.* **30**, 441-445.

Tarpey, P., Parnau, J., Blow, M., Woffendin, H., Bignell, G., Cox, C., Cox, J., Davies, H., Edkins, S., Holden, S., Korny, A., Mallya, U., Moon, J., O'Meara, S., Parker, A., Stephens, P., Stevens, C., Teague, J., Donnelly, A., Mangelsdorf, M., Mulley, J., Partington, M., Turner, G., Stevenson, R., Schwartz, C., Young, I., Easton, D., Bobrow, M., Futreal, P.A., Stratton, M.R., Gecz, J., Wooster, R. & Raymond, F.L. (2004): Mutations in the DLG3 gene cause nonsyndromic X-linked mental retardation. *Am. J. Hum. Genet.* **75**, 318-324.

Tarpey, P.S., Stevens, C., Teague, J., Edkins, S., O'Meara, S., Avis, T., Barthorpe, S., Buck, G., Butler, A., Cole, J., Dicks, E., Gray, K., Halliday, K., Harrison R., Hills, K., Hinton, J., Jones, D., Menzies, A., Mironenko, T., Perry, J., Raine, K., Richardson, D., Shepherd, R., Small, A., Tofts, C., Varian, J., West, S., Widaa, S., Yates, A., Catford, R., Butler, J., Mallya, U., Moon, J., Luo, Y., Dorkins, H., Thompson, D., Easton, D.F., Wooster, R., Bobrow, M., Carpenter, N., Simensen, R.J., Schwartz, C.E., Stevenson, R.E., Turner, G., Partington, M., Gecz, J., Stratton, M.R., Futreal, P.A. & Raymond, F.L. (2006): Mutations in the gene encoding the Sigma 2 subunit of the adaptor protein 1 complex, AP1S2, cause X-linked mental retardation. *Am. J. Hum. Genet.* **79,** 1119-1124.

Turner, G. & Partington, M.W. (1991): Genes for intelligence on the X chromosome. *J. Med. Genet.* **28,** 429.

Van Bohlen, O., Walther, T., Bader, M. & Albrecht, D. (2001): Genetic deletion of angiotensin AT2 receptor leads to increased cell numbers in different brain structures. *Regulatory Peptides* **99,** 209-216.

Vervoort, V.S., Beachem, M.A., Edwards, P.S., Ladd, S., Miller, K.E., de Mollerat, X., Clarkson, K., DuPont, B., Schwartz, C.E., Stevenson, R.E., Boyd, E. & Srivastava, A.K. (2002): AGTR2 mutations in X-linked mental retardation. *Science* **296,** 2401-2403.

Yntema, H., Poppelaars, F., Derksen, E., Oudakker, A., Van Roosmalen, T., Jacobs, A., Obbema, H., Brunner, H., Hamel, B. & Van Bokhoven, H. (2002): Expanding phenotype of XNP mutations: mild to moderate mental retardation. *Am. J. Med. Genet.* **110,** 243-247.

Zemni, R., Bienvenu, T., Vinet, M., Sefiani, A., Carrie, A., Billuart, P., McDonell, N., Couvert, P., Francis, F., Chafey, P., Fauchereau, F., Friocourt, G., Portes, V., Cardona, A., Frints, S., Meindl, A., Brandau, O., Ronce, N., Moraine, C., Bokhoven, H., Ropers, H., Sudbrak, R., Kahn, A., Fryns, J., Beldjord, C. & et al. (2000): A new gene involved in X-linked mental retardation identified by analysis of an X;2 balanced translocation. *Nat. Genet.* **24,** 167-170.

Chapter 8

Phenotypes of Smith-Magenis syndrome

Stefano D'Arrigo, Sara Bulgheroni and Chiara Pantaleoni

*Department of Developmental Neurology, Fondazione IRCCS Istituto Neurologico 'C. Besta',
via Celoria 11, 20133 Milan, Italy*
darrigo@istituto-besta.it

Summary

Smith-Magenis syndrome is a clinically recognizable syndrome caused by an interstitial deletion on the short arm of chromosome 17 (17p11.2) – probably a contiguous genes syndrome – which is characterized by multiple malformations and mental delay. Its frequency is estimated to be 1/25,000.
The diagnosis is based on the identification of an absolutely characteristic clinical phenotype, in terms of its somatic aspects and neurological, cognitive and behavioural features, correlated with the patient's age. The diagnosis is confirmed by fluorescence *in situ* hybridization (FISH) study in 95 per cent of cases. Around 5–10 per cent of patients with the clinical phenotype of Smith-Magenis syndrome but no deletion identifiable by FISH have revealed a point mutation in the RAI1 gene, contained in the same critical region.

Introduction

Smith-Magenis syndrome was first described in 1982 by Ann Smith, a medical geneticist, and Ellen Magenis, a cytogeneticist, who went on to outline its clinical spectrum in 1986, thanks to the description of other patients. This is a clinically recognizable syndrome caused by an interstitial deletion on the short arm of chromosome 17 (17p11.2), probably a contiguous genes syndrome, which is characterized by multiple malformations and mental delay. Its frequency is estimated to be 1/25,000, with no distinction between ethnic groups.

The diagnosis is based on the identification of an absolutely characteristic unique clinical phenotype, in terms of its somatic aspects and neurological, cognitive, and behavioural features. The diagnosis is confirmed by fluorescence *in situ* hybridization (FISH) study in 95 per cent of cases; it is only in a minority of cases that the deletion can be identified by cytogenetic investigations. Around 5–10 per cent of patients with the clinical phenotype of Smith-Magenis syndrome but no deletion identifiable by FISH have a point mutation in the RAI1 gene, contained in the same critical region, which codifies for a new protein of unknown function but believed to have a role in neuron differentiation.

In this chapter we describe the various somatic, neurological, cognitive, and behavioural phenotypes of Smith-Magenis syndrome and how they evolve in relation to the patient's age, particularly during the first 18 months of life (infants), in early and late childhood (18 months to 12 years), and in adolescence. A few paragraphs are also dedicated to a description of the genotype.

Somatic phenotype

The craniofacial characteristics of the somatic phenotype in Smith-Magenis syndrome are hard to recognize in the first 18 months of life (infants): the dysmorphic facial features are very mild, with the face acquiring 'cherub-like' features, with prominent and fleshy cheeks, upslanting eyelid fissures, a flattened root of the nose and micrognathia; the mouth has a typical shape, with a Cupid's bow upper lip and a pronounced philtrum. A gestaltic diagnosis is extremely difficult at this stage (Gropman et al., 2006).

During early and later childhood (18 months to 12 years), the face takes on a coarser appearance, developing 'Down-like' characteristics due to a hypotonic facial musculature and brachycephaly with a pronounced forehead, a flat, wide, square face, epicanthus, a short wide nose with an ample root, and auricular anomalies. In adolescence, the facial features become characteristic and clearly recognizable: they are very coarse, to the point of being defined as 'boxer-like', the eyes are sunken, with synophrys and hypertelorism, the lips become fleshy with evidence of prognathism, and the voice becomes particularly hoarse.

With regard to somatic growth, patients with Smith-Magenis syndrome have normal anthropometric indices at birth, but their subsequent growth rate is slow and this can lead to small stature in adolescence. Obesity is also a characteristic of this syndrome and becomes manifest in later childhood; microcephaly is seen in 20 per cent of cases.

Individuals with Smith-Magenis syndrome also have systemic problems secondary to malformations which may affect various parts of the body. The most common problems involve the ear, nose, and throat (in 94 per cent of cases) and include recurrent otitis media, which can lead to transmissive hypoacusia in 40 per cent of cases, while 20 per cent of patients have neurosensory hypoacusia, and eight per cent have a mixed form. Laryngeal anomalies (polyps, nodules, oedema, and vocal cord paralysis) also occur, as do cleft palate and velopharyngeal insufficiency.

Ophthalmological problems are very common (in 85 per cent of cases), and can manifest with mild disorders such as strabismus and refraction defects (myopia), but also with more complex conditions – for example, microcornea, iris dysplasia, coloboma, hamartoma (Wolfflin-Kruckmann spots), macula hypopigmentation, and even microphthalmia.

Numerous cardiac malformations are encountered in just under 50 per cent of patients with the syndrome. The most common are mild tricuspid valve or mitral valve insufficiency, subvalvar aortic stenosis, supravalvar pulmonary stenosis, and interatrial and interventricular septal defects.

There may also be evidence of kidney malformations, albeit in a smaller percentage of cases (35 per cent), usually in the form of renal collection system duplication, unilateral renal agenesis, and ectopic kidney.

Finally, the immune system may be affected, with immunoglobulin and endocrine system deficiencies, including altered thyroid hormone levels (fT4 deficiency and an increase in TSH), hypercholesterolaemia, hypertriglyceridaemia, and early puberty (Smith & Gropman, 2001).

Neurological phenotype

The neurological features of Smith-Magenis syndrome also correlate with the patient's age. In infants, the most characteristic element is delayed psychomotor development, with deficiencies mainly in terms of expressive language. Retrospective reviews of patients' clinical records have shown that the only significant element emerging during the pregnancy is a reduced intensity and frequency of active fetal movements – which is a non-specific finding. The neonate may also have a mild hypotonic-hyporeflexive syndrome and hypomotility of the buccolingual region.

In childhood and adolescence, symptoms and signs of central and peripheral nervous system involvement become apparent. First, mental delay emerges with a very variable degree of severity, as explained below. Clinical signs of peripheral neuropathy are reported in 55 to 75 per cent of cases, with hypotonia and hyporeflexia in the younger children, while older children show reduced sensitivity to heat and pain, distal hypotrophy of the limbs, flat foot or claw foot, and scoliosis. The motor conduction rates are generally normal, but a few cases reveal a markedly slower than normal motor conduction. Anatomopathological studies in these latter patients identify a segmental demyelinization and remyelinization similar to the picture seen in Charcot-Marie-Tooth 1A hereditary sensorimotor neuropathy (CMT1A), in which there is a contiguous deletion of the PMP22 gene located distally to the region that is critical for Smith-Magenis syndrome (Chevillard et al., 1993).

Epileptic seizures occur in 10 to 30 per cent of cases, while electroencephalographic (EEG) anomalies in the absence of seizures are documented in approximately 25 per cent. There is no specific clinical or EEG pattern, though complex partial seizures seem to be more frequent; sporadic cases of infantile spasms have also been reported. Diagnosing and treating the epileptic condition is important and can lead to behavioural improvements as well.

Structural central nervous system anomalies identifiable at neuroradiological assessment are described in approximately 50 per cent of cases and are non-specific, including ventriculomegaly and posterior fossa malformations such as mega cisterna magna and cerebellar vermis hypoplasia. A recent study by Boddaert et al., using brain magnetic resonance imaging on five patients aged between 11 and 16 years, revealed a modest dilatation of the lateral ventricles in all five cases and a retrocerebellar cyst in four; voxel-based morphometry was also conducted and showed a significant bilateral reduction in the grey matter of the insula and lenticular nucleus in comparison with controls. Positron emission tomography confirmed that these areas were hypoperfused (Boddaert et al., 2004). We might only hazard a guess, given the limited sample size of the study, but it is tempting to hypothesize an anatomofunctional correlation: the insula is implicated in temperature regulation processes so a functional alteration at this level might explain these patients' altered sensitivity to heat and cold; and the lenticular nucleus is known to be implicated in attention deficit hyperactivity disorder, which is also a feature of the Smith-Magenis syndrome, as discussed below.

A significant aspect to consider in the neurological phenotype is the sleep disorder characteristic of and peculiar to Smith-Magenis syndrome. Infants up to 18 months old tend to be excessively sleepy during the daytime: parents describe them as 'perfect babies', saying they cause no trouble during the day because they are usually asleep. In fact, they sleep less than normal in the 24 hours of the day. In childhood the sleep disorder becomes more evident, as the children's sleeping cycles become more fragmented and reduced: they spend lengthy periods awake at night, and wake up early in the morning, while they are excessively drowsy during the day. In adolescence, the disorder is unmistakable: the patient sleeps very little in quantitative terms during the night, waking frequently; then during the day they have a considerably increased need to sleep and have difficulty waking from their daytime 'naps'. Although other neurological mechanisms may be implicated in this dysfunction, the acknowledged principal reason is an inversion of the circadian pattern of melatonin secretion. In mammals, melatonin release follows a precise circadian rhythm, with plasma levels beginning to rise in the evenings and peaking during the night, as a consequence of the noradrenergic stimulation of the β-receptors in the pineal cells. Melatonin levels then fall in the morning and become minimal during the day. In patients with Smith-Magenis syndrome this pattern is reversed: melatonin reaches its peak during the day and falls to minimum levels at night. This inversion seems to be secondary to an altered direct control of melatonin release by the pineal cells. The suprachiasmatic nucleus of the hypothalamus does not appear to be involved, as lesions in this latter area reverse the circadian rhythm not only of melatonin secretion, but also of other hormones – for example, cortisol and growth hormone – while these continue to have a regular pattern in patients with Smith-Magenis syndrome.

The sleep disorder needs to be diagnosed to establish suitable treatment, which involves proper sleep training for a start, progressively limiting and eventually eliminating daily naps, especially in the afternoons. Pharmaceutical treatment has also proved effective. This involves administering melatonin up to a maximum dose of 6 mg at 8.00 p.m. and the β1-adrenergic antagonist acebutol at a dose of 10 mg/kg at 8.00 a.m. to reduce daytime melatonin secretion. It is clearly important to keep strictly to the schedule and it is also preferable to maintain a low dosage of melatonin (0.5–2.5 mg), because high doses induce an increase in daytime melatonin levels as well, causing drowsiness during the day (De Leersnyder, 2006).

Cognitive-behavioural phenotype

Mental retardation is characteristic of the Smith-Magenis syndrome and is seen in all patients suffering from this condition, though its severity varies considerably: 44 per cent of affected individuals have moderate mental delay, while mental defect is mild in 24 per cent, severe in 16 per cent, and profound in 12 per cent; four per cent have been described as having a borderline intelligence quotient (IQ). The majority of patients are reportedly most affected in terms of expressive language. In particular, as reported by Sarismki, in a group of 20 children aged between 5 and 12 years there was a deficient pragmatic use of language: patients continuously asked questions to which they knew the answer, ignoring the conversational context, bringing the conversation back to their favourite topics and disregarding the other party's interest in the conversation; they are tireless, often repetitive talkers (Sarismki, 2004).

In a study on 10 patients aged between 14 and 51 years, Dykens found that the weaknesses in cognitive profile concerned short-term memory and sequential processing, while these patients' strengths are long-term memory, participation in the environmental, attention to visual detail, and reading (Dykens *et al.*, 1997). Udwin conducted a study in 2001 on a group of 29 children between 6 and 16 years old and 21 adults between 16 and 52 years old, finding that the majority of the subjects had moderate harmonic cognitive delays, with no discrepancy between verbal abilities and performance. Here again, the study identified the patients' strong points as memory for biographical events and computer expertise, while response rate, visuomotor coordination, short-term memory and sequential activities were weak (Udwin *et al.*, 2001).

In relation to adaptive behaviour, Dykens could find no significant differences in the three domains on the Vineland scales (socialisation, communication, daily abilities) (Dykens *et al.*, 1997), while Udwin recorded a particularly deficient adaptive behaviour in the domain for independence, given the patients' marked dependence on their caregivers and the social difficulties deriving from their behavioural problems (Udwin et al., 2001). In a recent study, however, Martin applied the Vineland scales to 19 children from 2 to 12 years old and found that the scores in the domain for socialisation were higher than expected for the patient's IQ, whereas the scores in the domains for communication and daily abilities were consistent with the child's IQ (Martin et al., 2006).

The behavioural phenotype in the Smith-Magenis syndrome is highly characteristic, with aspects peculiar to this condition that often suggest the diagnosis to the clinician. The behavioural phenotype is also age-related. In infants the signs are very mild and hardly recognizable. These babies are often defined by the parents as 'perfect' because they sleep a lot during the day and, when awake, they are very tranquil and gratify their caregivers. They generally have a limited vocal output and rarely cry. In childhood there is a progressive escalation in the behavioural problems: with the onset of maladaptive behaviour, the children have fits of rage and aggressiveness, anxiety attacks, poor control over their impulses, and react negatively to changes in their routines. There is often a frank attention deficit, sometimes associated with hyperactivity. They can also have episodes of enuresis and encopresis. In their relationships with adults, they become very demanding and dependent. In a comparative analysis, Dykens demonstrated maladaptive behaviour, and particularly disobedience, impulsiveness, demands for attention, and destructive behaviour in significantly higher percentages of Smith-Magenis patients than among those with Prader-Willi syndrome or with mixed mental delay, matched for age and sex (Dykens & Smith, 1998).

Self-injurious behaviour is also very typical and common – the children bite their hands and wrists, bang their heads, puncture their skin, pull out their hair, slap themselves, and pick at their finger and toe nails. Another self-injurious behaviour typical of the condition is polyembolokoilamania, the compulsive tendency to insert objects in the bodily orifices (ears, nose, rectum, vagina), partly correlated with the children's more limited sensitivity to pain. In a study on 29 patients aged from 18 months to 49 years, Finucane recorded a variable number of self-injurious episodes from 0 (in only one patient) to eight per patient, and 55 per cent of the sample had a history of at least five such episodes. The numbers involved were directly age-related, as was the type of episode. While biting the hands and fingers and banging the head had already developed in the second year of life, other types of behaviour such as nail picking were rare before 5 years of age (Finucane et al., 2001). Moreover, such episodes are always associated with repetitive and stereotyped behaviour, including shaking of the trunk, or repeatedly and pointlessly moving objects (for example, object spinning). Among these, it is particularly worth noting that affected children hug themselves – that is, they repeatedly and spasmodically embrace the upper part of the trunk (spasmodic upper body squeeze) – and this represents a pathognomonic feature of the syndrome, so Smith-Magenis syndrome should always be suspected in patients seen hugging themselves in this way.

It is important to emphasize that these patients also have some positive behavioural features and some strengths. They are extremely affectionate and sociable, they have a good sense of humour, and they love music, water games, and electronic equipment. They respond well to various types of verbal reinforcement and learn well if they are guided by a visual stimulus. These strengths, and their good social interaction in particular, make them clearly distinguishable from cases of classic autism, though they share certain features, such as communication deficiencies and restricted, stereotyped behaviour patterns.

The behavioural issues often warrant pharmacological treatment, which is basically symptomatic. For the related attention deficit hyperactivity disorder, classic psychostimulants (methylphenidate) have proved minimally effective, while preliminary studies on atomoxetine have reported a higher incidence of psychotic symptoms, so this should not be used as a drug of first choice. The behavioural problems are well controlled by mood stabilizers (lithium, valproic acid) and atypical neuroleptics (low dose risperidone), and the latter is also effective at controlling aggressiveness and impulsiveness. It is nonetheless important to emphasize that valproic acid and risperidone must be used with caution in adolescence because they induce a further increase in obesity and affect the lipid profile. Selective serotonin reuptake inhibitors can be used to treat anxiety – particularly fluoxetine, which has proved useful in controlling episodes of explosive behaviour.

Of course, educational strategies and behavioural measures are also necessary. At school, it is particularly important to include the children in numerically small, very tranquil classes, with a large proportion of teachers to children, in order to cope with the children's attention deficit and avoid them competing for the adult's attention. It is also important to use visual prompts to guide these children in performing multistep tasks, and to organize the activities and switches from one activity to another, minimizing novelty and preparing for changes. Finally, it is always useful to exploit these children's passion for electronic games and computers.

Genetic aspects

Smith-Magenis syndrome is caused by an interstitial deletion on the short arm of chromosome 17 (17p11.2). With a very few exceptions, the deletion is *de novo* so the risk of recurrence is low; cytogenetic-molecular studies with FISH are nonetheless warranted in the parents of new cases. The syndrome is unrelated to the parents' age and the parental origin of the deletion is random, so there is no imprinting mechanism involved. Although the molecular reason for the syndrome is uncertain, it is thought to be a contiguous gene syndrome in which the haplo-insufficiency of multiple genes in the critical region contributes to determining the phenotype.

Approximately 70 per cent of patients have a 'classic' 17p11.2 deletion of approximately 3.5 Mb, while the remainder have more extensive or lesser deletions. The region of the deletion's minimum overlap was recently reduced to approximately 650 kb, thanks to the analysis of patients with atypical deletions. Intragenic mutations in heterozygosis have also been identified in the gene that codifies the retinoic acid induced 1 (RAI1) protein in patients with Smith-Magenis syndrome, with no deletion revealed, suggesting that the haplo-insufficiency of the RAI1 gene is responsible for the prevalent phenotypic signs of the syndrome (Bi *et al.*, 2006). Girirajan *et al.* (2006) recently showed that certain clinical characteristics are common both to patients with the deletion and to those with an intragenic RAI1 mutation, thus confirming the direct involvement of this gene: these characteristics include the dysmorphic facial features, the neurological pattern, the sleep disorder, and the behavioural phenotype. On the other hand, other characteristics – particularly small stature, cardiac and renal anomalies, and scoliosis – were not encountered in patients with intragenic RAI1 mutation and without the deletion (suggesting the involvement of other contiguous genes), while obesity was reported in patients with the RAI1 mutation, but not in those with the deletion. When they analysed the implication of other contiguous genes, the same investigators emphasized the role of the *TNFRSF13B* gene in the class A immunoglobulin deficiency, the *ALDH3A* gene (responsible for Sjögren-Larson syndrome) in determining dry skin, and the *PEMT* gene in the lipid anomalies (Girirajan *et al.*, 2006).

Conclusions

Smith-Magenis syndrome is rare but can be recognized by the clinician from its unique phenotypic pattern, characterized not only by peculiar somatic traits but also by a particular neurological pattern, with a frank sleep disorder and a cognitive-behavioural phenotype that may even be pathognomonic.

In the past, patients with Smith-Magenis syndrome have been erroneously diagnosed as suffering from autism or Down syndrome, Prader-Willi syndrome, DiGeorge syndrome, or fragile-X syndrome, all conditions that have certain clinical features in common. Certainly the abundance of recent contributions in the genetic and molecular field have contributed to a better definition of Smith-Magenis syndrome, but it is only by understanding and recognizing the phenotype – which is strictly the clinician's duty – that further diagnostic errors can be avoided. Proper diagnosis, especially if achieved early, enables a more suitable rehabilitation process to be implemented.

References

Bi, W., Saifi, G.M., Girirajan, S., Shi, X., Szomju, B., Firth, H., Magenis, R.E., Potocki, L., Elsea, S.H. & Lupski, J.R. (2006): RAI1 point mutations, CAG repeat variation, and SNP analysis in non-deletion Smith-Magenis syndrome. *Am. J. Med. Genet. A* **140,** 2454–2463.

Boddaert, N., De Leersnyder, H., Bourgeois, M., Munnich, A., Brunelle, F. & Zilbovicius, M. (2004): Anatomical and functional brain imaging evidence of lenticulo-insular anomalies in Smith-Magenis syndrome. *Neuroimage* **21,** 1021–1025.

Chevillard, C., Le Paslier, D., Passarge, E., Ougen, P., Billault, A., Boyer, S., Mazan, S., Bachellerie, J.P., Vignal, A., Cohen, D. & Fontes, M. (1993): Relationship between Charcot-Marie-Tooth 1A and Smith-Magenis regions: snU3 may be a candidate gene for the Smith-Magenis syndrome. *Hum. Mol. Genet.* **2,** 1235–1243.

De Leersnyder, H. (2006): Inverted rhythm of melatonin secretion in Smith-Magenis syndrome: from symptoms to treatment. *Trends Endocrinol. Metab.* **17,** 291–298.

Dykens, E.M. & Smith, A.C. (1998): Distinctiveness and correlates of maladaptive behaviour in children and adolescents with Smith-Magenis syndrome. *J. Intellect. Disabil. Res.* **42,** 481–489.

Dykens, E.M., Finucane, B.M. & Gayley, C. (1997): Cognitive and behavioural profiles in persons with Smith-Magenis syndrome. *J. Autism Dev. Disord.* **27,** 203–211.

Finucane, B.M., Dirrigl, K.H. & Simon, E.W. (2001): Characterization of self-injurious behaviours in children and adults with Smith-Magenis syndrome. *Am. J. Ment. Retard.* **106,** 52–58.

Girirajan, S., Vlangos, C.N., Szomju, B.B., Edelman, E., Trevors, C.D., Dupuis, M.S., Nezarati, M., Bunyan, D.J. & Elsea, S.H. (2006): Genotype-phenotype correlation in Smith-Magenis syndrome: evidence that multiple genes in 17p11.2 contribute to the clinical spectrum. *Genet. Med.* **8,** 417–427.

Gropman, A.L., Duncan, W.C. & Smith, A.C.M. (2006): Neurologic and developmental features of the Smith-Magenis syndrome (del 17p11.2). *Pediatr. Neurol.* **34,** 337–350.

Martin, S.C., Wolters, P.L. & Smith, A.C. (2006): Adaptive and maladaptive behaviour in children with Smith-Magenis syndrome. *J. Autism Dev. Disord.* **36,** 541–552.

Sarismki, K. (2004): Communicative competence and behavioural phenotype in children with Smith-Magenis syndrome. *Genet. Couns.* **15,** 347–355.

Smith, A.C. & Gropman, A. (2001): Smith-Magenis syndrome. In: *Management of genetic syndromes*, eds. S.B Cassidy & J.E. Allanson, pp. 363–387. New York: Wiley-Liss.

Udwin, O., Webber, C. & Horn, I. (2001): Abilities and attainment in Smith-Magenis syndrome. *Dev. Med. Child Neurol.* **43,** 823–828.

Chapter 9

Rett syndrome and its variants

Michele Zappella

Unit of Child Neuropsichiatry, Siena General Hospital, viale Bracci 2, 53100 Siena, Italy
M.Zappella@ao-siena.toscana.it

Summary

Rett syndrome is a genetic disease almost entirely affecting girls and caused by a mutation of *MECP2* gene situated on the X chromosome in more than 80 per cent of the cases. After a preclinical stage the disease has its onset in the second semester of life or later and follows four stages. The most notable clinical symptoms are hand apraxia and hand-washing stereotypies accompanied by alalya, acquired microcephaly, microsomia, breathing abnormalities, and stypsis. Epilepsy and scoliosis are often part of the clinical picture in the classical form. There are a few variants, such as precocious or, alternatively, late onset. Convulsions may begin in the first months of life and these rare cases represent another variant. In a preserved speech variant there is late improvement which allows some girls to speak, sometimes in long phrases, and to recover some of their manual abilities; these girls have usually a normal head circumference and an adequate somatic structure.

History

Rett syndrome was discovered in this way. In the middle of the sixties a young Viennese paediatric neurologist, Andreas Rett, while returning to his office after his rounds, noticed two mothers keeping their hands over their daughters' hands. He went up to them and asked them to leave their daughters' hands free, which they did it. He then saw that both girls had a form of repetitive stereotypic activity as if they were washing their hands. On entering his office he remarked to his secretary that he had seen this behaviour in other girls. His secretary promptly made a provisional list of girls with the same features, the initial core feature of the syndrome. Rett then published his observations in a short book and in an Austrian journal, *Wiener Medizinische Wochenschrift* (Rett 1966a; Rett 1966b), though he placed an inappropriate emphasis on hyperammonaemia, a metabolic disorder which can occasionally be found in affected girls. This approach may be explained by the 'spirit of the times': in the 1960s there was a tendency to place little diagnostic value on stereotypic activities in syndromes of congenital brain damage – stereotypic movements with similar features had been reported in different metabolic diseases such as phenylketonuria and maple syrup urine disease, as well as in tuberous sclerosis, non-specific severe mental retardation and other serious brain disorders. In fact, in the same decade other child neurologists were tempted to make a differential diagnosis of girls with hand-washing activities, but after the negative result of fairly extensive metabolic and chromosomal studies they decided not to publish their observations*. Rett's merit lay in recognizing that the stereotypic activity he had observed was a marker of a well defined disease, and in keeping faith with this observation despite the inappropriate prejudice of his colleagues. In the ensuing years he attended conferences and showed a film of the girls to colleagues on many occasions. He also wrote a chapter on the subject in a prestigious textbook of neurology (Rett, 1977). However, there was no consensus on his syndrome for almost 20 years. In the early eighties, while in Canada, he met by chance Dr. B. Hagberg, who had been working on similar girls for many years. Subsequently (in the interval of a conference in Lisbon) Hagberg exchanged his observations on this topic with other European child neurologists. They decided to publish their similar cases jointly and gave the name of Rett to the new syndrome (Hagberg et al., 1983).

Later it became clear that in the previous decades most of these girls had been inappropriately diagnosed as having autism (Witt-Engerstrom & Gillberg, 1987), and criteria were proposed to distinguish the two syndromes (Olsson & Rett, 1987). In the subsequent decade Rett syndrome was included among pervasive developmental disorders in the *Diagnostic and Statistical Manual of Mental Disorders* (DSM-IV), as autistic symptoms are consistently present only in stage 2 of the disease and may be absent in the later stages. A consensus paper (The Rett Syndrome Criteria Work Group, 1988) included complete alalia among the other symptoms, but it subsequently became clear that some girls were able to speak (Zappella, 1992); these probably have the more frequent Rett syndrome variant. In 1999 Amir and colleagues described a mutation of *MECP2* gene.

The history of how Rett syndrome was discovered teaches us that a precise description of the essential types and sequences of neurological symptoms was essential in defining this disorder, and this step in knowledge opened the way to genetic discoveries, which in turn have been and are of help in confirming and explaining the clinical observations.

Occurrence

The prevalence of Rett syndrome is estimated to be 1:10,000. There have been reports of increased local prevalence (Zappella & Cerioli, 1987; Hagberg & Hagberg, 1997). Most cases are sporadic but there is a rare occurrence of familial cases which may include a classical Rett syndrome girl, a variant, and a normal mother (with X skewed mutation) (Zappella et al., 2001). The vast majority of cases are female.

Clinical features

Pregnancy and birth are usually uneventful. Subsequently the baby is often placid, slow to move around, and has a low tone of voice. The child often sits in an unusual frog-like position, and bottom shuffling takes the place of crawling. In spite of these subtle abnormalities she passes the usual developmental screening tests. By the end of the first year she can take the bottle in her hands: in most cases she is considered normal by her parents. A period of developmental stagnation (stage 1) follows, with a slowing of general psychomotor development

---

* These included Bengt Hagberg and Michel Philippart. Something similar occurred to me when I was junior medical officer in the Fountain Hospital in London in 1962.

and loss of supporting reaction. This is followed by a stage of regression (stage 2), which is often dramatic with a rapid loss of social contact, communication, and use of the hands. Within a few days or weeks the infant appears frightened, with loss of contact with her parents and a lack of response to them. She often wakes up in the night, screaming or laughing. Regression may occur between the end of the first year (8–9 months) and 3 years of age, lasting from a few months to 1–2 years. The use of hands declines, with eventual complete apraxia; in parallel, recurring circular movements appear more and more frequently, during which the hands touch the hair, are brought to the mouth, or are clapped together. In the ensuing months, hand-washing stereotypies become constant, and towards the end of this stage abnormalities of breathing become evident. These stereotypies – or similar repetitive movements such as hand-wringing, hand-squeezing, clapping, or rubbing – occur in the midline and only when the girls are awake.

At the same time as these symptoms develop, the gait becomes dyspraxic. Eighty per cent of affected girls learn to walk and one-quarter of these will subsequently lose this ability (Percy & Lane, 2005). Head circumference growth rate declines by 4–6 months of life and by the end of the second year the occipito-frontal circumference is usually at the third centile or below.

Constant features of classical Rett syndrome are: (1) hand dyspraxia (or full apraxia) accompanied by stereotypic hand movements; (2) head growth deceleration; (3) normal pregnancy and childbirth, and normal development during the first months of life; (4) consistent disease staging, which in all cases includes stages 1 to 3, and often a fourth stage. Items (1) and (4) are also present in Rett syndrome variants, but head growth may be normal in less severe cases, and in some other variants the overt onset of the disease occurs at birth or shortly afterwards.

Other less constant features may or may not be present. In stage 3 there is a clear improvement in socialisation, with eye contact and smiling. In the following years there is usually some improvement in the child's general condition: affected girls develop an active interest in people and enjoy staying with them, are capable of interacting with other children and taking turns, and like listening to simple talk and stories. They have a good memory for people and places and are able to make choices. In some cases their interest in specific objects is shown by their response to images: the child will look with greatest intensity at a photograph of the object she is particularly interested in. The use of the hands may improve slightly in some girls, and certain manoeuvres may favour this – for example, giving support the elbow while the child is eating can be helpful.

Physical activity is essential for health, and walking, horse riding and swimming are generally enjoyed. Unfortunately other comorbidities often interfere with the wellbeing of the girls in this stage, which may be prolonged for many years and in some cases for decades or for the remainder of the patient's life. Epilepsy, involving grand mal seizures, partial seizures, myoclonic seizures, and all kinds of epileptic attacks except petit mal, may be hard to treat and in 50 to 80 per cent of affected children remains a persistent problem until late adolescence. Scoliosis of increasing severity may require surgery. Gallbladder disease should be suspected in Rett girls with abdominal pain. Muscle tone evolves over time from hypotonia to slight hypertonia, often with increased tendon reflexes and occasionally ankle clonus. These abnormalities can represent the start of stage 4, which is not universal but occurs in a proportion of Rett girls, usually beginning in adolescence but sometimes even before that or much later, with a progressive reduction in the ability to walk until the patient becomes wheelchair dependent, with muscular wasting and distal contractures. Epilepsy, if present, often diminishes at this stage.

The electroencephalogram (EEG) is usually normal in stage 1, but in stage 2 there is a slowing of background activity during waking periods, while during sleep spindles can be absent and focal, or multifocal spikes and sharp waves appear. In stage 3, multifocal spikes and sharp wave discharges are often present (Glaze, 2005). Intermittent delta or theta bursts are common. Continuous generalized rhythmic spikes are usual in stage 4 (Bader & Hagne, 1993).

Abnormalities of the autonomic system are an important feature of Rett syndrome. These include a flushed face and dilated pupils, accompanied by a state of agitation or distress; such episodes may recur at different periods over the lifespan. The feet are often small and cold in winter. Gastro-oesophageal reflux is frequent and constipation is the rule. Abdominal distension with air while awake is frequent, though it disappears during sleep; it may be painful and at times reaches huge proportions. Periods of hyperventilation and breath holding are often present and occur only while the patient is awake. They may alternate and cause abnormalities in CO_2 levels, with hypocapnoea (tachypnoea) or hypercapnoea (breath holding), producing dizziness and vacant spells (Yulu, 2001). On some occasions these breathing abnormalities can be prolonged, lasting for many hours, with epileptic seizures or status epilepticus. Deficient parasympathetic restraint is a feature of the autonomic imbalance in this disorder. The heart is affected, showing reduced heart rate variability and prolonged QTc. Sleep difficulties are common, especially in the early years of life.

Neuropathology

The brain in Rett syndrome is small and the weight reduction may as much as 40 per cent compared with a normal brain of the same age (Oldfords et al., 1993). Increasing age does not entail a change in brain weight, which has an average value of around 900 g. The external appearance of the brain is normal, though the cerebral hemispheres are comparatively smaller than the cerebellum. Dendritic branching is decreased in the frontal, motor and subicular regions. Decreased neuronal size can be seen in the cortex and in other subcortical structures, while in the hippocampus there is increased neuronal packing (Armstrong, 1992; Jellinger, 2003; Armstrong, 2005). Hypopigmentation of the zona compacta of the substantia nigra, caused by reduction in neuromelanin, had already been noticed by Rett (1977) and was confirmed in other studies (Jellinger & Seitelberger, 1986). Cortical minicolumns are reduced in size in the speech area, possibly reflecting a reduction in dendritic branching of the neurons (Casanova et al., 2003). The grey matter is diminished in volume – Rett syndrome appears to be a disorder of synaptic proliferation, and it has been suggested that the *MECP2* deficit disturbs the formation of synapses (Johnston et al., 2005). There is no evidence of nerve cell loss, and this is the main reason why Rett syndrome is not considered a neurodegenerative disorder but is included instead among the neurodevelopmental disorders such as autism, Angelman syndrome and so on. It is of interest that small minicolumns and reduced dendritic branching are also observed in the cortex in autism, with cell packing in some subcortical areas (Kemper & Bauman, 1993; Casanova, 2002), although the brain is heavier than normal and the cerebellum is smaller. *MECP2* deletion or other targeted mutations of *MECP2* in the mouse have been developed as models designed to reproduce Rett syndrome. These animals show normal development in the first month of life with the subsequent appearance of tremor, hypertonus, hypoactivity, ataxia, hind-limb clapping, reduced weight, and kyphosis.

There is substantial variation in the timing of the disease onset in Rett syndrome: overt disease may be present at birth or it may not appear until the child is several years old. Severity is also quite variable, some cases having a relatively benign course and others being associated with certain specific features. This has led to the recognition of several Rett syndrome variants.

Preserved speech variant

In the late eighties a consensus paper by The Rett Syndrome Criteria Work Group (1988) included among other symptoms complete alalia, and it was not until the early nineties (Zappella, 1992) that the possibility was considered that some girls could say words and enunciate fully formed phrases. These cases represent the *Preserved Speech Variant (PSV)*, possibly the most frequent of the variants, with distinctive and benign features compared with classical Rett syndrome. Thus somatic development and the neurovegetative system are normal or close to normal, while neurological aspects include an improvement in language and manual abilities which is specifically delayed until the second part of the first decade of life. In centres that are referral points for both autism and Rett syndrome, girls with this variant are over-represented: this is the case in Siena where 16 per cent of the female patients have Rett syndrome and the *MECP2* mutation. In fact many girls with PSV are autistic and they are often initially referred for autism; only after a careful evaluation is the diagnosis of PSV obtained. In most cases (close to 90 per cent), an *MECP2* mutation is found in these girls, with missense (for example, R133C) or late truncating mutations leading to a protein with some preserved domains that is capable of translocating to the nucleus, where it may exert some residual function (Zappella *et al.*, 2001; Zappella *et al.*, 2003). In this variant the somatic features are often within the normal range, including normal head circumference, height, and weight, although some girls are obese, and kyphosis, moderate scoliosis, genu valgum, and flat feet may occur.

Neurovegetative symptoms are limited or absent: prolongation of QTc is rare (20 per cent), normal power of heart rate variability (HRV) is the rule (Guideri *et al.*, 1999; Guideri *et al.*, 2001), and sudden death is not reported. The neurological disorder is analogous to classical Rett syndrome in the early years but it subsequently has a more benign course. The four stages typical of Rett syndrome are usually reported, but stages 1 and 2 may be less evident and dramatic, and the history must be careful and detailed to reveal them. The initial picture is analogous to the classical syndrome, with hand-washing or hand-clapping stereotypies, hand apraxia, non-existent linguistic communication (or limited to couple of words), ataxic-apraxic gait, and a strong interest in music. At 2–4 years the only difference from classical Rett syndrome is the normality of the somatic features, suggesting a better outcome – especially if coupled with the appropriate mutations. Improvements usually occur around 4–6 years, with a progressive increase in single word production and better use of the hands. In the ensuing years some of these girls will not go beyond the ability to say 15–20 words and a few two-word sentences, with limited use of the hands and retaining most of the features of classical Rett syndrome – including epilepsy in around 50 per cent, an EEG appearance similar to that of classical Rett, and often a marked scoliosis. Others will have a more marked improvement, but they may also have an unusual course. Thus, at 5–6 years they start to make slow but constant progress whereby they learn to speak in short but subsequently more complex phrases; in parallel, other functions improve, especially an increasing ability to use the hands, allowing them to built a tower of cubes, feed themselves with a spoon and fork, and draw complex objects, while hand-washing stereotypies diminish and may disappear. Their general mental abilities, which are especially poor in the early years, start to improve, and in some cases an IQ close to or slightly above 50 is achieved. They may lose ataxic features and also most of the symptoms of the autistic series if present. This late-onset improvement is a specific feature of these cases and suggest the possibility that an as yet unknown modifying factor may contribute to the unexpected improvement (Zappella *et al.*, 2003).

Autistic symptoms are often present in this variant of Rett syndrome, whereas cardiac dysautonomia, dysfunction affecting breathing, constipation and gastro-oesophageal reflux are usually absent or considerably reduced. Epilepsy is rare but it can be severe in some cases.

Formes frustes

Formes frustes (Goutières & Aicardi, 1986) represent 10 to 15 per cent of all the cases (Hagberg & Rasmussen, 1986; Hagberg & Gillberg, 1993). These girls show a later the onset of the first stages, their hand-washing stereotypic activities are less intense, the use of hands is better preserved, and in general the disease is less severe.

Congenital Rett syndrome

The congenital form of Rett syndrome (Rolando, 1985) is very rare. Affected infants show severe symptoms in the neonatal period, with severe hypotonia and very marked delay in developmental progress. The usual stages and symptoms of Rett syndrome appear later during the second year of life.

Infantile seizure onset

In the variant with infantile seizure onset (Hanefeld, 1985), infantile spasms with hypsarrhythmia, myoclonic seizures or other epileptic fits mark the overt beginning of the disorder while the classical symptoms and stages appear later. These rare cases are caused by mutations of *CDKL5*, coding for a kinase which is able to phosphorylate itself and mediates MeCP2 phosphorylation in the central nervous system (Mari *et al.*, 2005). Mutations of this gene can also cause early-onset seizures and severe mental retardation in females without any overlap with Rett syndrome, and these cases are possibly more numerous than the infantile seizure variant of Rett syndrome (Archer *et al.*, 2006).

Late-childhood regression onset

The late-childhood regression onset (Gillberg, 1989) involves girls with intellectual disability of medium degree who show mental deterioration in the second part of the first decade, with autistic behaviour and hand-washing or other similar stereotypic activities associated with hand dyspraxia.

Male variant

Very rarely Rett syndrome may occur in boys, with mutations similar to those in girls and often with a sister affected by the same disease. The clinical picture is similar to the severe form of classic Rett syndrome and includes epilepsy, apnoeic fits, and death in the first two years of life (Maiwald *et al.*, 2004).

Other variants

MECP2 mutations have also been observed in some boys with mental retardation of various degrees (Moog *et al.*, 2003), in boys with a neonatal encephalopathy (Leuzzi *et al.*, 2004), in girls with intrauterine microcephaly (Erlandson & Hagberg, 2005), and in boys and girls with an Angelman phenotype (Watson *et al.*, 2001).

Medical treatment

There is no cure for Rett syndrome, but various treatments can ameliorate some symptoms and the co-morbid disorders.

L-carnitine (50–100 mg/kg/d) has been observed to improve sleep, energy level, and communication (Ellaway et al., 1999; Ellaway et al., 2001) and, in a dose of 50 mg/kg/d, to improve cardiac dysautonomia, producing a significant increase in HRV total power and a slight reduction in sympathetic overactivity (Guideri et al., 2004; Guideri et al., 2005). β-blockers have been recommended for Rett girls with long QT (Glaze, 2006).

For sleep disturbances, melatonin given for a few weeks (McArthur & Budden, 1998) is often a useful treatment (2.5–7.5 mg one hour before bedtime). Its positive effects can be prolonged for several months.

Topiramate and magnesium citrate may have a beneficial effect on breathing irregularities.

For epileptic seizures the usual drugs are normally effective and well tolerated. Uncontrolled seizures and status epilepticus may occur. Non-epileptic behaviours such as inadequate control of cardiorespiratory rhythms by the brain stem may lead to vacant spells with irregular breathing, fluctuations in heart and blood pressure, and sudden reduction in consciousness. In these situations prolonged video-EEG and autonomic (brain stem) monitoring may help in making the correct diagnosis. If a child has low levels of carbon dioxide as a result of repeated hyperventilation, the administration of CO_2 and oxygen may reduce the breathing disorder (Smeets et al., 2006).

Dystonic movements are frequent and can be helped by the use of trihexyphenidyl (Artane). These movements are often associated with face flushing and other autonomic symptoms. They can be triggered by the extrapyramidal system but a hyperexcitable brain stem may also be the cause, as may a dystonic storm, leading to true epileptic seizures in the form of status epilepticus.

Gastro-oesophageal reflux is common and usually responds well to ranitidine and other appropriate drugs. Constipation is also common. Feeding may be difficult and a Mediterranean diet and olive oil appear useful in maintaining an adequate weight (Zappella et al., 1992). Alternative forms of feeding may be necessary in a few cases, usually in the fourth stage – for example, by gastrostomy. In some cases, self aggression, a sad appearance, profound sleep disturbance, and a decreased interest in food are features of depression, which should be treated with selective serotonin reuptake inhibitors (SSRIs).

Scoliosis may require surgery, especially if it progresses beyond 40 per cent.

P.S. Some months following the meeting on Mental Retardation interesting advances were reported in the field of experimental engineering concerning MECP2 gene. It was found that in the experimental mouse the neurologic symptoms related to MECP2 deficiency could be reversed by the subsequent activation of this gene [Giacometti E., Luikenhuis S., Beard C., Jaenisch R. (2007): Partial rescue of MECP2 deficiency by postnatal activation of MECP2. *Proceedings of the National Academy of Science USA* **104**, 1931-1936; Guy J, Gan J, Selfridge J, Cobb S, Bird A (2007): Reversal of neurological defect in a mouse model of Rett syndrome. *Science*, **315**, 1143-1147].

References

Amir, R.E., Van den Veyver, I.B., Wan, M., Tran, C.Q., Francke, U. & Zoghbi, H.Y. (1999): Rett syndrome is caused by mutations in X-linked MECP2, encoding methyl-CpG-binding protein 2. *Nat. Genet.* **23**, 185–188. Comment: **23**, 127–128.

Armstrong, D.D. (1992): The neuropathology of Rett syndrome. *Brain Dev.* **14** (Suppl.), S89-S98.

Armstrong, D.D. (2005): Neuropathology of Rett syndrome. *J. Child Neurol.* **20**, 747–752.

Archer, H.L., Evans, J., Edwards, S., Colley, J., Newbury-Ecob, R., O'Callaghan, F., Huyton, M., O'Reagan, M., Tolmie, J., Sampson, J., Clarke, A. & Osborne, J. (2006): CDKL5 mutations cause infantile spasms, early onset seizures, and severe mental retardation in female patients. *J. Med. Genet.* **43**, 729–734.

Bader, G. & Hagne, I. (1993): Neurophysiological diagnosis. In: *Rett syndrome – clinical and biological aspects*, ed. B. Hagberg. London: MacKeith Press.

Casanova, M.F. (2002): Asperger's syndrome and cortical neuropathology. *J. Child Neurol.* **17**, 142–145.

Casanova, M.F., Buxhoeveden, D., Switala, A. & Roy, E. (2003): Rett syndrome as a minicolumnopathy. *Clin. Neuropathol.* **22**, 163–168.

Ellaway, C.J., Williams, K., Leonard, H., Higgins, G., Wilcken, B. & Christodoulou, J. (1999): Rett syndrome: randomized controlled trial of L-carnitine. *J. Child Neurol.* **14**, 62–67.

Ellaway, C.J., Peat, J., Williams, K., Leonard, H. & Christodoulou, J. (2001): Medium term open label trial of L-carnitine in Rett syndrome. *Brain Dev.* **23** (Suppl. 1), S85-S89.

Erlandson, A. & Hagberg, B. (2005): MECP2 abnormality phenotypes: clinicopathologic area with broad variability. *J. Child Neurol.* **20**, 727–732.

Gillberg, C. (1989): The borderland of autism and Rett syndrome: five case histories to highlight diagnostic difficulties. *J. Autism Dev. Disord.* **19**, 545–549.

Glaze, D.G. (2005): Neurophysiology of Rett syndrome. *J. Child Neurol.* **20**, 740–746.

Glaze, D.G. (2006): Rett syndrome: therapeutic interventions and prognosis. Proceedings of VII National Conference of the Italian Society of Pediatric Nutrition, Milan, 23–25 November.

Goutières, F. & Aicardi, J. (1986): Atypical forms of Rett syndrome. *Am. J. Med. Genet.* **24**, 183–186.

Guideri, F., Acampa, M., Hayek, G., Zappella, M. & Di Perri, T. (1999): Reduced heart variability in patients affected with Rett syndrome. A possible explanation for sudden death. *Neuropediatrics* **30**, 146–148.

Guideri, F., Acampa, M., Di Perri, T., Zappella, M. & Hayek, G. (2001): Progressive cardiac dysautonomia observed in patients affected by classic Rett syndrome and not in the preserved speech variant. *J. Child Neurol.* **16**, 370–373.

Guideri, F., Acampa, M., Blardi, P., de Lalla, A., Zappella, M. & Hayek, Y. (2004): Cardiac dysautonomia and serotonin plasma levels in Rett syndrome. *Neuropediatrics* **35**, 36–38.

Guideri, F., Acampa, M., Blardi, P., DeLalla, A., Zappella, M. & Hayek, G. (2005): Effects of acetyl-L-carnitine on cardiac dysautonomia in Rett syndrome: prevention of sudden death? *Pediatr. Cardiol.* **26**, 574–577.

Hagberg, B. & Rasmussen, P. (1986): Forme fruste of Rett syndrome: a case report. *Am. J. Med. Genet.* **24**, 175–177.

Hagberg, B. & Gillberg, C. (1993): Rett variants – Rettoid phenotypes. In: *Rett syndrome – clinical and biological aspects*, ed. B. Hagberg. London: MacKeith Press.

Hagberg, B. & Hagberg, G. (1997): Rett syndrome: epidemiology and geographical variability, *Eur. Child Adolesc. Psychiatry* **6**, 5–7.

Hagberg, B., Aicardi, J., Dias, K. & Ramos, O. (1983): A progressive syndrome of autism, dementia, ataxia and loss of purposeful hand use in girls: Rett's syndrome – report of 35 cases. *Ann. Neurol.* **14**, 471–479.

Hanefeld, F. (1985): The clinical pattern of the Rett syndrome. *Brain Dev.* **7**, 320–325.

Jellinger, K. (2003): Rett syndrome – an update. *J. Neural Transm.* **110**, 681–701.

Jellinger, K. & Seitelberger, F. (1986): Neuropathology of Rett syndrome. *Am. J. Med. Genet. Suppl.* **1**, 259–288.

Johnston, M.V., Blue, M. & Naidu, S. (2005): Rett syndrome and neuronal development. *J. Child Neurol.* **20**, 759–763.

Kemper, T.L. & Bauman, M.L. (1993): The contribution of neuropathologic studies to the understanding of autism. *Neurol. Clin.* **11**, 175–178.

Leuzzi, V., Di Sabato, M.L., Zollino, M., Montanaro, M.L. & Seri, S. (2004): Early-onset encephalopathy and cortical myoclonus in a boy with MECP2 gene mutation. *Neurology* **63**, 1968–1970.

Maiwald, R., Bonte, A., Jung, H., Bitter, P., Storm, Z., Laccone, F. & Herkenrath, P. (2002): De novo MECP2 mutation in a 46,XX male patient with Rett syndrome. *Neurogenetics* **4**, 107–108.

Mari, F., Azimonti, S., Bertani, I., Bolognese, F., Colombo, E., Caselli, R., Scala, E., Longo, I., Grosso, S., Pescucci C., Ariani, F., Hayek, G., Balestri, P., Bergo, A., Badaracco, G., Zappella, M., Broccoli, V., Renieri, A., Kilstrup-Nielsen, C. & Landsberger, N. (2005): CDKL5 belongs to the same molecular pathway of MECP2 and it is responsible for the early-onset seizure variant of Rett syndrome. *Hum. Mol. Genet.* **14,** 1935–1946.

McArthur, A.J. & Budden, S.S (1998): Sleep dysfunction in Rett syndrome a trial of exogenous melatonin treatment. *Dev. Med. Child Neurol.* **40,** 186–192.

Moog, U., Smeets, E.E., von Roozendaal, K.E., Schoenmakers, S., Herbergs, J., Schoonbrood-Lenssen, A.M. & Schrander-Stumpel, C.T. (2003): Neurodevelopmental disorders in males related to the gene causing Rett syndrome in females (MECP2). *Eur. J. Paediatr. Neurol.* **7,** 5–12.

Oldfords, A., Sopurander, P. & Percy, A.K. (1993): Neuropathology and neurochemistry. In: *Rett syndrome – clinical and biological aspects*, ed. B. Hagberg. London: MacKeith Press.

Olsson, B. & Rett, A. (1987): Autism and Rett syndrome: behavioural investigations and differential diagnosis. *Dev. Med. Child Neurol.* **29,** 429–441.

Percy, A. & Lane, J. (2005): Rett syndrome: model of neurodevelopmental disorder. *J. Child Neurol.* **20,** 718–721.

Rett, A. (1966a): *Über ein zerebral-atrophisches Syndrom bei Hyperammonaemie*. Vienna: Brueder Hollinek.

Rett, A. (1966b): Über ein eigenartiges hirnatrophisches Syndrom im Kindesalter. *Wien. Med. Wochenschr.* **116,** 723–726.

Rett, A. (1977): Cerebral atrophy associated with hyperammonaemia. In: *Handbook of clinical neurology*, vol. 29: *Metabolic and deficiency diseases of the nervous system*, ed. P.J. Vinken. Amsterdam: North Holland.

Rolando, S. (1985): Rett syndrome: report of eight cases. *Brain Dev.* **7,** 290–296.

Smeets, E.E., Julu, P.O., van Waardenburg, D., Engerstrom, I.W., Hansen, S., Apartopoulos, F., Curfs, L.M. & Schrander-Stumpel, C.T. (2006): Management of a severe forceful breather with Rett using carbogen. *Brain Dev.* **28,** 625–632.

The Rett Syndrome Criteria Work Group (1988): Diagnostic criteria for Rett syndrome. *Ann. Neurol.* **23,** 425–428.

Watson, P., Black, G., Ramsden, S., Barrow, M., Super, M., Kerr, B. & Clayton-Smith, J. (2001): Angelman syndrome phenotype associated with mutation in MECP2, a gene encoding a methyl CpG binding protein. *J. Med. Genet.* **39,** 132–136.

Witt-Engerstrom, I. & Gillberg, C. (1987): Rett syndrome in Sweden. *J. Autism Dev. Disord.* **17,** 149–150.

Yulu, P.O.O. (2001): The central autonomic disturbance in Rett syndrome. In: *Rett disorder and the developing brain*, eds. A. Kerr & I. Witt-Engerstrom. New York: Oxford University Press.

Zappella, M. (1992): The Rett girls with preserved speech. *Brain Dev.* **14,** 98–101.

Zappella, M. & Cerioli, M. (1987): High prevalence of Rett syndrome in a small area. *Brain Dev.* **9,** 479–480.

Zappella, M., Menchetti, M.G. & Pini, G. (1992): Italian girls have better auxologic features. *Rassegna di Studi Psichiatrici* **81,** 273–277.

Zappella, M., Meloni, I., Longo, I., Hayek, G. & Renieri, A. (2001): Preserved speech variant of the Rett syndrome: molecular and clinical analysis. *Am. J. Med. Genet.* **104,** 14–22.

Zappella, M., Meloni, I., Longo, L., Canitano, R., Hayek, G., Rosaia, L., Mari, F. & Renieri, A. (2003): Study of MECP2 gene in Rett syndrome variants and autistic girls. *Am. J. Med. Genet. Neuropsychiatr. Genet.* **119B,** 102–107.

Chapter 10

Phenotypes in chromosome 15-linked syndromes

Agatino Battaglia

Stella Maris Clinical Research Institute for Child and Adolescent Neurology and Psychiatry, via dei Giacinti 2, 56018 Calambrone, Pisa, Italy, and Division of Medical Genetics, Department of Paediatrics, University of Utah, Salt Lake City, Utah, USA
abattaglia@inpe.unipi.it

Summary

The chromosome region 15q11-q13 is known for its instability resulting from the presence of repeated DNA elements, and many rearrangements may occur in this imprinted segment. These are represented by deletions, interstitial duplications, supernumerary marker chromosomes, and, less often, by triplications, translocations, and inversions. Deletions on the maternal chromosome 15q11.2-q13 are associated with Angelman syndrome, which is characterized by developmental delay/mental retardation (DD/MR), microcephaly, ataxic gait, absent or very poor speech, seizures/epilepsy with distinctive EEG findings, and a happy demeanour. Deletions on the paternal chromosome 15q11.2-q13 are associated with Prader-Willi syndrome, which is characterized by DD/MR, infantile central hypotonia and feeding problems, rapid weight gain between 1 and 6 years, characteristic face, hypogonadism, and a distinctive behaviour disorder. Duplication on the maternal chromosome 15q11-q13 is found in one per cent of individuals with autism spectrum. The syndrome phenotype is characterized by a lack of distinctive dysmorphic features, hypotonia, and mild mental retardation. Inv dup(15) is the most common of the structurally abnormal supernumerary marker chromosomes, resulting in tetrasomy 15p and partial tetrasomy 15q. The syndrome phenotype is characterized by early central hypotonia, minor dysmorphic features, DD/MR, autism or autistic-like behaviour, and severe seizures/epilepsy (Lennox-Gastaut type).

Introduction

Some disease genes may be expressed differently when inherited from one sex compared with the other. This is 'genomic imprinting.' It is associated with, and possibly caused by, methylation of DNA. The attachment of methyl groups to DNA may inhibit the binding of proteins that promote transcription.

The imprinted chromosome region 15q11-q13 is known for its instability, owing to the presence of repeated DNA elements. Many rearrangements may occur in this segment. These are represented by deletions, interstitial duplications, supernumerary marker chromosomes (formed by the **inverted dup**lication of proximal chromosome 15), and, less often, by triplications, translocations, and inversions.

Deletions on the maternal chromosome 15q11.2-q13 are associated with Angelman syndrome, whereas deletions on the paternal chromosome 15q11.2-q13 are associated with Prader-Willi syndrome. Duplication on the maternal chromosome 15q11-q13 is found in one per cent of individuals with autistic spectrum disorders, whereas **inv**erted **dup**lication of the maternal proximal chromosome 15 causes the inv dup(15) or idic(15) syndrome (Fig. 1).

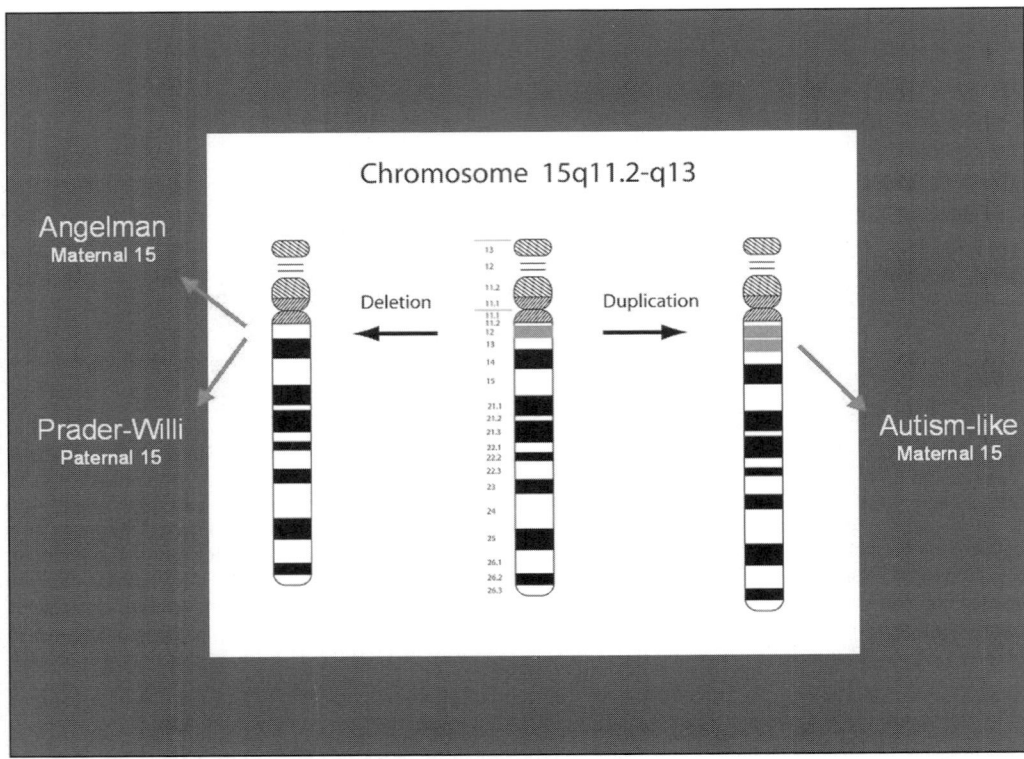

Fig. 1. Ideograms of G-banding patterns for human chromosome 15, showing some of the rearrangements that may occur in the 15q11.2-q13 imprinted segment.

Angelman syndrome

Angelman syndrome (AS) is caused by loss of the maternal segment 15q11.2-q13, either by 'deletion' in the maternal homologue (70–75 per cent of cases), or by paternal 'disomy' 15 (two to five per cent), thereby leading to functional nullisomy of a gene or genes whose paternal copies are switched off (imprinted). The minimal genetic alteration is 'mutation' or 'deletion' within the imprinted *UBE3A* gene (20–25 per cent of cases), or the imprinting centre (IC) (two to five per cent). The syndrome has been reported throughout the world among different racial groups. The estimate incidence is 1 in 12,000 to 1 in 20,000, and life span seems to be similar to the general population (Williams, 2005a). Angelman syndrome is characterized by severe developmental delay/mental retardation (DD/MR), microcephaly, ataxic gait, absent or very poor speech, seizures/epilepsy with distinctive EEG findings, and a happy demeanour. Microcephaly is more pronounced in children with 15q11.2-q13 deletions, and becomes evident by 2 years of age. Developmental delay, evident by age 6–12 months, is often associated with truncal hypotonia. On formal testing, the ceiling for psychomotor development achievement is around the 24–30 months range (Andersen et al., 2001; Thompson & Bolton, 2003). Imdividuals with Angelman syndrome have relative strengths in visual skills and social interaction that are based on non-verbal events. Expressive language is absent or very poor, and more impaired than receptive language. However, some cases with a mosaic form of an 'imprinting defect' can use many words and a few of them can even speak in simple sentences. The movement disorder of Angelman syndrome is characterized by an ataxic gait or forward lurching, unsteadiness, clumsiness or quick, jerky motions, and tremulousness of limbs. The latter has been shown to be caused by a quasi-continuous 11-Hz multifocal, rhythmic cortical myoclonus, mainly involving hands and face, responsible for mild jerking or twitching, easily mistaken for a tremor (Guerrini et al., 1996). Individuals with Angelman syndrome show a unique behaviour pattern with unprovoked and frequent laughter/smiling, apparently happy demeanour, an easily excitable personality often with uplifted hand flapping or waving movements, hyperactivity, and fascination with water and crinkly items. Associated clinical features – present in 20–80 per cent of individuals – are represented by a flat occiput, protruding tongue or tongue thrusting, prognathia with a wide mouth and frequent drooling, hypopigmentation (deletion cases), an abnormal sleep/wake cycle, scoliosis, and constipation (Williams et al., 2006). Epilepsy affects 90 per cent of children with Angelman syndrome, mostly starting before the age of 3. The first seizures are often triggered by fever. The main ictal patterns are represented by atypical absences, myoclonic seizures, generalized tonic-clonic seizures, and unilateral seizures (Battaglia & Gurrieri, 1999). Complex partial seizures with eye deviation and vomiting, possibly indicating occipital lobe origin, seem to occur frequently. Over 50 per cent of patients suffer from episodes of decreased alertness and hypotonia lasting for days or weeks (non-convulsive status epilepticus), often with a concomitant mild jerking. Video-EEG-polygraphy, carried out during myoclonic status or short myoclonic seizures, shows diffuse, irregular, 2 Hz spike/wave complexes, at times accompanied by EEG spikes that are time-locked to myoclonic potentials. Rather distinctive EEG patterns are characterized by the following:

- Prolonged runs of 200–500 μV, rhythmic 1–3 Hz activity mainly over both frontal regions, with superimposed interictal spikes/sharp waves, as ill-defined complexes, not disappearing during sleep. Such findings have been observed in almost 50 per cent of alert and responsive children and adults before the clinical diagnosis of Angelman syndrome was made.

- Persistent, often generalized, rhythmic 3–4 Hz activity larger than 200 μV, independent of eye closure (observed in children with Angelman syndrome under age 12).

- Spikes/sharp waves mixed with 3–4 Hz waves larger than 200 μV, mainly over the posterior temporo-parieto-occipital regions, facilitated by eye closure (Boyd et al., 1988; Battaglia & Guerrini, 2005; Laan & Vein, 2005).

The usual phasic sleep organization appears to be disrupted in children with Angelman syndrome. The AS gene, *UBE3A*, is imprinted in brain but not in other tissues, a finding compatible with the brain being the most affected organ in this syndrome (Rougelle et al., 1997). The electro-clinical picture is more severe in those individuals with a 15q11.2-q13 deletion than in those where the syndrome is caused by uniparental disomy (UPD), *UBE3A*, or IC mutation (Williams et al., 2006). This observation suggests that one or more genes in the deleted region, including the GABA receptor subunit genes, may modify the AS phenotype caused by the lack of maternal *UBE3A* function. A possible mechanism for seizures is dysfunction of inhibition owing to deletion or other genetic disruption of $GABA_A$ receptor subunits.

DNA methylation testing of blood is a sensitive and specific screening for three (deletion, UPD, IC defects) of the four known genetic mechanisms underlying Angelman syndrome. Diagnosis is confirmed if the test is abnormal, but to determine which of the three mechanisms is operative, it is suggested that one should perform, as a second step, chromosome 15 q11.2-q13 fluorescence *in situ* hybridization (FISH). This test allows sensitive detection of 15 q11.2-q13 microdeletions. If there is no deletion, the next step would be the analysis of microsatellites in parents and the affected subject in search for a UPD. If this test also turns out to be negative, then the proband has an IC defect. If DNA methylation testing of blood is normal, the next step would be to carry out mutation analysis of *UBE3A* (testing now available in clinical laboratories) (Williams, 2005b).

Prader-Willi syndrome

Prader-Willi syndrome (PWS) is caused by loss of the paternal segment 15q11.2-q13, either by deletion (4 Mb) in the paternal homologue (70–75 per cent of cases), or by maternal disomy 15 (20–25 per cent of cases). In fewer than five per cent of cases there is an abnormality in the imprinting process. The incidence is estimated to be 1 in 10,000 to 1 in 15,000 (Cassidy & McCandless, 2005). Major diagnostic criteria are neonatal/infantile central hypotonia, infantile feeding problems, rapid weight gain between the ages of 1 and 6 years, hyperphagia, narrow bifrontal diameter, almond-shaped palpebral fissures, down-turned mouth, hypogonadism, developmental delay, mild to moderate mental retardation, and multiple learning disabilities. Minor diagnostic criteria are decreased fetal movements and infantile lethargy, behaviour disorder, sleep disturbances, short stature for the family by age 15, small hands and feet, hypopigmentation, esotropia, myopia, and skin picking (Holm *et al.*, 1993). The behaviour profile is distinctive, including temper tantrums, controlling and manipulative behaviour, obsessive-compulsive characteristics, stubbornness, difficulty with change in routine, stealing, and lying. This behaviour disorder increases with age and body mass index (Steinhausen *et al.*, 2004). Behavioural problems interfere greatly with the quality of life in adolescence and adulthood, though they diminish considerably in older adults (Dykens *et al.*, 2004).

DNA methylation testing of blood is diagnostic in 99 per cent of cases of Prader-Willi syndrome, and it is justified in the presence of the following:

Birth to 2 years: hypotonia with poor suck in the neonatal period.

2 to 6 years: hypotonia with history of poor suck; global developmental delay.

6 to 12 years: history of hypotonia with poor suck; global developmental delay; excessive eating with central obesity if uncontrolled.

13 years to adulthood: cognitive deficit, usually of mild degree; excessive eating with central obesity if uncontrolled; hypothalamic hypogonadism and/or distinctive behaviour disorder.

Of note, regardless of measured IQ, most children with Prader-Willi syndrome have multiple severe learning disabilities and poor academic performance for their mental skills. However, they show unusual skill with jigsaw puzzles. Excessive eating is believed to be caused by a hypothalamic abnormality, resulting in lack of satiety and subsequent food-seeking behaviour. Obesity ensues from such behaviours and a low metabolic rate causing decreased total energy requirements.

Individuals with UPD have a somewhat higher IQ and milder behaviour problems, are less likely to have the typical facial appearance, hypopigmentation, or skill with jigsaw puzzles, but are more likely to suffer from psychosis and autism spectrum disorders (Cassidy & Schwartz, 2006).

Duplication 15q syndrome

Duplication on the maternal chromosome 15q11-q13 is found in one per cent of individuals with autism spectrum disorders (Schroer et al., 1998). The syndrome phenotype is characterized by a lack of dysmorphic features (Ludowese et al., 1991) or only rare minor anomalies, mild hypotonia, mild mental retardation, hyperactivity, and some degree of clumsiness (Gurrieri et al., 1999). Some dup(15) individuals show a peculiar language impairment with an associated language-based learning disability (Boyar et al., 2001). The dup(15q) can be inherited from a normal mother, and can be missed by routine chromosome study, requiring FISH analysis for diagnosis. The breakpoints on 15q11-q13 are identical or close to those found in PWS/AS deletions, and the precise genes have not yet been identified. The phenotypic expression is influenced by the parental origin of the duplication, and the paternally inherited cases may show only a borderline cognitive impairment. Seizures/epilepsy rarely occur.

Inv-dup (15) or Idic (15) syndrome

The inv dup(15) is the most common of the heterogeneous group of the extra structurally abnormal chromosomes (ESACs), and accounts for about 50 per cent of supernumerary marker chromosomes (Hook & Cross, 1987). Of the two identified cytogenetic types of inv dup(15) marker chromosomes, one is similar to a G group chromosome, not containing the PWS/AS critical region, and is found in children with a normal phenotype (Cheng et al., 1994). The second type of inv dup(15) is as large as or larger than a G group chromosome, contains the PWS/AS critical region (Robinson et al., 1993; Blennow et al., 1995), and is associated with an abnormal phenotype (Battaglia et al., 1997). Its cytogenetic description is dic(15)(q12 or q13). Most dic(15)(q12 or q13) cases derive from the two homologous maternal chromosomes at meiosis, and are associated with increased maternal age at conception. The presence of large inv dup(15) results in tetrasomy 15p and partial tetrasomy 15q. The incidence at birth is estimated to be 1 to 30,000, with a sex ratio of 1 (Schinzel & Niedrist, 2001). In order to detect the rearrangement, standard cytogenetics must be associated with FISH analysis, with probes both from proximal chromosome 15 and from the PWS/AS critical region (Luke et al., 1994; Webb et al., 1998). For detection of parent-of-origin, microsatellite analysis on parental DNA or methylation analysis on the proband DNA are also needed (Luke et al., 1994; Webb et al., 1998). The most consistent clinical findings are represented by moderate to profound developmental delay/mental retardation with absent or very poor expressive language, severe epilepsy, hypotonia, and autistic behaviour (Battaglia et al., 1997; Cabrera et al., 1998; Takeda et al., 2000; Borgatti et al., 2001; Battaglia, 2005). There may be either no dysmorphic features or only 'minor anomalies' such as epicanthus, downslanting of the palpebral fissures, low-set ears, and skin pigmentary changes. In the majority of individuals, epilepsy shows the characteristics of the Lennox-Gastaut or Lennox-Gastaut-like syndrome, with onset between the ages of 4 and 8 years and a poor outcome. West syndrome has been reported in a few patients (Battaglia et al., 1997; Cabrera et al., 1998; Takeda et al., 2000; Torrisi et al , 2001; Battaglia, 2005). Myoclonic and complex partial seizures have also been observed (Gillberg et al., 1991; Aguglia et al., 1999). A milder clinical presentation with adult-onset generalized epilepsy has occasionally been reported (Chifari et al., 2002). Various genetic mechanisms have been hypothesized to explain the clinical heterogeneity, beyond the size of chromosomal duplication, including dosage effect of genes located within the duplicated region and the imprinting mechanism (Bolton et al., 2001; Torrisi et al., 2001; Battaglia, 2005). Many inv dup (15) patients meet the clinical criteria for the diagnosis of autistic disorder by DSM-IV. They usually show gaze avoidance and shun body contact, stare at people as though looking through them, prefer being left alone lying on their back looking at their fingers and taking up bizarre postures, show no interest in their peers, and have a variety of stereotypies (Rineer *et al.*, 1998; Battaglia, 2005).

Conclusion

It is now clear that one or more genes within the PWS/AS critical region, showing imprinting, with selective activity of the maternally derived copy at least in the brain, have a deleterious effect on mental development, when an additional functional copy is present.

References

Aguglia, U., Le Piane, E., Gambardella, A., Messina, D., Russo, C., Sirchia, S.M., Porta, G. & Quattrone, A. (1999): Emotion-induced myoclonic absence-like seizures in a patient with inv-dup(15) syndrome: a clinical, EEG, and molecular genetic study. *Epilepsia* **40**, 1316–1319.

Andersen, W.H., Rasmussen, R.K. & Stromme, P. (2001): Levels of cognitive and linguistic development in Angelman syndrome: a study of 20 children. *Logoped. Phoniatr. Vocol.* **26**, 2–9.

Battaglia, A. (2005): The inv dup(15) or idic(15) syndrome: a clinically recognisable neurogenetic disorder. *Brain Dev.* **27**, 365–369.

Battaglia, A. & Gurrieri, F. (1999): Case of apparent Gurrieri syndrome showing molecular findings of Angelman syndrome. *Am. J. Med. Genet.* **82**, 100.

Battaglia, A. & Guerrini, R. (2005): Chromosomal disorders associated with epilepsy. *Epileptic Disord.* **7**, 181–192.

Battaglia, A., Gurrieri, F., Bertini, E., Bellacosa, A., Pomponi, M.G., Paravatou-Petsotas, M., Mazza, S. & Neri, G. (1997): The inv dup(15) syndrome: a clinically recognizable syndrome with altered behaviour, mental retardation and epilepsy. *Neurology* **48**, 1081–1086.

Blennow, E., Nielsen, K.B., Telenius, H., Carter, N.P., Kristoffersson, U., Holmberg, E., Gillberg, C. & Nordenskjold, M. (1995): Fifty probands with extra structurally abnormal chromosomes characterized by fluorescence in situ hybridization. *Am. J. Med. Genet.* **55**, 85–94.

Bolton, P.F., Dennis, N.R., Browne, C.E., Thomas, N.S., Veltman, M.W.M., Thompson, R.J. & Jacobs, P. (2001): The phenotypic manifestations of interstitial duplications of proximal 15q with special reference to the autistic spectrum disorders. *Am. J. Med. Genet. B Neuropsychiatr. Genet.* **105**, 675–685.

Borgatti, R., Piccinelli, P., Passoni, D., Dalprà, L., Miozzo, M., Micheli, R., Gagliardi, C. & Balottin, U. (2001): Relationship between clinical and genetic features in 'inverted duplicated chromosome 15' patients. *Pediatr. Neurol.* **24**, 111–116.

Boyar, F.Z., Whitney, M.M., Lossie, A.C., Gray, B.A., Keller, K.L., Stalker, H.J., Zori, R.T., Geffken, G., Mutch, J., Edge, P.J., Voeller, K.S., Williams, C.A. & Driscoll, D.J. (2001): A family with a grand-maternally derived interstitial duplication of proximal 15q. *Clin. Genet.* **60**, 421–430.

Boyd, S.G., Harden, A. & Patton, M.A. (1988): The EEG in early diagnosis of the Angelman (happy puppet) syndrome. *Eur. J. Pediatr.* **147**, 508–513.

Cabrera, J.C., Marti, M., Toledo, L., Gine, R. & Vazquez, C. (1998): West's syndrome associated with inversion duplication of chromosome 15. *Rev. Neurol. (Spain)* **26**, 77–79.

Cassidy, S.B. & McCandless, S.E. (2005): Prader-Willi syndrome. In: *Management of genetic syndromes*, 2nd ed., eds. S.B. Cassidy & J.E. Allanson, pp. 429–448. Hoboken, NJ: John Wiley & Sons.

Cassidy, S.B. & Schwartz, S. (2006): Prader-Willi syndrome. In: *Gene reviews at GeneTests: Medical Genetics Information Resource.* Seattle: University of Washington, Seattle. Available at http://www.genetests.org

Cheng, S.D., Spinner, N.B., Zackai, E.H. & Knoll, J.H. (1994): Cytogenetic and molecular characterization of inverted duplicated chromosomes 15 from 11 patients. *Am. J. Hum. Genet.* **55**, 753–759.

Chifari, R., Guerrini, R., Pierluigi, M., Cavani, S., Sgro, V., Elia, M., Canger, R. & Canevini, M.P. (2002): Mild generalized epilepsy and developmental disorder associated with large inv dup(15). *Epilepsia* **43**, 1096–1100.

Dykens, E.M., Sutcliffe, J.S. & Levitt, P. (2004): Autism and 15q11-q13 disorders: behavioral, genetic, and pathophysiological issues. *Ment. Retard. Dev. Disabil. Res. Rev.* **10**, 284–291.

Gillberg, C., Steffenburg, S., Wahlstrom, J., Gillberg, I.C., Sjostedt, A., Martinsson, T., Liedgren, S. & Olofsson, O. (1991): Autism associated with marker chromosome. *J. Am. Acad. Child. Adolesc. Psychiatry* **30**, 489–494.

Guerrini, R., De Lorey, T.M., Bonanni P., Moncla, A., Dravet, C., Suisse, G., Livet, M.O., Bureau, M., Malzac, P., Genton, P., Thomas, P., Sartucci, F., Simi, P. & Serratosa, J.M. (1996): Cortical myoclonus in Angelman syndrome. *Ann. Neurol.* **40**, 39–48.

Guerrini, R., Battaglia, A., Carrozzo, R., Gobbi, G., Parrini, E., Pramparo, T. & Zuffardi, O. (in press): Chromosomal abnormalities. In: *Epilepsy: a comprehensive textbook*, eds. J. Engel Jr. & T.A. Pedley, chapter 263. Philadelphia: Lippincott-Raven.

Gurrieri, F., Battaglia, A., Torrisi, L., Tancredi, R., Cavallaro, C., Sangiorgi, E. & Neri, G. (1999): Pervasive developmental disorder and epilepsy due to maternally derived duplication of 15q11-q13. *Neurology* **52**, 1694–1697.

Holm, V.A., Cassidy, S.B., Butler, M.G., Hanchett, J.M., Greenswag, L.R., Whitman, B.Y. & Greenberg, F. (1993): Prader-Willi syndrome: consensus diagnostic criteria. *Pediatrics* **91**, 398–402.

Hook, E.B. & Cross, K. (1987): Extra structurally abnormal chromosomes (ESAC) detected at amniocentesis: frequency in approximately 75,000 prenatal cytogenic diagnoses and associations with maternal and paternal age. *Am. J. Hum. Genet.* **54**, 748–756.

Laan, L.A. & Vein, A.A. (2005): Angelman syndrome: is there a characteristic EEG? *Brain Dev.* **27**, 80–87.

Ludowese, C.J., Thompson, K.J., Sekhon, G.S. & Pauli, R.M. (1991): Absence of predictable phenotypic expression in proximal 15q duplications *Clin. Genet.* **40**, 194–201.

Luke, S., Verma, R.S., Giricharan, R., Conte, R.A. & Macera, M.J. (1994): Two Prader-Willi/Angelman syndrome loci present in an isodicentric marker chromosome. *Am. J. Med. Genet.* **51**, 232–233.

Rineer, S., Finucane, B. & Simon, E.W. (1998): Autistic symptoms among children and young adults with isodicentric chromosome 15. *Am. J. Med. Genet. B Neuropsychiatr. Genet.* **81**, 428–438.

Robinson, W.P., Binkert, F., Gine, R., Vazquez, C., Muller, W., Rosenkranz, W. & Schinzel, A. (1993): Clinical and molecular analysis of five inv dup (15) patients. *Eur. J. Hum. Genet.* **1**, 37–50.

Rougelle, C., Glatt, H. & Lalande, M. (1997): The Angelman syndrome candidate gene, UBE3A/E6-AP, is imprinted in brain [letter]. *Nat. Genet.* **17**, 14–15.

Schinzel, A. & Niedrist, D. (2001): Chromosome imbalances associated with epilepsy. *Am. J. Med. Genet. (Semin. Med. Genet.)* **106**, 119–124.

Schroer, R.J., Phelan, M.C., Michaelis, R.C., Crawford, E., Skinner, S.A., Cuccaro, M., Simensen, R., Bishop, J., Skinner, C., Fender, D. & Stevenson, R.E. (1998): Autism and maternally derived aberrations of chromosome 15q. *Am. J. Med. Genet.* **76**, 327–336.

Steinhausen, H.C., Eiholzer, U., Hauffa, B.P. & Malin, Z. (2004): Behavioural and emotional disturbances in people with Prader-Willi Syndrome. *J. Intellect. Disabil. Res.* **48**, 47–52.

Takeda, Y., Baba, A., Nakamura, F., Ito, M., Honma, H. & Koyama, T. (2000): Symptomatic generalized epilepsy associated with an inverted duplication of chromosome 15. *Seizure* **9**, 145–150.

Thompson, R.J. & Bolton, P.F. (2003): Case report: Angelman syndrome in an individual with a small SMC(15) and paternal uniparental disomy: a case report with reference to the assessment of cognitive functioning and autistic symptomatology. *J. Autism Dev. Disord.* **33**, 171–176.

Torrisi, L., Sangiorgi, E., Russo, L. & Gurrieri, F. (2001): Rearrangements of chromosome 15 in epilepsy. *Am. J. Med. Genet. (Semin. Med. Genet.)* **106**, 125–128.

Webb, T., Hardy, C.A., King, M., Watkiss, E., Mitchell, C. & Cole, T. (1998): A clinical, cytogenetic and molecular study of ten probands with inv dup (15) marker chromosomes. *Clin. Genet.* **53**, 34–43.

Williams, C.A. (2005a): Angelman syndrome. In: *Management of genetic syndromes*, 2nd ed., eds. S.B. Cassidy & J.E. Allanson, pp. 53–62. Hoboken, NJ.: John Wiley & Sons.

Williams, C.A. (2005b): Neurological aspects of the Angelman syndrome. *Brain Dev.* **27**, 88–94.

Williams, C.A., Beaudet, A.L., Clayton-Smith, J., Knoll, J.H., Kyllermann, M., Laan, L.A., Magenis, R.E., Moncla, A., Schinzel, A.A., Summers J.A. & Wagstaff, J. (2006): Conference report. Angelman syndrome 2005: updated consensus for diagnostic criteria. *Am. J. Med. Genet.* **140A**, 413–418.

Chapter 11

The psychopathological structure of the child with mental retardation

Pietro Pfanner and Mara Marcheschi

Scientific Institute 'Stella Maris', viale del Tirreno 331, 56018 Calambrone, Pisa, Italy
Pietro.Pfanner@inpe.unipi.it

Summary

The clinical picture of mental retardation is the prime example of a defect that reveals itself principally at the highest levels of functioning – cognitive, critical, and socially adaptive. Mental retardation is always a very serious problem, even when defined as 'mild' by psychometrics. It prevents the achievement of the standards expected by the biological machine in its full complexity. These are conditioned by the interactive needs of the environment which have been determined by civilisation and culture over the long development of the human species.
A psychopathological and structural evaluation of mental retardation includes the following: definition of the severity of the global cognitive deficit and of the quality of thought, especially the presence or not (during adolescence) of logical concrete thought; characterization of the cognitive structure, strengths and weaknesses, strategies, blocks, heterochrony, and use of knowledge; assessment of the internal world (fantasies, fears and anxieties which the weak cognitive tools are unable to control) and level of development of self; and specification of interaction between the individual and the environment. Psychopathological disorders in mental retardation seem to have a peculiar specificity, both intrinsic to retardation and secondary to environmental factors, or frequently linked to a specific comorbidity.

The expression 'mental retardation' is a vague, ambiguous, and euphemistic way of naming a serious mental disorder that deserves to be better analysed from a psychopathological perspective.
It is the family that usually discovers their child's mental retardation, by observing the child's intrinsic inability to learn through play and by having evidence of a deficiency of integration, comprehension and adaptation. This difficulty reveals itself in the first years of life and is seen as a developmental slowing of psychological functions. During the school years it becomes clear that there is a serious and global learning difficulty, and by the beginning of adolescence this stabilizes as an established disability in developing formal and abstract thoughts – that is to say, building hypotheses, anticipating actions, and planning behaviours in an original way (Pfanner & Marcheschi, 2000).

'Not understanding' is often mistaken for 'not wanting to understand', because of indifference to the problem or unwillingness to accept it. The child's behaviour appears to be exceptional and differs greatly from that of his age group. This sets in motion the sequence of misunderstandings that determines the lack of acceptance of people with mental disorders: fear and hostility from adults, censure, stress, estrangement, and sometimes overprotection, which can also cause educational problems. Abilities and desires seem to be impoverished and distorted, while linguistic, perceptive and psychomotor retardation is highlighted. Playmates at school will soon confirm these judgements, often by cruel and offensive attitudes. Educators and teachers may also show discriminating behaviour, as may the other children's parents, who consider themselves luckier and more capable.

Mental retardation is a complex and global psychopathological syndrome, more 'categorical' than 'dimensional', linked to a severe deficiency of abstractive and adaptive functions. It reveals itself precociously during childhood and tends to remain fixed over the lifespan (especially if there is no proper supporting stimulation). As the appearance of human intelligence determines the development of the human species – that is, the *Homo sapiens* category – so the non-appearance of intelligence suggests a different biological category that is seriously pathological (Zazzo, 1979).

Mental retardation is not just an isolated defect of cognitive performance, revealed by psychometric tests and IQ, but a psychopathological syndrome in which the structure of the mind is dominated by a cognitive deficit, just as a neurotic persona is dominated by anxiety, or a psychopathic persona by impulsiveness. It should not be regarded as an accessory symptom related to other somatic or mental disorders, as it always constitutes the most important phenotypical aspect of the many syndromes with which it may be associated.

Exploring the psychopathology of mental retardation, which is modulated by age and social experience, needs an intuitive approach along with formal analytical observations. Evaluation of the core aspects of mental retardation appears to be influenced by psychiatric culture and experience. In fact, mental retardation is a diagnosis which belongs to clinical psychiatry rather than to other medical or psychological disciplines, although these may be complementary – for example, psychology, neurology and paediatrics.

We consider mental retardation to be the most important example of a type of psychopathology involving associated and reactive defects. It is wrong – though this is still seen in some textbooks – to place the pathology of mental retardation among malformational or cerebral lesion syndromes and to confuse its main symptom (the pathology of the mind) with the secondary symptoms (associated with metabolic or neurological diseases). In fact, quite a frequent mistake in medicine is to confuse the symptomatology (the best known aspect) with the pathogenesis (the least known or unknown). In descriptions of multi-symptomatic and multi-dimensional syndromes it is common to consider mental retardation as a complementary or accessory symptom having only social importance (Marcheschi & Cipriani, 1993; Masi *et al.*, 1999).

Another frequent mistake in psychiatry is to confuse mental retardation symptoms with other psychological diseases (depression, anxiety, excitement, hyperactivity, pervasivity, and so on). In the individual with mental retardation these symptoms, although having a specific phenomenology, may have very different origins and mechanisms (see below). The *Diagnostic and Statistical Manual of Mental Disorders* (DSM-IV) has given important help to clinicians to avoid this mistake. It suggests classifying mental retardation on a different basis from psychopathological symptoms (American Psychiatric Association, 1996). To clarify this concept, let us underline two terminological objections:

(1) Though the term 'mental retardation' remains, despite many subsequent definitions, the one most commonly used, it is incorrect as it appears to refer to a temporary slowdown in

mental development as if this were just a matter of timing. Currently, however, the more correct Anglo-Saxon definition 'intellectual disability' is making headway. This term substitutes the concept of 'disability' for the more pejorative 'handicap', a term which has been used with different and discriminating connotations now made illegal in many countries (we hope that the arguable expression of 'differently able' will not survive) (Luckasson et al., 1992).

(2) A contradiction in terms occurs when we consider mental retardation to be among the most pathological human conditions but then allow the description 'mild' (as suggested by the psychometric classifications, which are dictated by statistical criteria) for those kinds of mental retardation with an IQ test score between 50 and 70. Intellectual disability of this degree limits abstractive functioning, which is the absolute privilege of our species. We must avoid the use of this confusing expression in our clinical reports (Pfanner & Marcheschi, 2003; Pfanner & Marcheschi, 2005).

The most important phenotypical aspect of mental retardation remains the impossibility of developing abstract thought, the highest human function, which is conditioned by a long phylogeny and prepared in the individual ontogenesis. It is the severest pathological human state (though unfortunately very frequent), upon which modern medicine should polarize its attention for prophylaxis and cure. Many other psychopathological, cognitive, and affective symptoms of varying typology are associated with the primary symptom of mental retardation and can modify the subject's self-consciousness and adaptive skills.

Published scientific reports (in particular the DSMs) have now defined the psychosocial disorders of mentally retarded individuals as essential symptoms, in addition to the above-mentioned cognitive symptoms – that is, disorders of adaptive skills which play a leading role in the origins of the psychopathology of mental retardation (Dosen, 2005). An impairment of adaptation to their own culture by affected individuals is an essential aspect of clinical diagnosis, separate from the pathogenesis. The main causes of maladjustment can be cognitive, affective, or environmental (Cannao, 2003).

Adaptive behaviour is a set of conceptual, social, and practical skills which people have learned in order to function normally in their daily lives. Limitations of this behaviour that are typical of mental retardation influence everyday living in all its aspects, including the ability to adapt to the environmental demands (AAMR, 2002). These limitations to adaptive behaviour should be assessed by standardized measurements and validated on the general population.

Mental retardation is multiform, but there are many reasons to justify the view that it is a unitary system:

- It can be associated with other disorders, yet represents the most important symptom.
- It affects the moulding factors of a developing personality.
- It has early onset with progressive slowing of intellectual development and generally tends to stabilize.
- It prevents the achievement of the goals typical of normal development – logical abstract thought linked to intelligence, self-consciousness to personality, and adaptive skills to autonomy.
- It shows particular qualitative defects in the progression and transformation of intellectual abilities which distinguish normal development: 'genetic viscosity' (Inhelder, 1963); 'intellectual inertia' (Luria, 1963), and 'mental stiffness' (Lewin, 1936).

Thus mental retardation not only has a varied clinical expression but also a core symptomatology (nucleus) which is common to many forms. Moreover, we should recall that it also shows structural evolution in its behavioural and affective aspects. For some French investigators (Lang, 1973; Misès *et al.*, 1994; Gibello, 1995), mental retardation is a prolonged evolutionary and psychodynamic process throughout which the deficient structure organizes and progressively remodels itself. In addition, the compromised intelligence coexists with other positive and negative aspects of intellectual functioning, with different modes of mutual investment from the environmental side to the child side, and *vice versa* from the child to the environment.

Let us consider metal retardation symptoms. We can distinguish different kinds of manifestations, which can be classified as:

- intrinsic symptoms, linked to the pathology of intellectual functioning and its correlated affective function (therefore 'nuclear');
- extrinsic symptoms, linked to the pathology of non-nuclear functioning that can originate from both the specific co-morbid condition and the environment.

Principally, the intrinsic symptoms are caused by weakness of the entire cognitive process – abstraction, generalization of experience, psycholinguistics and perceptive-motor synthesis, attention and memory (involved in different ways), reversibility of thought, classification and assessment processes, cognitive control of behaviour, construction of self, and identity dispersion, but also ideo-affective synthesis, originality, and autonomy. Deficiency and distortion of these various functions determine the nuclear outline, 'the core' of mental retardation, with a varied pathogenesis (genetic, neurological, and environmental).

In addition, when the development of the components matures over different time periods (heterochronia), the biological and social 'appointments' are difficult or impossible to achieve – for example, gene expressivity, brain development processes, and relations with a pre-organized environment which offer stimuli (incentives and frustrations) typical of any chronological age. This leads to loss of parallelism and of the synergies expected among the various genetic, cultural, and environmental factors (all of which are necessary for cognitive development). It also leads to the introduction of substitution – unpredictable and inappropriate reactions – which are major factors generating commotion and chaos. Examples are cognitive interests without operative abilities; adaptation to social rules without the ability to generalise and without abstract thought; reactive, depressive or self-injurious behaviour caused by defective self-esteem and therefore without any repairing ability; and so on. It seems that the whole personality is subverted and tries reparation, substitutions, and compensation – that is, an alternative organisation.

There are also the extrinsic symptoms, which are neither strictly cognitive nor correlated with cognition. These symptoms can be associated with mood expression, intensity of emotions, basic abilities of coping, and with 'resilience' towards social attitudes (introversion and extroversion), anxiety levels, and so on. They have their roots in temperament but are modulated by the environment and therefore by the family and school.

The scarcity or abundance of received stimuli (for example, stress from the environment, failure in competition and thus loss of self-esteem, disharmony at home or at school, and developmental crises) can be conditioning factors for environmental modulation. They comprise a set of risk factors that can affect psychological development in its affective and relational aspects. In an individual with mental retardation many life experiences are regarded as failures (Moravia, 1984). This often leads these individuals to build up a mental representation of reality that is dominated by a constant expectation of failure. This pervades every action, and profoundly affects both intrinsic and extrinsic psychodynamic processes with respect to cognitive functioning – for example, instinctual inhibition, negative social interaction, depression, and so on.

The French investigators mentioned above, along with others, have emphasized some aspects of mental retardation that need to be considered. These include the following:

- An early disorder of the so-called epistemophilic drive (knowledge instinct).

- The particular relation between the 'primary process' (of fantasies and emotions) and the 'secondary process' (of thought), with infiltration of the secondary processes into the primary ones (Lang, 1973). The result of this is a lack of differentiation between reality and imagery, with an intrusion of fantasies into the thought processes. Even interactions with people (relatives, educators) are primitive and often involve tyrannical affections.

- Disorders of meaning that are related to symbol construction, leading to an inability to give meaning to different behaviours.

- The weakness of cognitive tools – the difficulties in controlling fear lead to anxiety and ideas of persecution.

Other affective aspects often found in children with mental retardation are depression, apathy, asthenia, fatiguability, inhibition, impairment of self-esteem, and excessive requests for attention and support. These modes of functioning may imply rejection or withdrawal in the face of situations considered dangerous, which might generate overwhelming experiences. The child with mental retardation defends himself against these experiences, reducing the range of stimuli and their significance, and thus impoverishing his experience (Misés et al., 1994). As a result the child will resort to reassuring behaviours, impulsive actions, and 'magic' thought.

In the relationships with others, the child with mental retardation may perceive a threat to his integrity and security. The mother can perpetuate a symbiotic relationship or enforce separation anxiety (Mannoni, 1964).

Extrinsic symptoms can have a different origin and may be linked to a specific comorbidity, responsible for various relationship disorders but also for anxiety and mood swings or personality and behavioural disorders. It is well known that the incidence of psychopathological disorders is four or five times greater than in individuals without mental retardation, but the pathogenesis of this association has not been clarified up to now and needs further specific research. On the other hand we know that 25 per cent of people with mental retardation present with important psychiatric problems (Dykens et al., 2002; Volkmar & Dykens, 2002; Emerson, 2003).

To conclude this complex subject we propose that affective disorders in mental retardation can be divided into three categories:

(1) Those that are intrinsic to mental retardation (even though they may differ in the various well known mental deficiency syndromes), and which are studied by dynamic psychiatry.

(2) Those occurring as a comorbidity disorder, with a predominant genetic component and not related to the mental retardation.

(3) Those that are reactive to the environment.

The individual with mental retardation can suffer, for example, from pathological anxiety for different reasons: to defend himself from his cognitive chaos, or because of an inherited anxiety, or to protect himself from environmental abuse.

A particular terminological question deals with the so-called dual diagnosis. The Anglo-Saxon literature has emphasized the distinction between intellectual and extra-intellectual disability, proposing the term and concept of 'dual diagnosis'. This term can be confusing because its pathogenesis – the relation between the classes of symptoms – remains obscure, and it is unclear whether the extra-intellectual disability (affective disorder) is really autonomous or is a consequence of the intellectual disability. It should be recalled that judgements about psychopathological comorbidity are based on the recognizable autonomy of two kinds of disability and exclude a causative relation between them. We should also remember that genetic advances have revealed interesting correlations between genotype and mental retardation (Pfanner et al., 1993; Battaglia & Carey, 2003). They have also shown significant relations between genetic anomalies and the type of retardation, especially those related to linguistic, perceptive-spatial, practical, and behavioural functioning, and other aspects of cognitive function (Moldavsky et al., 2001). Research into the so-called 'behavioural phenotypes' has developed in this way. For example, fragile-X syndrome, Prader-Willi syndrome (Dykens & Shah, 2003) and Down syndrome seem associated with specific manifestations of behaviour (Bargagna et al., 2000). Individuals affected by fragile-X syndrome have a severe deficit of attention with hyperactivity. Prader-Willi syndrome is almost always associated with compulsive feeding behaviour, hyperphagia (and consequently obesity), and rebellious behaviour. In Down syndrome, language is a relatively weak area, whereas social abilities and interpersonal behaviours are better preserved. In Williams syndrome, spatial abilities are compromised whereas language is well developed and nuclei of anxiety and specific phobias are present (Giannotti & Vicari, 1994).

Conclusions

In conclusion, a psychopathological and structural evaluation of mental retardation includes the following:

• A definition of the severity of the global cognitive deficit and of the quality of thought, especially the presence or absence (during adolescence) of logical concrete thought (using Piaget's terminology) – an essential condition for social interaction (without abstract thought, social life may be nearly normal in an undemanding environment, but such a life is characterized by dependency).

• The characterisation of cognitive structure, strengths and weaknesses, strategies, blocks, heterochrony, and the use of knowledge (Cornoldi, 1995).

• Assessment of the internal world: the fantasies, fears, and anxieties that weak cognitive tools cannot control; and assessment of the level of development of self.

• Specification of the interactive modes between the individual and the environment, in particular between the child and the family, relating to tasks at different phases of development and to mutual interactions.

Psychopathological disorders in mental retardation – both intrinsic to retardation and secondary to environmental factors or linked to a specific comorbidity – seem to have a particular specificity. The disorders occur because of a loss of organization of the ego which determines a specific way of assimilating emotions and stress, and an equally specific integration of emotions, mood, and anxiety. All of this has been underestimated in both the diagnostic and the therapeutic phases, and for this reason a major effort to achieve methodological adaptation and integration is necessary (Soresi, 2003).

Our hope is to develop on a methodological basis the rehabilitative treatment of people with mental retardation, starting from the more complex psycho-educative aspects. We expect to achieve a better understanding of the psychopathological disorders associated with mental retardation, so that we can elaborate increasingly specific techniques of treatment.

References

AAMR (2002): *Mental retardation*, 10th ed. Washington DC: American Association on Mental Retardation.

American Psychiatric Association (1996): *Diagnostic and statistical manual of mental disorders*, 4th ed. (DSM-IV). Washington DC: American Psychiatric Association.

Bargagna, S. (2000): *La sindrome di Down*. Tirrenia: Del Cerro.

Battaglia, A. & Carey, J.C. (2003): Diagnostic evaluation of developmental delay/mental retardation. *Am. J. Med. Genet.* **117C**, 3–14.

Cannao, M. (2003): Disabilità e integrazione nel pensiero di Giorgio Moretti. *Saggi* **4**, 7–92.

Cornoldi, C. (1995): *Metacognizione ed apprendimento*. Bologna: Il Mulino.

Dosen, A. (2005): Applying the developmental perspective in the psychiatric assessment and diagnosis of persons with intellectual disability: part I – assessment. *J. Intellect. Disabil. Res.* **49**, 1–8.

Dykens, E.M. & Shah, B. (2003): Psychiatric disorders in Prader-Willi syndrome: epidemiology and management. *CNS Drugs* **17**, 167–178.

Dykens, E.M., Shah, B., Sagun, J., Beck, T. & King, B.H. (2002): Maladaptive behaviour in children and adolescents with Down's syndrome. *J. Intellect. Disabil. Res.* **46**, 484–492.

Emerson, E. (2003): Prevalence of psychiatric disorders in children and adolescents with and without intellectual disability. *J. Intellect. Disabil. Res.* **47**, 51–58.

Giannotti, A. & Vicari, S. (1994): *Il bambino con sindrome di Williams*. Milan: FrancoAngeli.

Gibello, B. (1995): *La pensée décontenancée: essai sur la pensée et ses perturbations*. Paris: Bayard.

Inhelder, B. (1963): *Le diagnostic du raisonnement chez les débiles mentaux*. Paris: Delachaux et Niestlé.

Lang, J.L. (1973): Esquisse d une abord structural des états déficitaires. *Confront. Psychiatr.* **10**, 30–52.

Lewin, K. (1936): *Dynamic theory of personality*. New York: McGraw-Hill.

Luckasson, R., Coulter, D., Followay, E., Reiss, S., Schalock, R., Snell, M., Spitalnik & Stark, J. (1992): *Mental retardation: definition, classification and systems of support*, 9th ed. Washington DC: American Association on Mental Retardation.

Luria, A.R. (1963): *The mentally retarded child*. Oxford: Pergamon Press.

Mannoni, M. (1964): *L'enfant arriéré et sa mère*. Paris: Le Seuil.

Marcheschi, M. & Cipriani, P. (1993): Il ritardo mentale. In: *Diagnosi differenziale in pediatria*, vol. 3, Torino: C.G Edizioni Medico Scientifiche.

Masi, G., Marcheschi, M. & Pfanner, P. (1999): Ritardo mentale. In: *Trattato Italiano di psichiatria*, eds. G.B. Cassano & P. Pancheri. Milan: Masson

Misés, R., Perron, R. & Salbreux, R. (1994): *Retards et troubles de l'intelligence de l'enfant*. Paris: ESF.

Moldavsky, M., Lev, D. & Lerman-Sagie, T. (2001): Behavioural phenotypes of genetic syndromes: a reference guide for psychiatrists. *J. Am. Acad. Child Adolesc. Psychiatry* **40**, 749–761.

Moravia, S. (1984): *L'enigma della mente. Il 'mind-body problem' nel pensiero contemporaneo*. Bari: Laterza.

Pfanner, P. & Marcheschi, M. (2000): I segni precoci del ritardo mentale. *Sistema Nervoso e Riabilitazione* **2**, 15–21.

Pfanner, P. & Marcheschi, M. (2003): Una difficile diagnosi psichiatrica. *Giorn. Neuropsic. Età Evol.* **23**, 271–286.

Pfanner, P. & Marcheschi, M. (2005): *Il ritardo mentale*. Bologna: Il Mulino.

Pfanner, P., Marcheschi, M., Battaglia, A. & Tosi, B. (1993): Aspetti psicologici del bambino plurimalformato e della sua famiglia. *Riv. Ital. Pediatr.* **19**, 349–354.

Soresi, S. (2003): *Disabilità, trattamento, integrazione*. Pordenone: ERIP.

Volkmar, F. & Dykens, E.M. (2002): Mental retardation. In: *Child and adolescent psychiatry: modern approaches*, 4th ed., eds. M. Rutter & E. Taylor, pp. 697–710. Oxford: Blackwell Scientific Publications.

Zazzo, R. (1979): *Les débilités mentales*. Paris: Armand Colin.

Chapter 12

Psychiatric comorbidity in intellectual disability (mental retardation)

Carlo Cianchetti, Marta Meloni and Giorgio Gaspa

Clinic of Child and Adolescent Neuropsychiatry, University of Cagliari, via Ospedale 119, 09124 Cagliari, Italy
cianchet@unica.it

Summary

Intellectual disability, or mental retardation, is caused by a deficiency in the functional ability of the brain cortex. In most cases this deficiency probably involves large areas if not the whole of the cortex, but with various degrees of deficit or potentiality in different areas or functions. This is presumed to be the cause of the differences in intelligence characteristics found in the several pathological conditions producing intellectual disability (for example, the varying cognitive phenotypes in fragile-X syndrome, Williams syndrome, and so on).

An intellectual disability, even when caused by pathologies not implying neurological or neuropsychological dysfunctions, predisposes to a psychiatric comorbidity. Two main mechanisms probably underlie this. The first is psychological-relational: subjects with intellectual disability find it hard to activate adequate coping mechanisms when facing daily stress, a condition in which their reduced critical ability and emotional control probably plays a role. The second is genetic and structural: it is known that there is an increase in psychic disorders in intellectual disability, linked to specific genetic anomalies. Moreover, a higher incidence of specific psychiatric disorders is present in some forms of genetic intellectual disability – for example, attention deficit hyperactivity disorder and pervasive developmental disorders in fragile-X syndrome. It is probable that the altered genes become decisive if inserted in a particular genetic constellation, with modification of functions causing greater sensitivity to environmental pathogenic factors. This chapter also reports published data on the incidence of different psychiatric disorders in specific chromosomal and single-gene disorders.

Introduction

People suffering from mental retardation are subject to psychiatric disorders. This chapter deals with the various psychiatric disorders that may arise in mentally retarded subjects and the mechanisms causing them.

As regards terminology, we now tend to substitute 'intellectual disability' for 'mental retardation.' Aside from the inaccuracy of the term 'retardation,' which suggests a condition that can be overcome with the passing of time, the term 'disability' is more in keeping with the way we currently evaluate incurable disorders on the basis of their functional consequences. We will therefore use the new terminology in this chapter.

Another problem is that some people use the term 'dual diagnosis,' which was introduced by English-speaking investigators to indicate the presence of psychiatric pathology associated with a substance-abuse disorder. The term is now commonly used to indicate such an association. We therefore prefer to use the term 'comorbidity' for all other conditions, as we do in this chapter.

Epidemiology

A study by Rutter *et al.* (1976) on the Isle of Wight on the prevalence of psychiatric disorders found a 30 to 42 per cent frequency of psychiatric pathologies in children and adolescents with intellectual disability, compared with only seven per cent in those without such disability. Recent studies have identified significant levels of psychopathology in children with intellectual disability: in 40 per cent of a population-based sample of 454 Australian children (Einfeld & Tonge, 1996a; 1996b); in 38 per cent of a sample of 143 children with severe impairment in Lothian, Scotland (Hoare *et al.*, 1998); in 50 per cent of a sample of 123 children attending schools for children with severe intellectual disability in Southampton and the New Forest area of England (Cormack *et al.*, 2000); and in 31 per cent of a sample of children attending special schools in Cape Town, South Africa (Molteno *et al.*, 2001).

The most recent study by Dekker *et al.* (2002) assessed the prevalence, comorbidity, and impact of DSM-IV disorders in 474 children with intellectual disability selected from Dutch schools for the intellectually disabled. In all, 21.9 per cent of the children met the DSM-IV symptom criteria for anxiety disorder, 4.4 per cent for mood disorder, and 25.1 per cent for disruptive disorder. More than half the children meeting the criteria for a DSM-IV disorder were severely impaired in everyday functioning, and about 37 per cent had a comorbid disorder.

Mechanisms and causes

On the basis of the above epidemiological data, it is evident that intellectual disability, even if caused by pathologies not involving other neurological and neuropsychological dysfunctions, predisposes to comorbidity of a psychological nature. The reasons for this predisposition, and therefore for the not uncommon association with psychiatric disturbances, are probably attributable to two types of mechanism: genetic-structural and psychological-relational.

Genetic and structural causes

There is an increase of psychiatric disorders in conditions causing intellectual disability linked to specific genetic anomalies. It is hypothesized that genes linked to psychiatric disorders are involved in these pathologies or at least in functions favouring the appearance of psychiatric disorders. It is probable that these genes become decisive if inserted in a particular genetic constellation; this leads to a modification of function causing greater sensitivity to environmental pathogenic factors.

Intellectual disability is caused by a deficiency in the functional ability of the cerebral cortex. This deficiency – at least in most cases – probably involves large areas if not the whole of the neocortex, but with various degrees of deficit or potentiality in different areas or functions. This must be presumed to be the cause of the differences in the intelligence characteristics of several conditions causing intellectual disability (for example, the varying cognitive phenotypes in Down syndrome, fragile-X syndrome, Williams syndrome, and so on).

There are also predispositions to specific psychiatric pathologies typically more frequent in some forms of intellectual disability: for example, the greater frequency of conditions such as attention deficit hyperactivity disorder (ADHD) and pervasive developmental disorder (PDD) in subjects with fragile-X syndrome. In these cases, it is justified to maintain that the genetic anomaly itself predisposes to the psychiatric pathology which, however, only emerges in patients in whom there is a particular genotypic combination or epigenetic situation.

Psychological-relational causes

Subjects with reduced intellectual capabilities are less able to organize and control their emotions. This creates unfavourable conditions with regard to the environment, starting from the first dual relationship (mother-child), but probably above all in the subsequent broader social interrelationships. These subjects find it difficult to activate adequate coping mechanisms when facing daily stress, a condition in which reduced critical ability and emotional control probably play a role. The end result is an objectively greater difficulty in facing relationships, caused by the discomfort and insecurity the subject feels with other people as a result of his cognitive problems.

Evaluation tools

The use of proper evaluation tools helps in detecting and characterizing psychiatric disturbances in subjects with intellectual disability. In fact, as Reiss et al. (1992) pointed out, a clinician is more prone to diagnose a psychic disorder in a subject without intellectual disability than in one with intellectual disability with the same clinical symptoms. This is probably related to the difficulty in expressing these mainly subjective symptoms by persons with intellectual disability, the degree of difficulty being directly in proportion to the severity of the intellectual deficit.

In people with intellectual disability it is advisable to use evaluation tools such as the semi-structured psychiatric scales of the Child Behavior Checklist (CBCL; Achenbach, 1991). The youth self-report form of the CBCL is applicable in adolescents with an IQ > 48 (Douma et al., 2006). When some type of autistic disorder is suspected, the Pervasive Developmental Disorder in Mentally Retarded Persons (PDD-MRS) test can be applied. The PDD-MRS assesses social interaction (with adults and peers), language and speech (stereotypes, echolalia, incorrect use of pronouns, neologisms, and modulation), and other behaviour (outstanding and obsessive interests, stereotypes, unusual handling of objects, stereotyped manipulation of own body, strong dependence on fixed patterns, routines or rituals, self-injurious behaviour, highly erratic/unpredictable behaviour, unusual, unreasonable and excessive anxiety or panic) (Kraijer & de Bildt, 2005).

Individual pathologies and their frequency

In patients with intellectual disability there is a greater frequency of behavioural disorders and disruptive behaviour. In cases of severe disability, greater comorbidity with pervasive developmental disorders is evident. On the other hand, individuals with extremely serious disability are less likely to develop psychiatric symptoms, as they lack sufficient awareness of their own condition. This may protect them from excessive mental discomfort.

There are no specific habits or personality traits in subjects with intellectual disability; however, they generally display an excess of negative self-image, low self-esteem, low tolerance of frustration, interpersonal dependence, and rigidity in problem solving.

Table 1 shows the frequency of the principal psychiatric disorders in patients with and without intellectual disability.

Let us now examine the psychiatric disorders that may appear in intellectual disability, and their distinguishing characteristics.

Table 1. Frequency of the principal psychiatric disorders in patients with and without intellectual disability (ID); modified by Emerson (2003)

Psychiatric disorder	Prevalence in ID	Prevalence in non-ID	Odds ratio
Any diagnosed disorder	39%	8.1%	7.3
Any anxiety disorder	8.7%	3.6%	2.5
Depression	1.5%	0.9%	1.7
Oppositional defiant disorder	13.3%	2.3%	6.5
Unsocialized conduct disorder	3.4%	0.3%	10.4
Hyperkinesis	8.7%	0.9%	10.0
Pervasive developmental disorder	7.6%	0.1%	74.7
Two diagnosed disorders	16%	2%	14.0

Mood disorders

Mood disorders are not uncommon in people with intellectual disability. Depressive disorders may be reactive (adaptive disorder) because of awareness of their own problems in social interaction, usually in less severe cases. There is generally a profile of low self-esteem and a sense of inability or inadequacy.

Recognizing depressive illness in those with severe or profound mental retardation is difficult because of their inability to express their emotional state. It is therefore necessary to consider mimicry, crying, social isolation, lack of interest, apathy, behavioural regression, and ultimately the presence of self-harm and aggressive behaviour towards others.

We should also recall that depressive disorders may be induced by treatment with neuroleptic drugs.

Bipolar disorders are rare during development (one to five per cent) and are often characterized by rapid cycling and mixed states.

Anxiety disorders

People with intellectual disability have a greater percentage of anxiety disorders than those without such disability – 8.7 per cent *vs.* 3.6 per cent according to Emerson (2003). However, they often find it difficult to express and interpret their anxieties. Therefore, anxiety crises or panic attacks may appear as episodes of sudden anger or flight.

People with intellectual disability may have phobias, which are often peculiar and changeable. They commonly exhibit compulsions and rituals. In subjects with non-verbal intellectual disability, repetitive or self-injurious behaviour suggests this diagnosis, as it is a way of controlling anxiety. On the other hand, obsessions are rare or inadequately expressed.

Post-traumatic stress disorder is frequent in intellectual disability, according to the AACAP Practice Parameters (Szymanski & King, 1999), as there is a greater risk of exposure and greater vulnerability to abuse and neglect, owing to difficulties in reporting such problems and a tendency to want to please others (Costello et al., 1996; Verhulst & van der Ende, 1997). However, according to Newman et al. (2000), there is no evidence of a higher prevalence or incidence of trauma exposure and post-traumatic stress disorder (PTSD) among people with developmental disabilities.

Eating disorders

Some patients with severe or profound intellectual disability show rumination, regurgitation, pica, and food faddiness or refusal. A younger age and male sex seem to be risk factors for pica and rumination/regurgitation (Danford & Huber, 1982; McAlpine & Singh, 1986). Pica is the most common eating disorder seen in individuals with intellectual disability, although often unrecognized and underreported. Pica severity increases as intellectual disability becomes more serious (McAdam et al., 2004).

Behaviour disorders

A three- to fourfold increased risk was found in intellectual disability for general problem behaviour, with about 50 per cent scoring in the deviant range on the Total Problem Score Scale, compared with about 18 per cent of children without intellectual disability (Dekker et al., 2002).

Also increased in intellectual disability are conduct disorders (25 vs. 4.2 per cent), oppositional defiant disorder (13.3 vs. 2.3 per cent), unsocialized conduct disorders (3.4 vs. 0.3 per cent), socialized conduct disorders (3.8 vs. 0.3 per cent), and other conduct disorders (4.9 vs. 1.6 per cent) (Emerson, 2003).

Self-aggressive behaviour is present in 10–15 per cent of patients with intellectual disability, the percentage increasing with the severity of the disability.

Attention deficit hyperactivity disorder

Fox & Wade (1998) investigated the prevalence of ADHD in a sample of adults with profound intellectual disability drawn from a residential facility and found it to be at least 15 per cent – significantly higher than estimates reported for the general population.

Pervasive development disorder

There is a close relation between intellectual disability and PDD: 40 per cent of people with intellectual disability also present PDD; on the other hand, nearly 70 per cent of those with PDD also have intellectual disability (La Malfa et al., 2004). The prevalence of autism in the general population is 0.1–0.15 per cent according to DSM-IV.

We must bear in mind that in published reports autism is sometimes diagnosed in intellectual disability (essentially in the more severe cases) only on the basis of secondary non-specific elements, particularly those in the third group of diagnostic criteria on DSM-IV (behaviour, interests and activities that are limited, repetitive and stereotyped).

Schizophrenia

The incidence of schizophrenia in subjects with intellectual disability is greater than in the general population (~1 *vs.* ~3 per cent). It is characterized by more negative symptoms with mixed clinical features often present, especially those of a disorganized or catatonic nature.

Psychiatric disorders in definite genetic anomalies

As stated above, some genetic anomalies causing intellectual disability are associated with an increased frequency of specific psychiatric disorders. This is important not only for the clinician, who has to keep in mind the increased risk of these pathologies, but also for the researcher, as they could be of value in singling out the genes involved in psychiatric disorders.

We will now consider some of the most frequent genetically determined intellectual disability syndromes, subdividing them into 'chromosomal disorders' and 'single-gene disorders'.

Chromosomal disorders

Down syndrome

Ninety-five per cent of cases of Down syndrome are caused by trisomy 21. In the other five per cent, one copy is translocated to another acrocentric chromosome, most often chromosome 14 or 21. In 2–4 per cent of cases with free trisomy 21, there is recognizable mosaicism for a trisomic and a normal cell line. In Europe, the average prevalence is 18.9 per 10,000 births.

Down syndrome patients have traditionally been described as friendly, affectionate and extroverted (Gibbs & Thorpe, 1983). Adults with Down syndrome show a lower prevalence of maladaptive behaviour compared with those with intellectual disability of other cause (Collacot *et al.*, 1998). However, there is evidence that not all individuals with Down syndrome possess these personality traits. Kent *et al.* (1999) describe the comorbid occurrence of autism and Down syndrome in at least seven per cent of cases (4/58 patients) and the comorbid occurrence of obsessive compulsive disorder (OCD) and Down syndrome in 19 per cent (11/58).

Angelman syndrome

Angelman syndrome results from an abnormality at site q11-13 on chromosome 15. Its prevalence is 1/12,000 to 1/20,000 births.

Language impairment is severe, with receptive language skills always more advanced than expressive skills. Most older children and adults with Angelman syndrome are able to communicate by pointing, gestures, and using communication boards.

Behaviourally, affected individuals are characterized by a generally happy disposition, impulsivity, and hyperactivity (Gillberg, 1995; Summers *et al.*, 1995; Steffenburg *et al.*, 1996; Andersen *et al.*, 2001; Lossie *et al.*, 2001).

All children with Angelman syndrome show some hyperactivity, equally present in boys and girls. Infants and toddlers may have seemingly ceaseless activity, constantly keeping their hands or toys in their mouth, moving from object to object. Most have a short attention span (Clayton-Smith *et al.*, 1993). A decreased need for sleep and abnormal sleep/wake cycles are also characteristic of Angelman syndrome (Summers *et al.*, 1992).

Comorbidity between Angelman syndrome and autism has been found in many studies. Trillingsgaard & Østergaard (2004) studied 16 children with Angelman syndrome with the Autism Diagnostic Observation Schedule-Generic (ADOS-G): 10 were found to be autistic and three more were in the autism spectrum. In a review of 12 studies by Veltman *et al.* (2005), a 1.9 per cent rate of autism spectrum disorders (2/104) was found in Angelman syndrome.

Prader-Willi syndrome

Prader-Willi syndrome is a disorder caused by a paternally-derived deletion at chromosome 15 (q11-q13) in about 70 per cent of cases, and by maternal uniparental disomy in most of the remainder. The incidence is approximately 1 in 20,000 births.

Individuals with Prader-Willi syndrome are prone to severe behaviour problems, as many as 85 per cent showing clinically raised scores on standardized behavioural checklists. In 100 patients aged 4 to 46 years studied with CBCL, Dykens & Cassidy (1999) found the following types of salient maladaptive behaviour: skin picking, temper tantrums, impulsivity, stubbornness, arguing with others, disobedience, stealing food or money to buy food, compulsions, withdrawal and anxiety.

Dykens *et al.* (1996) found high rates of specific symptoms on the Yale-Brown Obsessive Compulsive Scale in 91 children and adults with Prader-Willi syndrome, suggesting high rates of obsessive-compulsive disorder.

Twelve studies on autism spectrum disorders (ASD) in Prader-Willi syndrome were reviewed by Veltman *et al.* (2005); the ASD rate was 25.3 per cent (38/150).

Beardsmore *et al.* (1998) found that 17.4 per cent of 25 young adults with Prader-Willi syndrome met formal criteria for affective disorders, all with psychotic components.

Chromosome 15q11-q13 duplication (dup15q11-q13)

Dup15q11-q13 is located in the Angelman-Prader-Willi region. The clinical phenotype usually includes severe intellectual disability, seizures, hypotonia, language disorders, and autism (Kwasnicka-Crawford *et al.*, 2006; Jacquemont *et al.*, 2006). Most of the reported cases with autism had duplications inherited from the mother (Cook *et al.*, 1997).

Inversion-duplication of chromosome 15 (inv-dup15)

Inv-dup15 is a rare disorder in which the most evident findings are dysmorphic features with frontal bossing, genital abnormalities, seizures, intellectual disability and autistic behaviour (Schroer *et al.*, 1998).

Williams syndrome

Williams syndrome is caused by a chromosomal microdeletion in the 7q11.23 region. The incidence is 1/10,000 to 1/20,000 births. It is characterized by intellectual disability, short stature, an 'elfin' face, stellate pattern of the iris, dental abnormalities, hoarse voice, and cardiovascular anomalies, mainly supravalvar aortic stenosis.

Anxiety, hyperactivity, and hypersociability are frequent. In the study by Leyfer *et al.* (2006), 80.7 per cent of children with Williams syndrome (96/119) met criteria for at least one DSM-IV diagnosis: ADHD in 64.7 per cent, specific phobias in 53.3 per cent, OCD in 2.5 per cent, and oppositional defiant disorder (ODD) in 3.4 per cent.

According to Korenberger (2006), individuals with an atypically small deletion in 7q11.23 show some but not all Williams syndrome characteristics – for example, hypersociability is absent.

22q11.2 microdeletion syndrome (22q11DS)

This microdeletion occurs at a rate of 0.025 per cent in the general population. It leads to variable physical phenotypes, including DiGeorge syndrome (OMIM 188400), velocardiofacial syndrome (OMIM 192430), conotruncal anomaly face syndrome (OMIM 188400), Opitz G/BBB syndrome (OMIM 145410), and Cayler cardiofacial syndrome (OMIM 125520).

The various phenotypes are not always associated with intellectual disability; one study comprising 37 individuals aged between 8 months and 20 years showed IQ < 70 in 45 per cent of cases (Swillen *et al.*, 1997).

Individuals with 22q11DS represent a particularly high-risk group for schizophrenia (Bassett *et al.*, 2000). According to Murphy *et al.* (1999), 25 per cent or more patients are estimated to develop schizophrenia, and according to Liu *et al.* (2002) one third to one quarter develop schizophrenia or schizoaffective disorder. This microdeletion has been found in up to two per cent of adult schizophrenic patients (Karayiorgou *et al.*, 1995) and in up to six per cent of cases with childhood onset schizophrenia (Usiskin *et al.*, 1999).

The 22q11DS cases with childhood onset schizophrenia did not differ from other patients in onset age, IQ, premorbid functioning, or psychosis severity, but had fewer negative symptoms and a good clinical response to atypical narcoleptics (Sporn *et al.*, 2004).

Niklasson *et al.* (2001) studied 32 children and young adults with 22q11DS and found a neuropsychiatric disorder in 56 per cent (intellectual disability in 53 per cent, ADHD in 44 per cent, and autism spectrum disorder in 31 per cent).

Chromosome 22q13.3 deletion

This deletion has been reported to be associated with PDD in 31 per cent of cases (10/32), ADHD in 44 per cent (14/32), and schizophrenia in 25 per cent (11/45).

Smith-Magenis syndrome

Smith-Magenis syndrome is associated with an interstitial deletion on 17p11.2. The prevalence is 1 in 25,000 children. It is characterized by distinctive facial features progressing with age, intellectual disability, and behavioural abnormalities. Characteristic of Smith-Magenis syndrome are two types of stereotyped behaviour: spasmodic upper body squeezing ('self-hug'), and hand licking and page flipping ('lick and flip') (Finucane *et al.*, 1994; Dykens & Smith, 1998; Smith *et al.*, 1998; Finucane *et al.*, 2001).

Other reported symptoms are inattention, hyperactivity, maladaptive behaviour including frequent outbursts/temper tantrums, attention seeking, impulsivity, distractibility, disobedience, aggression, toilet difficulties and self-injurious behaviour, including self-hitting, self-biting, and skin picking, inserting foreign objects into body orifices (polyembolokoilamania) and yanking fingernails and toenails (onychotillomania).

Rubinstein-Taybi syndrome

Rubinstein-Taybi syndrome is a syndrome of multiple congenital anomalies mapped to 16p13.3. The birth incidence is 1/125,000. Studying psychiatric phenotypes in 13 individuals with this disorder, Levitas & Reid (1998) found mood disorders in eight, tic/OCD spectrum in four, and PDD-NOS in one. No association between intellectual disability severity and psychiatric diagnosis was found.

Single-gene disorders

Fragile-X syndrome

In most cases, this disorder is caused by the unstable expansion of a CGG repeat in the FMR1 gene and abnormal methylation, resulting in suppression of FMR1 transcription and decreased protein levels in the brain. Fragile-X syndrome is found in approximately 1/4,000 males; in females, the prevalence of the permutation carrier is 1/260 in the general population.

Fragile-X syndrome is characterized by moderate to severe mental retardation, macroorchidism, and distinct facial features, including long face, large ears, and prominent jaw.

Affected boys show a high prevalence of ADHD symptoms (between 54 and 59 per cent) (Sullivan et al., 2006), higher than rates found in individuals with other genetic conditions (Backes et al., 2000) or in individuals with non-specific intellectual disability (Borghgraef et al., 1987). Moreover, 16 per cent of affected boys meet DSM criteria for autism (Hagerman & Sobesky,1989).

In females heterozygous for fragile-X syndrome, chronic affective disorders were seen in 40 per cent and schizotypal features in 31 per cent (Reiss et al., 1988).

Tuberous sclerosis complex

Genetic mutations in tuberous sclerosis complex 1 (TSC1 on chromosome 9q34) and TSC2 (on chromosome 16p13.3) lead to abnormalities in cell proliferation, differentiation, and migration. The prevalence of tuberous sclerosis is estimated at 1/6000 to 1/9000 births.

Approximately 55 per cent of individuals have an IQ within the normal range, 44 per cent have an IQ below 70, and about 31 per cent below 21. Problems in attention and executive functioning predominate.

ADHD was the most common comorbid diagnosis (44 per cent), followed by oppositional defiant disorder (25 per cent) and separation anxiety disorder (19 per cent) (Steinhausen et al., 2002).

Prevalence rates of autism in tuberous sclerosis vary from 50 per cent (Bolton & Griffiths, 1997; Hunt & Dennis, 1987) to 60 per cent (Gillberg et al., 1994).

Lewis et al. (2004) found more frequent reports of autism in patients with TSC2 mutations than in those with TSC1 mutations.

Neurofibromatosis

The main forms of neurofibromatosis are NF-1 and NF-2; the latter is not associated with psychiatric morbidity.

The NF1 gene responsible for the disease is located on the long arm of chromosome 17 at 17q11.2, with a prevalence of 1/3000 births and autosomal dominant inheritance. Learning disabilities occur in 30 to 60 per cent of cases of NF-1 (North et al., 1997).

Three subtypes of learning disability were noted (Eliason, 1986). A primarily visual-perceptual subtype was most common, occurring in 56 per cent. A mixed type was noted in 30 per cent, compared with a primarily verbal type in only four per cent.

ADHD behaviour is more frequent in individuals with NF-1 than in the general population (Riccardi, 1981; Eliason, 1986; Moore et al., 1996, Schrimsher et al., 2003) with an estimated rate of 33 per cent (Kayl & Moore, 2000).

α-mannosidosis

α-mannosidosis is an autosomal recessive lysosomal storage disease caused by mutations of the gene (in 19cen-q12) encoding α-mannosidase, causing the deficient activity of this lysosomal enzyme. Its incidence is believed to be about 1/500,000 births.

It is characterized by mild to moderate intellectual disability, moderate to severe neurosensory hearing loss, psychomotor disturbances, and skeletal dysmorphism associated with immunodeficiency, leading to frequent infections. α-mannosidosis is associated with depressive or psychotic symptoms in 25 per cent of patients (Malm & Nilssen, 2001).

Smith-Lemli-Opitz syndrome

Smith-Lemli-Opitz syndrome (SLOS) is caused by a mutation of the 7-dehydrocholesterol reductase gene (DHCR7) in 11q12-q13. Its incidence is 1/10,000 to 1/30,000 births. SLOS carries microcephaly, facial anomalies, intellectual disability, growth retardation, feeding problems, incomplete development of male genitalia, and syndactyly of the second and third toes.

Approximately 71 to 86 per cent of children with SLOS have an autism spectrum disorder, about 50 per cent of which are autistic disorders (Sikora et al., 2006).

Adenylosuccinate lyase (adenylosuccinase) deficiency

This is a rare single-gene disorder in 22q13.1, altering purine synthesis. It comprises a variable association of intellectual disability, autism spectrum disorder, epilepsy, and axial hypotonia with peripheral hypertonia (Stone et al., 1992).

Other conditions

The following single-gene disorders have been described in individuals with PDD disorder.

- Cohen syndrome (COH1, 8q22-23): Howlin et al. (2005), using standardized diagnostic assessments, found that 49 per cent of affected children (22/45) met criteria for autism.
- Sanfilippo syndromes: Ritvo et al. (1990) reported this disorder in one per cent of a series of autistic patients.
- Rett syndrome, affecting girls with mutations of MECP2 in Xq28 or of CDKL5 in Xp22, is characterized by a peculiar behavioural phenotype belonging to the PDD spectrum.

Conclusions

Knowledge of an increased possibility of psychiatric problems in subjects with intellectual disability suggests the need to evaluate them more carefully and to identify problems at an early stage, permitting more effective treatment. This should especially be taken into account in patients with intellectual disability caused by specific chromosomal or single-gene disorders, in which certain psychiatric disorders are reported to be particularly common.

From a research point of view, knowledge of the more frequent associations could suggest the location of genes relevant to the causation of psychiatric disorders.

References

Achenbach, T.M. (1991): *Manual for the Child Behavior Check-List 14–18 and 1991 profile*, Burlington, VT: University of Vermont – Department of Psychiatry.

Andersen, W.H., Rasmussen, R.K. & Stromme, P. (2001): Levels of cognitive and linguistic development in Angelman syndrome: a study of 20 children. *Logoped. Phoniatr. Vocol.* **26**, 2–9.

Backes, M., Genc, B., Schreck, J., Doerfler, W., Lehmkuhl, G. & von Gontard, A. (2000): Cognitive and behavioral profile of fragile-X boys: correlations to molecular data. *Am. J. Med. Genet.* **95**, 150–156.

Bassett, A.S., Chow, E.W.C. & Weksberg, R. (2000): Chromosomal abnormalities and schizophrenia. *Am. J. Med Genet. Semin. Med. Genet.* **97**, 45–51.

Beardsmore, A., Dorman, T., Cooper, S.A. & Webb, T. (1998): Affective psychosis and Prader-Willi syndrome. *J Intellect. Disabil. Res.* **42**, 463–471.

Bolton, P.F. & Griffiths, P.D. (1997): Association of tuberous sclerosis of temporal lobes with autism and atypical autism. *Lancet* **349**, 392–395.

Borghgraef, M., Fryns, J.P. Dielkens, A., Pyck, K. & Van den Berghe, H. (1987): Fragile X syndrome: a study of the psychological profile in 23 prepuberta. patients. *Clin Genet.* **32**, 179–186.

Clayton-Smith, J., Driscoll, D.J., Waters, M.F., Webb, T., Andrews, T., Malcolm, S., Pembrey, M.E. & Nicholls, E.D (1993): Difference in methylation patterns within the D15S9 region of chromosome 15q11-13 in first cousins with Angelman syndrome and Prader-Willi syndrome. *Am. J. Med. Genet.* **47**, 683–686.

Collacot, R.A., Cooper, S.A., Branford, D. & McGrother, C. (1998): Behavior phenotype for Down syndrome. *Br. J Psychiatry* **172**, 85–89.

Cook, E.H., Lindgren, V., Leventhal, B.L., Courehesnes, R., Lincoln, A., Shulman, C., Lord, C. & Courehesnes E.(1997): Autism or atypical autism in maternally but not paternally derived proximal 15q duplication. *Am. J. Hum Gen.* **60**, 928–934.

Cormack, K.F.M., Brown, A.C. & Hastings, R.P. (2000): Behavioural and emotional difficulties in students attending schools for children and adolescents with severe intellectual disability. *J. Intellect. Disabil. Res.* **44**, 124–129.

Costello, E.J., Angold, A., Burns, B.J., Stangl, D.K., Tweed, D.L., Erkanli, A. & Worthman, C.M. (1996): The Great Smokey Mountains Study of Youth: goals, design, methods, and the prevalence of *DSM-III-R* disorders. *Arch. Gen. Psychiatry* **53**, 1129–1136.

Danford, D.E. & Huber, A.M. (1982): Pica among mentally retarded adults. *Am. J. Ment. Defic.* **87**, 141–146.

Dekker, M.C., Koot, H.M., van der Ende, J. & Verhulst, F.C. (2002): Emotional and behavioral problems in children and adolescents with and without intellectual disability. *J. Child Psychol. Psychiatry* **43**, 1087–1098.

Douma, J.C., Dekker, M.C., Verhulst, F.C. & Koot, H.M. (2006): Self-reports on mental health problems of youth with moderate to borderline intellectual disabilities. *J. Am. Acad. Child. Adolesc. Psychiatry* **45**, 1224–1231.

Dykens, E.M. & Smith, A.C. (1998): Distinctiveness and correlates of maladaptive behaviour in children and adolescents with Smith-Magenis syndrome. *J. Intellect. Disabil. Res.* **42**, 481–489.

Dykens, E.M. & Cassidy, S.B. (1999): Prader-Willi syndrome. In: *Handbook of neurobehavioral and genetic disorders in children*, eds. S. Goldstein & C.R. Reynolds, pp. 525–554. New York: Guilford Press.

Dykens, E.M., Leckman, J.F. & Cassidy, S.B. (1996): Obsessions and compulsions in Prader-Willi syndrome. *J. Child. Psychol. Psychiatry* **37**, 995–1002.

Einfeld, S. & Tonge, B.J. (1996a): Population prevalence of psychopathology in children and adolescents with intellectual disability I. Rationale and methods. *J. Intellect. Disabil. Res.* **40**, 91–98.

Einfeld, S. & Tonge, B.J. (1996b): Population prevalence of psychopathology in children and adolescents with intellectual disability I. Epidemiological findings. *J. Intellect. Disabil. Res.* **40**, 99–109.

Eliason, M.J. (1986): Neurofibromatosis: implications for learning and behavior. *J. Dev. Behav. Pediatr.* **7**, 175–179.

Emerson, E. (2003): Prevalence of psychiatric disorders in children and adolescents with and without intellectual disability. *J. Intellect. Disabil. Res.* **1**, 51–58.

Finucane, B.M., Konar, D., Haas-Givler, B., Kurtz, M.B. & Scott, C.I. (1994): The spasmodic upper-body squeeze: a characteristic behavior in Smith-Magenis syndrome. *Dev. Med. Child Neurol.* **36**, 78–83.

Finucane, B., Dirrigl, K.H. & Simon, E.W. (2001): Characterization of self-injurious behaviors in children and adults with Smith-Magenis syndrome. *Am. J. Ment. Retard.* **106**, 52–58.

Fox, R.A. & Wade, E.J. (1998): Attention deficit hyperactivity disorder among adults with severe and profound mental retardation. *Res. Dev. Disabil.* **19**, 275–280.

Gibbs, M.V. & Thorpe, J.G. (1983): Personality stereotype of noninstitutionalized Down syndrome children. *Am. J. Ment. Defic.* **87**, 601–605.

Gillberg, C. (1995): *Clinical child neuropsychiatry*. Cambridge: Cambridge University Press.

Gillberg, I.C., Gillberg, C. & Ahlsen, G. (1994): Autistic behaviour and attention deficits in tuberous sclerosis: a population-based study. *Dev. Med. Child. Neurol.* **36**, 50–56.

Hagerman, R.J. & Sobesky, W.E. (1989): Psychopathology in fragile X syndrome. *Am. J. Orthopsychiatry* **59**, 142–152.

Hoare, P., Harris, M., Jackson, P. & Kerley, S. (1998): A community survey of children with severe intellectual disability and their families: psychological adjustment, carer distress and the effect of respite care. *J. Intellect. Disabil. Res.* **42**, 218–227.

Howlin, P., Karpf, J. & Turk, J. (2005): Behavioural characteristics and autistic features in individuals with Cohen Syndrome. *Eur. Child Adolesc. Psychiatry* **14**, 57–64.

Hunt, A. & Dennis, J. (1987): Psychiatric disorder among children with tuberous sclerosis. *Dev. Med. Child Neurol.* **29**, 190–198.

Jacquemont, M.L., Sanlaville, D., Redon, R., Raoul, O., Cormier-Daire, V., Lyonnet, S., Amiel, J., Le Merrer, M., Heron, D., de Blois, M.C., Prieur, M., Vekemans, M., Carter, N.P., Munnich, A., Colleaux, L. & Philippe, A. (2006): Array-based comparative genomic hybridisation identifies high frequency of cryptic chromosomal rearrangements in patients with syndromic autism spectrum disorders. *J. Med. Genet.* **43**, 843–849.

Karayiorgou, M., Morris, M.A., Morrow, B., Shprintzeni, R.J., Goldberg, R., Borrow, J., Gos, A., Nestadt, G., Wolyniec, P.S., Lasseter, V.K., Eisen, H., Childs, B., Kazazian, H.H., Kucherlapati, R., Antonarakis, S.E., Pulver, A.E. & Housman, D.E. (1995): Schizophrenia susceptibility associated with interstitial deletions of chromosome 22q11. *Proc. Natl. Acad. Sci. USA* **92**, 7612–7616.

Kayl, A.E. & Moore, B.D. (2000): Behavioral phenotype of neurofibromatosis, type 1. *Ment. Retard. Dev. Disabil. Res. Rev.* **6**, 117–124.

Kent, L., Evans, J., Paul, M. & Sharp, M. (1999): Comorbidity of autistic spectrum disorders in children with Down syndrome. *Dev. Med. Child Neurol.* **41**, 153–158.

Korenberger, J.R. (2006): The impact of Williams syndrome mutations on neural organization and brain function: a window into social cognition. *Am. J. Med. Genet.* **141**, 768.

Kraijer, D.W. & de Bildt, A.A. (2005): The PDD-MRS: an instrument for identification of autism spectrum disorders in persons with mental retardation. *J. Autism Dev. Disord.* **35**, 499–513.

Kwasnicka-Crawford, D.A., Roberts, W. & Scherer, S.W. (2007): Characterization of an autism-associated segmental maternal heterodisomy of the chromosome 15q11-13 region. *J. Autism Dev. Disord.* **37**, 694–702.

La Malfa, G., Lassi, S., Bertelli, M., Salvini, R. & Placidi, G.F. (2004): Autism and intellectual disability: a study of prevalence on a sample of the Italian population. *J. Intellect. Disabil. Res.* **48**, 262–267.

Levitas, A.S. & Reid, C.S. (1998): Rubinstein-Taybi syndrome and psychiatric disorders. *J. Intellect. Disabil. Res.* **42**, 284–292.

Lewis, J.C., Thomas, H.V., Murphy, K.C. & Sampson, J.R. (2004): Genotype and psychological phenotype in tuberous sclerosis. *J. Med. Genet.* **41**, 203–207.

Leyfer, O.T., Woodruff-Borden, J., Klein-Tasman, B.P., Fricke, J.S. & Mervis, C.B. (2006): Prevalence of psychiatric disorders in 4- to 16-year-olds with Williams syndrome. *Am. J. Med. Genet. B Neuropsychiatr. Genet.* **141**, 615–622.

Liu, H., Heath, S.C., Sobin, C., Roos, J.L., Galke, B.L., Blundell, M.L., Lenane, M., Robertson, B., Wijsman, E.M., Rapoport, J.L., Gogos, J.A. & Karayiorgou, M. (2002): Genetic variation at the 22q11 PRODH2/DGCR6 locus presents an unusual pattern and increases susceptibility to schizophrenia. *Proc. Natl. Acad. Sci. USA* **99**, 3717–3722.

Lossie, A.C., Whitney, M.M., Amidon, D., Dong, H.J., Chen, P., Theriaque, D., Hutson, A., Nicholls, R.D., Zori, R.T., Williams, C.A. & Driscoll, D.J. (2001): Distinct phenotypes distinguish the molecular classes of Angelman syndrome. *J. Med. Genet.* **38**, 834–845.

Malm, D. & Nilssen, O. (2001): Alpha-mannosidosis (October2001 through 2003). In: *Genereviews: clinical genetic information resource* [database online]. University of Washington, Seattle. Available at http://www.geneclinics.org/query?dz=a-mannosidosis.

McAdam, D.B., Sherman, J.A., Sheldon, J.B. & Napolitano, D.A. (2004): Behavioral interventions to reduce the pica of persons with developmental disabilities. *Behav. Modif.* **28**, 45–72.

McAlpine, C. & Singh, N.N. (1986): Pica in institutionalized mentally retarded persons. *J. Ment. Defic. Res.* **30**, 171–178.

Molteno, G., Molteno, C.D., Finchilescu, G. & Dawes, A.R.L. (2001): Behavioural and emotional problems in children with intellectual disability attending special schools in Cape Town South Africa. *J. Intellect. Disabil. Res.* **45**, 515–520.

Moore, B.D., Slopis, J.M., Schomer, D., Jackson, E.F. & Levy, B.M. (1996): Neuropsychological significance of areas of high-signal intensity on brain MRIs of children with neurofibromatosis. *Neurology* **46**, 1660–1668.

Murphy, K.C., Jones, L.A. & Owen, M.J. (1999): High rates of schizophrenia in adults with velo-cardio-facial syndrome. *Arch. Gen. Psychiatry* **56**, 940–945.

Newman, E., Christopher, S.R. & Berry, J.O. (2000): Developmental disabilities, trauma exposure, and post-traumatic stress disorder. *Trauma Violence Abuse* **1**, 154–170.

Niklasson, L., Rasmussen, P., Oskarsdottir, S. & Gillberg, C. (2001): Neuropsychiatric disorders in the 22q11 deletion syndrome. *Genet. Med.* **3**, 79–84.

North, K.N., Riccardi, V., Samango-Sprouse, C., Ferner, R., Moore, B., Legius, E., Ratner, N. & Denckla, M.B. (1997) Cognitive function and academic performance in neurofibromatosis: 1. Consensus statement from the NF1 Cognitive Disorders Task Force. *Neurology* **48**, 1121–1127.

Reiss, A.L., Hagerman, R.J , Vinogradov, S., Abrams, M. & King, R.J. (1988): Psychiatric disability in female carriers of the fragile X chromosome. *Arch. Gen. Psychiatry* **45**, 25–30.

Reiss, A.L., Cianchetti, C., Cohen, I.L. DeVries, B., Hagerman, R., Hinton, V., Froster, U., Lachiewicz, A., Mazzocco. M. & Sobesky, W. (1992): Brief screening questionnaire for determining affected state in fragile X syndrome: a consensus recommendation *Am. J. Med. Genet.* **43**, 61–64.

Riccardi, V.M. (1981): Neurofibromatosis: an overview and new directions in clinical investigations. *Adv. Neurol.* **29**, 1–9.

Ritvo, E.R., Mason-Brothers, A., Freeman, B.J., Pingree, C., Jenson, W.R., McMahon, W.M., Petersen, P.B., Jorde, L.B., Mo, A. & Ritvo, A. (1990): The UCLA-University of Utah epidemiologic survey of autism: the etiologic role of rare diseases. *Am. J. Psychiatry* **147**, 1614–1621.

Rutter, M., Tizard, J., Yule, W., Graham, P. & Whitmore, K. (1976): Research report: isle of Wight studies, 1964-1974. *Psychol. Med.* **6**, 313–332.

Schrimsher, G.W., Billingsley, R.L., Slopis, J.M. & Moore, B.D. (2003): Visual-spatial performance deficits in children with neurofibromatosis type-1. *Am. J. Med. Genet. A.* **120**, 326–330.

Schroer, R.J., Phelan, M.C., Michaelis, R.C., Crawford, E.C., Skinner, S.A., Cuccaro, M., Simensen, R.J., Bishop, J., Skinner, C., Fender, D. & Stevenson, R.E (1998): Autism and maternally derived aberrations of chromosome 15q. *Am. J. Med. Genet.* **76**, 327–336.

Sikora, D.M., Pettit-Kekel, K., Penfield, J., Merkens, L.S. & Steiner, R.D. (2006): The near universal presence of autism spectrum disorders in children with Smith-Lemli-Opitz syndrome. *Am. J. Med. Genet.* **140**, 1511–1518.

Smith, A.C., Dykens, E. & Greenberg, F. (1998): Behavioral phenotype of Smith-Magenis syndrome (del 17p11.2). *Am. J. Med. Genet.* **81**, 179–185.

Sporn, A., Addington, A., Reiss, A.L., Dean, M., Gogtay, N., Potocnik, U., Greenstein, D., Hallmayer, J., Gochman, P., Lenane, M., Baker, N., Tossell, J. & Rapoport, J.L. (2004): 22q11 deletion syndrome in childhood onset schizophrenia: an update. *Mol. Psychiatry* **9**, 225–226.

Steffenburg, S., Gillberg, C.L., Steffenburg, U. & Kyllerman, M. (1996): Autism in Angelman syndrome: a population-based study. *Pediatr. Neurol.* **14**, 131–136.

Steinhausen, H.C., Von Gontard, A., Spohr, H.L., Hauffa, B.P., Eiholzer, U., Backes, M., Willms, J. & Malin, Z. (2002): Behavioral phenotypes in four mental retardation syndromes: fetal alcohol syndrome, Prader-Willi syndrome, fragile X syndrome, and tuberous sclerosis. *Am. J. Med. Genet.* **111**, 381–387.

Stone, R.L., Aimi, J., Barshop, B.A., Jaeken, J., Van den Berghe, G., Zalkin, H. & Dixon, J.E. (1992): A mutation in adenylosuccinate lyase associated with mental retardation and autistic features. *Nat. Genet.* **1**, 59–63.

Sullivan, K., Hatton, D., Hammer, J., Siders, J., Hooper, S., Ornstein, P. & Bailey, D. (2006): ADHD symptoms in children with FXS. *Am. J. Med. Genet. A.* **140**, 2275–2288.

Summers, J.A., Lynch, P.S.Harris, J.C., Burke, J.C., Allison, D.B. & Sandler, L. (1992): A combined behavioral/pharmacological treatment of sleep-wake schedule disorder in Angelman syndrome. *J. Dev. Behav. Pediatr.* **13**, 284–287.

Summers, J.A., Allison, D.B., Lynch, P.S. & Sandler, L. (1995): Behaviour problems in Angelman syndrome. *J. Intellect. Disabil. Res.* **39**, 97–106.

Swillen, A., Devriendt, K., Legius, E. & Fryns, J.P. (1997): Intelligence and psychosocial adjustment in velocardiofacial syndrome: a study of 37 children and adolescents with WCFS. *J. Med. Genet.* **34**, 453–458.

Szymanski, L. & King, B.H. (1999): Practice parameters for the assessment and treatment of children, adolescents, and adults with mental retardation and comorbid mental disorders. American Academy of Child and Adolescent Psychiatry Working Group on Quality Issues. *J. Am. Acad. Child. Adolesc. Psychiatry* **38** (Suppl. 12), S5-S31.

Trillingsgaard, A. & Østergaard, J.R. (2004): Autism in Angelman syndrome: an exploration of comorbidity. *Autism* **8**, 163–174.

Usiskin, S.I., Nicolson, R., Krasnewich, D.M., Yan, W., Lenane, M., Wudarsky, M., Hamburger S.D. & Rapoport, J.L. (1999): Velocardiofacial syndrome in childhood-onset schizophrenia. *J. Am. Acad. Child Adolesc. Psychiatry* **38**, 1536–1543.

Veltman, M.W., Craig, E.E. & Bolton, P.F. (2005): Autism spectrum disorders in Prader-Willi and Angelman syndromes: a systematic review. *Psychiatr. Genet.* **15**, 243–254.

Verhulst, F.C. & van der Ende, J. (1997): Factors associated with child mental health service use in the community. *J. Am. Acad. Child Adolesc. Psychiatry* **36**, 901–909.

Chapter 13

Pharmacological treatment of psychiatric comorbidities in mental retardation

Gabriele Masi and Cinzia Pari

*IRCCS Stella Maris, Scientific Institute of Child Neurology and Psychiatry,
via dei Giacinti 2, 56018 Calambrone, Pisa, Italy*
gabriele.masi@inpe.unipi.it

Summary

Mental retardation is not simple cognitive impairment but a complex syndrome characterized by intellectual disability, a reduced ability to cope with daily activities, and a high psychiatric comorbidity, which strongly affects the current clinical picture and the natural history of the syndrome. The aim of this clinical review is to analyse critically the available literature and our personal experience of psychiatric comorbidity in children and adolescents with mental retardation, including pharmacological interventions. Mood disorders (both depression and bipolar disorder), anxiety disorders, obsessive-compulsive disorder, psychotic disorders, attention deficit hyperactivity disorder, pervasive developmental disorders, and disruptive behaviour disorders are included in our review. General principles of pharmacotherapy in mental retardation are also provided.

Introduction

Mental retardation has often been considered as an intelligence disorder requiring principally pedagogic or social interventions; hence the psychiatric dimension of the problem has been neglected (Potter, 1971). This is particularly true for mentally retarded children and adolescents (Masi, 1998). It is now well recognized that persons with mental retardation have an increased vulnerability for additional mental disorders ('dual diagnosis'). Rutter *et al.* (1970), in their epidemiological study in the Isle of Wight, found psychiatric problems in 30 to 42 per cent of retarded children and adolescents, as opposed to seven per cent in children with normal intelligence. Incidence rates were similar among non-institutionalized subjects in Sweden (Gillberg *et al.*, 1986). Similar rates of psychopathology were reported in an epidemiological sample from Australia (Einfeld & Tonge, 1996): 40.7 per cent of subjects with mental retardation aged between 4 and 18 years were classified as having severe emotional and behavioural disorder. An early diagnosis of psychopathology in subjects with normal IQ as well as in developmentally disabled persons is crucial, as it provides a window of opportunity for preventing psychosocial impairment, reduces the likelihood of institutionalization, and saves costs for the community.

According to the *Diagnostic and Statistical Manual of Mental Disorders* (DSM-IV; American Psychiatric Association, 1994), all types of mental disorder can be observed in these subjects, with a prevalence estimated to be at least three to four times higher than in the general population. One of the main reasons for the exclusion of people with mental retardation from psychiatric services – along with the paucity of research in the field of psychopathology – is the difficulty in making reliable diagnoses (Einfeld & Aman, 1995). Uniform methods for collecting diagnostic information should result in more homogeneous diagnostic groups and greater comparability among studies.

A crucial challenge in the psychiatric diagnosis is to apply reliable assessment instruments for psychopathology and to define their range of application, for example in terms of the severity of mental retardation (Masi *et al.*, 2000). Rating scales are good instruments for longitudinal assessment as they can quantify the severity of symptoms over time, but they have some limitations for the diagnosis and clinical description of the illness. Verbal interviewing techniques can be used in most patients with mild mental retardation, if examiners carefully establish the patient's comprehension of the questions. Clinical interviews allow the interviewer to undertake a deep exploration of the symptomatology and to make diagnoses according to the DSM diagnostic criteria. This clinical definition is crucial for epidemiological, prognostic, and therapeutic studies. Furthermore the use of structured diagnostic interviews can reduce the risk of diagnostic overshadowing (Reiss *et al.*, 1982) – that is, the tendency of clinicians to underdiagnose mental disorders when a patient has mental retardation.

The clinical characteristics of mental disorders are strongly influenced by the intellectual disability. Clinical features are often not well defined and symptoms become less specific as the intellectual impairment becomes more severe, so their diagnosis can be particularly difficult. The longitudinal course in subjects with intellectual impairment often differs from that of corresponding disorders in subjects with normal intelligence – for example, remission of symptomatology is less frequent in mental retardation. The role of traumatic life events is especially important, as these more often have a triggering effect than in subjects with normal intelligence.

Several diagnostic instruments for psychopathology have been developed or adapted in recent years, designed to improve the detection of psychiatric disorders in people with mental retardation, but further research is needed on screening tools and assessment instruments for dual diagnosis in all degrees of mental deficiency (Aman, 1991). For many people with mental retardation, reduced linguistic ability limits self-reports of what the individuals are experiencing; thus the diagnostic process relies on third-party reports and observations. Clinical structured interviews, such as the K-SADS (Kiddie-Schedule for Affective Disorders and Schizophrenia), can allow clinicians to carry out a comprehensive diagnosis, but their use in subjects with mental retardation is still preliminary (Masi *et al.*, 2002). General inventories of psychopathology and rating scales for more specific disorders have some limitations for the diagnosis and clinical description of the illness, but they are good instruments for identifying subjects needing further psychiatric consultation, for measuring the severity of illness, and for monitoring natural history (Aman, 1991). Some of these general instruments were developed specifically for people with mental retardation, such as the Psychopathology Instrument for Mentally Retarded Adults (PIMRA), while for others, such as the Child Behavior Checklist (CBCL), the use was extended from normal IQ to developmentally delayed subjects.

Research on the pharmacotherapy of mental disorders in intellectual impairment has traditionally been affected by the interpretation of the psychopathology. The scantness of studies of specific psychiatric disorders has resulted in a simplification of the aims of pharmacological treatments, which are often directed at suppressing non-specific aberrant behaviours such as aggression or self-harm. Only recently has new interest grown in the treatment of specific DSM-IV diagnoses. Unfortunately, most of the studies have relied on adult samples, and data on children and adolescents are often extrapolated from research into adults with mental retardation.

Depression

People with mental deficiency are considered to be at higher risk of mood disorders, both depressive and bipolar (Masi et al., 1999a). Diagnosis of a depressive disorder in these special populations is often difficult because of their deficits in language expression and comprehension and their lack of insight, together with the unusual clinical expression of depressive disorder in such cases (Moss et al., 1997). Although DSM diagnostic criteria and DSM-IV-inspired diagnostic instruments are considered adequate in people with mild mental retardation (Masi et al., 1999b), their reliability declines with the increasing of severity of mental retardation (Einfeld & Aman, 1995).

The pharmacological approach to depression changed dramatically in the 1980s, when the selective serotonin reuptake inhibitors (SSRI) replaced the tricyclic antidepressants (TCA) as first-line treatment for depression, as well as for anxiety and obsessive-compulsive disorders, because of their greater efficacy and more consistent tolerability. More recently, newer antidepressants have been marketed, but data on subjects with mental retardation are still not available. Most of the studies on SSRI included patients with pervasive developmental disorders (PDD), and will be reviewed in that section. There are far fewer studies that specifically consider children and adolescents with depression and mental retardation (Aman et al., 1999). As a whole, controlled studies with fluoxetine in children and adolescents with normal IQ support the use of this medication in mental retardation. Clinical experience in adult patients indicates that these types of drug can be effective in depressive symptoms as well as in irritability and self-injurious behaviours, which often co-occur in depressed mentally retarded children. In an open-label, 9-week study of adolescents with mental retardation treated with paroxetine, four of seven patients no longer met diagnostic criteria for depression, and there were only mild and transitory side effects (Masi et al., 1997).

Few studies with TCA are available in children and adolescents with mental retardation. However, besides their poor tolerability, there are no controlled studies supporting the efficacy of TCA in childhood depression. Recent concerns about the increased risk of suicidal tendencies in depressed adolescents treated with SSRI have led to the inclusion of a boxed warning about this. Published data on suicides in adolescents with mental retardation are not available. Despite this important concern, SSRI (mainly fluoxetine) are the treatment choice for children and adolescents with depression.

Bipolar disorder

Presentation of bipolar disorder is frequently different in childhood-onset as opposed to adult-onset disorder. While the adult type is usually characterized by euphoric, depressive, and euthimic phases, inflated self-esteem, and an episodic course, in early-onset bipolar disorder the course is often not clearly episodic but subcontinuous and erratic, and the most prominent symptoms are irritability, hostility, and aggressiveness, both verbal and physical (Masi et al., 2006b). This is particularly true in patients with mental retardation, in whom the affective phenomenology is often mixed – dysphoria, with affective storms, temper outbursts, aggression, and self-injurious behaviours are more frequent than euphoria (Venstraelen & Tyrer, 1999). For this reason, bipolar disorder in mental retardation often goes unrecognized and undertreated.

Mood stabilizers are the first choice of medication in bipolar disorder – namely lithium and antiepileptic agents (most often valproic acid), but they can also be used in disruptive behaviour disorders with aggression and impulsiveness (Masi, 2005). Lithium is approved for bipolar disorder in patients older than 12 years, but formal data on adolescents with mental retardation are not available. Despite its effectiveness, clinical experience suggests that some side effects may be more frequent, including tremor, slurred speech, and blurred vision.

According to certain reports, valproic acid may be more effective than lithium in rapid-cycling or mixed mania. Given that persons with mental retardation often present mixed features and rapid cycling, valproate may be particularly effective in these patients. The most frequent side effects are sedation, gastrointestinal upset, weight gain, tremor, and more rarely severe hepatotoxicity in younger patients.

When mood stabilizers, alone or in combination, are ineffective, or when severe behavioural disorders or psychotic symptoms co-occur, atypical antipsychotic agents can be added, at least during the acute manic phases (Masi, 2005).

Anxiety disorders

Anxiety symptoms are documented in persons with mental retardation, though prevalence reports are conflicting, with rates ranging between three per cent and 25 per cent (Ollendick *et al.*, 1993; Masi *et al.*, 2000). The frequency of anxiety disorders is increased in higher-IQ mentally retarded individuals (Einfeld & Tonge, 1996), while this diagnosis should be approached with greater caution in persons with severe and profound mental retardation. The prevalence of anxiety disorders is usually underestimated (mainly in children and adolescents), because the diagnosis stems from subjective reports. Furthermore, anxiety disorders in mental retardation are often considered to be a unique group, without distinction between different categories of anxiety syndromes (Masi *et al.*, 2000). Similarities between intellectually disabled patients and those with normal IQ in several items – such as feelings of tension, apprehension, need for reassurance, and above all negative self-image – are more significant than discrepancies, suggesting that the phenomenology of anxiety in persons with mild developmental delay roughly parallels that of people with normal IQ (Masi *et al.*, 2000). An accurate diagnosis of anxiety in adolescents affected by mental retardation is not just of academic importance. An early diagnosis of an anxiety disorder in developmentally disabled persons is crucial, as anxiety symptoms can cause disruption over and above that caused by the mental retardation. Hyperactivity, irritability, and self-injurious behaviours can be a manifestation of severe anxiety. An appropriate diagnosis can lead to appropriate treatment, sparing these patients neuroleptic drugs or other ineffective treatments.

Although SSRI have well known anti-anxiety properties, and controlled studies support their efficacy in children and adolescents, no studies are available on their value in adolescents with mental retardation. Benzodiazepines should be used carefully and only for limited periods, as they can cause a paradoxical increase in agitation and impulsivity in persons with mental retardation.

Obsessive-compulsive disorder

Obsessive-compulsive disorder (OCD) has been specifically described in mentally retarded persons (Vitiello et al., 1989). As with mood and anxiety disorders, a crucial problem relating to OCD in children and adolescents with mental retardation has to do with diagnostic criteria and clinical features. DSM-IV criteria seem to suggest reliable diagnoses in subjects with mild mental retardation. In severe mental retardation, modifications to the current diagnostic criteria are needed, as the boundaries among compulsions, tics, stereotypies, and other repetitive phenomena (including self-injurious behaviours) are often unclear. Whether all these manifestations share the same neurobiological basis, and consequently the same sensitivity to medication, is still debated (Aman et al., 1999).

The SSRIs and the TCA clomipramine have been proven effective in the pharmacological treatment of OCD in adults with mental retardation (Hellings et al., 1996). However, the severe repetitive phenomena can be poorly sensitive to serotonergic agents, which may also cause an increase in impulsiveness and aggression. In these cases – namely when aggression and self-injurious behaviours occur together – an atypical antipsychotic agent (for example, risperidone) in mono- or polypharmacy may be needed.

Psychotic disorders

Psychotic disorders are reported in about three per cent of persons with mental retardation, usually when CNS lesions are present. Negative symptoms are prevalent, delusions are usually poorly structured, hallucinations are elementary, verbal expression and behaviour are grossly disorganized, and the diagnosis 'psychotic disorder not otherwise specified' is most frequent. These disorders have traditionally been treated with conventional antipsychotic agents (neuroleptics), but there is a high rate of sedation and extrapyramidal side effects, especially akathisia, in children with mental retardation (Aman & Madrid, 1999; Madrid et al., 2000). A new generation of antipsychotic agents – named 'atypical antipsychotics' and including clozapine, risperidone, olanzapine, quetiapine, ziprasidone, and aripiprazole – is believed to carry a lower risk of extrapyramidal side effects and to have greater efficacy in patients who fail to respond to conventional antipsychotic drugs (Masi et al., 2006a). These features are mostly present in the prototypical drug of this category, clozapine, but are only partly shared by the other atypical antipsychotic agents. From a pharmacological point of view, all these compounds share a combined dopamine-serotonin antagonism and a lower affinity for dopamine receptors, except for aripiprazole which acts as a partial agonist of dopamine receptors. Their use, formerly limited to psychotic disorders and schizophrenia, has gradually expanded to other psychiatric disorders, PDD, mood disorders (mostly bipolar disorder), disruptive behaviour disorders, Tourette's syndrome, OCD, and eating disorders. Unfortunately, only risperidone has been approved for children with PDD in the USA, while all other atypical antipsychotic agents are used off-label. Studies on the use of atypical antipsychotic drugs in adolescents with psychotic disorders and mental retardation remain limited. Most studies have reported on the efficacy and tolerability of this class of drug in young patients with PDD and disruptive behaviour disorders, and they will be considered in those sections. Taken as a whole, the use of the most commonly employed atypical antipsychotic agents, risperidone and olanzapine, has resulted in good efficacy and tolerability both in adolescents with mental retardation (Friedlander et al., 2001) and in mentally retarded adults (Williams et al., 2000).

People with mental retardation are at risk of side effects, namely sedation, weight gain, and extrapyramidal symptoms (parkinsonism, dystonic reactions, akathisia). Persons with mental retardation are more prone than general population to the most troublesome side effect of antipsychotic treatment – namely neuroleptic malignant syndrome – which is characterized by hyperthermia, muscular rigidity, tachycardia, hyper- or hypotension, autonomic instability, meionecrosis, and altered mental state (Masi *et al.*, 2006a). When unrecognized and untreated, this condition can progress to loss of consciousness and death.

Attention deficit hyperactivity disorder

Attention deficit hyperactivity disorder (ADHD) is one of the most commonly diagnosed and best studied mental disorders in mentally retarded children and adolescents, with a prevalence of approximately eight per cent (Emerson, 2003). Methylphenidate and other psychostimulants have been assessed in ADHD in at least 20 well controlled studies in the past 15 years; in most of these, they have proven effective at reducing hyperactivity, inattention, and impulsiveness (Handen & Gilchrist, 2006). Improvement in social functioning, cognitive performance, and classroom behaviour has also been reported (Handen *et al.*, 1995; Aman, 1996), with a mean response rate of about 50 per cent and a reduced response as the IQ decreases (Aman *et al.*, 2003). It is important to note that this rate is significantly below the 75 per cent found in patients with normal IQ. Furthermore, beyond the common side effects of stimulants (reduced appetite, insomnia, growth suppression, abdominal pain, cephalalgia), children with mental retardation have a higher risk of specific side effects, including irritability, tics, stereotypies, and social withdrawal (Handen *et al.*, 1991). No studies are available with alternative non-stimulant drugs such as the TCA group or the more recent specific inhibitor of noradrenaline reuptake, atomoxetine – now considered the best alternative to stimulant treatments if they are ineffective or when side effects limit their use.

Pervasive developmental disorders

Pervasive developmental disorders (PDD) are severe and early-onset (in the first 3 years of life) psychiatric disorders which typically cause severe impairment of reciprocal social interaction, communication, and cognitive development. Mental retardation is associated with PDD in about 75 per cent of affected subjects (American Psychiatric Association, 1994). Although there is currently no cure for autism or other PDD, the appropriate use of medication can reduce many of the associated maladaptive behaviours and enhance the subject's ability to benefit from educational interventions, behavioural strategies, speech therapy, and occupational treatments. Primary behavioural targets of pharmacotherapy in autism include impaired social behaviour, interfering repetitive phenomena, and aggression towards self, others, and property (Masi, 2004). Antipsychotic agents (mainly atypical antipsychotics) and antidepressants (mainly serotonergic agents) are the most commonly used drugs.

Risperidone is currently the atypical antipsychotic agent most often used in PDD patients. One controlled study of risperidone has been published in children and adolescents (Research Units on Pediatric Psychopharmacology, 2002). This included 101 subjects (age range 5 to 17 years, mean age 8.8 years); 69 per cent of the patients in the risperidone group and 12 per cent in the placebo group were responders by the eighth week, but by the sixth month, the rate of response decreased to 47 per cent. Irritability, hyperactivity, and stereotypies were more sensitive to treatment than were social withdrawal and inappropriate speech. Increased appetite and weight gain, fatigue, and drowsiness were the most commonly reported side effects. Masi *et al.* (2001) described efficacy and tolerability of risperidone treatment in children aged 3.6 to 6.6 years (mean 4.6 years) in a 16-week open label trial. In an enlargement of that study (Masi *et al.*, 2003), describing systematic data from a further 3-year naturalistic study on 53 preschool children with PDD (age range 3.5 to 6.6 years, mean 4.5 years), 46.8 per cent of the subjects were considered responders. Behavioural disorders and affect dysregulation were more sensitive to treatment than interpersonal functioning. Increased prolactin levels without clinical signs and increased appetite were the most frequent side-effects.

There is less evidence for the efficacy of olanzapine. Kemner *et al.* (2002) explored efficacy and tolerability of olanzapine in 25 patients (age range 6 to 16 years) in an open-label study, with a significant improvement in irritability, hyperactivity, excessive speech, and some autistic symptoms, assessed by the Aberrant Behavior Checklist. More recently, Hollander *et al.* (2006) randomized 11 patients with PDD, aged 6 to 14 years: 50 per cent of those on olanzapine *vs.* 20 per cent on placebo were responders, but olanzapine was associated with significant weight gain.

Regarding antidepressant use in PDD, DeLong and coworkers (2002) have treated 129 autistic children (aged 2 to 8 years) with fluoxetine, with an excellent response in 22 subjects (17 per cent), a good response in 67 subjects (52 per cent), and a fair or poor response in 40 subjects (31 per cent). Treatment response correlated highly with familial major affective disorder (mainly bipolar disorder). Five children treated for more than 3 years developed bipolar disorder during the treatment.

Sertraline was used at low dosage (25–50 mg daily) in a case series of nine autistic children and resulted in a decrease in anxiety symptoms, irritability, and the need for sameness, though three of the eight responders had a recurrence of symptoms after 3 to 7 months (Steingard *et al.*, 1997). Two subjects showed behavioural activation when the sertraline dose was increased to 75 mg/day, suggesting a possible dose effect.

Promising results from a placebo-controlled study in autistic adults treated with fluvoxamine (276.7 mg daily) (McDougle *et al.*, 1996) were not confirmed in a 12-week double-blind, placebo-controlled study in 34 PDD children and adolescents from the same research group; the drug was ineffective (only one of the 18 treated patients improved significantly) and many subjects had side effects (insomnia, hyperactivity, agitation, aggression). Developmental changes in serotonin function across the life span may account for the striking differences in the efficacy and tolerability of treatment at different ages.

More recently, two open-label studies (Couturier & Nicolson, 2002; Namerow *et al.*, 2003) supported the efficacy and safety of citalopram in children and adolescents with PDD, with good tolerability, a response rate of approximately 60 per cent, and improvement in anxiety and mood (but less in social relatedness).

Finally, two studies have explored the efficacy of newer antidepressants that act on both serotonin and noradrenaline (venlafaxine and mirtazapine), based on the hypothesis that the noradrenergic action may improve hyperactive and inattentive symptoms (Hollander *et al.*, 2000; Posey *et al.*, 2001). Improvement in hyperactivity and inattention, and to a lesser degree in aggression, self-injury, and irritability, were found, while social impairment was not affected by treatment.

Disruptive behaviour disorders

Disruptive behaviour disorders (DBD) include the following: conduct disorder, characterized by aggressive behaviour towards other persons or animals or properties, as well as deceitfulness, theft, or other severe violations of rules; oppositional defiant disorder, with defiant, negativistic behaviour; and DBD not otherwise specified. In person with mental retardation a frequently associated core element is self-aggressive behaviour. DBD are among the most frequent reasons for referral in patients with mental retardation, and are commonly treated with drugs, mainly antipsychotic agents (Aman & Gharabawi, 2004).

Risperidone is the most studied drug used in the treatment of children and adolescents with co-morbid DBD, and it has proven effective at controlling hyperactivity, irritability, hostility, aggression, and self-injurious behaviour. Well-designed studies, both controlled and open label – including large samples of children and adolescents with mental retardation and severe behavioural disorders – support the efficacy of risperidone in DBD in the short and medium term (Aman *et al.*, 2002; Snyder *et al.*, 2002; Aman *et al.*, 2004; Findling *et al.*, 2004). The rate of response in patients taking risperidone was about 50 per cent (*vs.* 7.8 per cent in the placebo group), and the clinical response was apparent within the first week of treatment (Aman *et al.*, 2002). However, concerns about long term safety of these drugs have been raised more recently for the following reasons: weight gain, alterations of glucose metabolism (type II diabetes), and alterations of lipid metabolism (hyperlipidaemia, hypercholesterolaemia). Furthermore, at higher doses or with rapid titration, risperidone treatment can be associated with extrapyramidal side effects. Similar side effects have been found during olanzapine treatment (Handen *et al.*, 2006). Quetiapine and aripiprazole are associated with a significantly lower weight gain, but data on their efficacy in mental retardation are still lacking.

Given these concerns over safety, children and adolescents with mental retardation and DBD should first have a trial with a mood stabilizer (for example, valproic acid in children, lithium in adolescents), and an antipsychotic agent may be used in the most severe conditions, or in those with poor clinical response.

Conclusions

The pharmacotherapy of mental disorders in people with mental retardation is an understudied field. This is partly a consequence of diagnostic overshadowing – people with mental retardation are still considered less likely to be affected by these disorders. However, people with mental retardation are also usually excluded from participation in formal controlled studies aimed at exploring the efficacy and safety of new drugs. Only recently have studies specifically included children and adolescents with subaverage intelligence in order to address the issue of any peculiarities in their clinical responses (efficacy and safety). Most of the findings have relied on open-label studies and have involved small samples of patients, with limited potential for generalization. To date, the available research suggests that the same drug treatments can be effective in patients of normal IQ and in mentally retarded patients, though the response rate is lower and the risk of side effects greater in mental retardation (Handen & Gilchrist, 2006).

General principles for the use of psychotropic drugs in mental retardation are as follows:

- Pharmacotherapy should be used only after a careful evaluation of the severity of the symptoms, any concurrent psychosocial variables, and alternative non-pharmacological interventions.

- Treatment should be started only after a careful diagnostic process and after a psychiatric diagnosis, including target symptoms for the pharmacological intervention.
- The initial dose should be lower and titration should be slower than in patients with a normal IQ.
- The response to treatment and the evolution of the mental disorder should be monitored using a rigorously applied structured follow-up protocol.
- Close monitoring of side effects should be mandatory, given the greater risk of most of these events in people with mental retardation.
- The possibility of discontinuing the drug(s) should be considered periodically (though chronic treatment may be necessary in schizophrenia, in severe and recurrent mood disorders, in severe and recurrent OCD, or in chronic aggression).

References

Aman, M.G. (1991): *Assessing psychopathology and behavior problems in persons with mental retardation: a review of available instruments*. (DHHS Publication No. ADM 91–1712). Rockville, MD: US Department of Health and Human Services.

Aman, M.G. (1996): Stimulant drugs in the developmental disabilities revisited. *J. Dev. Phys. Disabil.* **8**, 347–355.

Aman, M.G. & Madrid, A. (1999): Atypical antipsychotics in persons with developmental disabilities. *Ment. Retard. Dev. Disabil. Res. Rev.* **5**, 253–263.

Aman, M.G. & Gharabawi, G.M. (2004): Treatment of behavior disorders in mental retardation: report on transition to atypical antipsychotics, with emphasis on risperidone. *J. Clin. Psychiatry* **65**, 1197–1210.

Aman, M.G., Arnold, L.E. & Armstrong, S.C. (1999): Review of serotonergic agents and perseverative behavior in patients with developmental disabilities. *Ment. Retard. Dev. Disabil.* **5**, 279–289.

Aman, M.G., De Smedt, G., Derivan, A., Lyons, B., Findling, R.L. & Risperidone Disruptive Behavior Study Group (2002): Risperidone treatment of children with disruptive behavior symptoms and subaverage IQ: a double-blind, placebo-controlled study. *Am. J. Psychiatry* **159**, 1337–1346.

Aman, M.G., Buican, B. & Arnold, L.E. (2003): Methylphenidate treatment in children with borderline IQ mental retardation: analysis of three aggregated studies. *J. Child. Adolesc. Psychopharmacol.* **13**, 29–40.

American Psychiatric Association (1994): *Diagnostic and Statistical Manual of mental disorders*, 4th ed. Washington, DC: American Psychiatric Association.

Couturier, J.L. & Nicolson, R. (2002): A retrospective assessment of citalopram in children and adolescents with pervasive developmental disorders. *J. Child Adolesc. Psychopharmacol.* **12**, 243–248.

DeLong, G.R., Ritch, C.R. & Burch, S. (2002): Fluoxetine response in children with autistic spectrum disorder: correlation with familial major affective disorder and intellectual achievement. *Dev. Med. Child Neurol.* **44**, 652–659.

Einfeld, S.L. & Aman, M. (1995): Issues in the taxonomy of psychopathology in mental retardation. *J. Autism Dev. Disord.* **25**, 143–167.

Einfeld, S.L. & Tonge, B.J. (1996): Population prevalence of psychopathology in children and adolescents with intellectual disability: II. Epidemiological findings. *J. Intellect. Disabil. Res.* **40**, 99–109.

Emerson, E. (2003): Prevalence of psychiatric disorders in children and adolescents with and without intellectual disability. *J. Intellect. Disabil. Res.* **47**, 51–58.

Findling, R.L., Aman, M.G., Eerdekens, M., Derivan, A., Lyons, B. & Risperidone Disruptive Behavior Study Group (2004): Long-term, open-label study of risperidone in children with severe disruptive behaviors and below-average IQ. *Am. J. Psychiatry* **161**, 677–684.

Friedlander, R., Lazar, S. & Klancnik, J (2001): Atypical antipsychotic use in treating adolescents and young adults with developmental disabilities. *Can. J. Psychiatry* **46**, 741–745.

Gillberg, C., Persson, E., Grufman, N. & Themmer, V. (1986): Psychiatric disorders in mildly and severely mentally retarded urban children and adolescents: epidemiological aspects. *Br. J. Psychiatry* **149**, 68–74.

Handen, B.L. & Gilchrist, R. (2006): Practitioner review: psychopharmacology in children and adolescents with mental retardation. *J. Child Psychol. Psychiatry* **47**, 871–882.

Handen, B.L., Feldman, H., Gosling, A., Breaux, A.M. & McAuliffe, S. (1991): Adverse side effects of Ritalin among mentally retarded children with ADHD. *J. Am. Acad. Child Adolesc. Psychiatry* **30**, 241–245.

Handen, B.L., McAuliffe, S., Janowski, J., Breaux, A.M. & Feldman, H. (1995): Methylphenidate in children with mental retardation and ADHD: effects on independent play and academic functioning. *J. Dev. Phys. Disabil.* **7**, 91–103.

Handen, B.L., Stahl, R. & Hardan, A. (2006): Open-label, prospective trial of olanzapine in adolescents with subaverage intelligence and disruptive behavioral disorders. *J. Am. Acad. Child Adolesc. Psychiatry* **45**, 928–935.

Hellings, J.A., Kelley, L.A., Gabrielli, W.F., Kilgore, E. & Shah, P. (1996): Sertraline response in adults with mental retardation and autistic disorder. *J. Clin. Psychiatry* **57**, 333–336.

Hollander, E., Kaplan, A., Cartwright, C. & Reichman, D. (2000): Venlafaxine in children, adolescents and young adults with autism spectrum disorders: an open retrospective clinical report. *J. Child Neurol.* **15**, 132–135.

Hollander, E., Wasserman, S., Swanson, E.N., Chaplin, W., Schapiro, M.L., Zagursky, K. & Novotny, S. (2006): A double-blind placebo-controlled pilot study of olanzapine in childhood/adolescent pervasive developmental disorder. *J. Child Adolesc. Psychopharmacol.* **16**, 541–548.

Kemner, C., Willemsen-Swinkels, S., de Jonge, M., Tuynman-Qua, H. & van Engeland, H. (2002): Open-label study of olanzapine in children with pervasive developmental disorders. *J. Clin. Psychopharmacol.* **22**, 455–460.

Madrid, A.L., State, M.W. & King, B.H. (2000): Pharmacological management of psychiatric and behavioral symptoms in mental retardation. *Child Adolesc. Psychiatr. Clin. North Am.* **9**, 225–243.

Masi, G. (1998): Psychiatric illness in mentally retarded adolescents. *Adolescence* **33**, 425–434.

Masi, G. (2004): Pharmacotherapy of pervasive developmental disorders in children and adolescents. *CNS Drugs* **18**, 1031–1052.

Masi, G. (2005): Prepubertal bipolar disorder: available pharmacological treatment options. *Expert Rev. Neurother.* **6**, 547–560.

Masi, G., Marcheschi, M. & Pfanner, P. (1997): Paroxetine in mentally retarded adolescents with depression: an open label study. *J. Intellect. Disabil. Res.* **41**, 268–272.

Masi, G., Mucci, M., Favilla, L. & Poli, P. (1999a): Dysthymic disorder in mild mentally retarded adolescents. *J. Intellect. Disabil. Res.* **43**, 80–87.

Masi, G., Mucci, M. & Favilla, L. (1999b): Depressive symptoms in adolescents with mild mental retardation. *Educ. Train. Ment. Retard. Dev. Disabil.* **34**, 223–226.

Masi, G., Favilla, L. & Mucci, M. (2000): Generalized anxiety disorder in adolescents and young adults with mild mental retardation. *Psychiatry* **63**, 54–64.

Masi, G., Cosenza, A. & Mucci, M. (2001): Open trial of risperidone in 24 young children with pervasive developmental disorders. *J. Am. Acad. Child Adolesc. Psychiatry* **40**, 1206–1214.

Masi, G., Brovedani, P., Mucci, M. & Favilla, L. (2002): Assessment of psychopathology in people with mental retardation. *Child Psychiatry Hum. Dev.* **32**, 227–237.

Masi, G., Cosenza, A., Mucci, M. & Brovedani, P. (2003): A three-year naturalistic study of 53 preschool children with pervasive developmental disorder treated with risperidone. *J. Clin. Psychiatry* **64**, 1039–1047.

Masi, G., Mucci, M. & Pari, C. (2006a): Children with schizophrenia: clinical picture and pharmacological treatment. *CNS Drugs* **20**, 841–866.

Masi, G., Perugi, G., Toni, C., Millepiedi, S., Mucci, M., Bertini, N. & Akiskal, H. (2006b): The clinical phenotypes of juvenile bipolar disorder: toward a validation of the episodic-chronic-distinction. *Biol. Psychiatry* **59**, 603–610.

McDougle, C.J., Naylor, S.T., Cohen, D.J., Volkmar, F.R., Heninger, G.R. & Price, L.H. (1996): A double-blind, placebo-controlled study of fluvoxamine in adults with autistic disorder. *Arch. Gen. Psychiatry* **53**, 1001–1008.

Moss, S., Emerson, E., Bouras, N. & Holland, A. (1997): Mental disorders and problematic behaviours in people with intellectual disability: future directions for research. *J. Intellect. Disabil. Res.* **41**, 440–447.

Namerow, L.B., Thomas, P., Bostic, J.Q., Prince, J. & Monuteaux, M.C. (2003): Use of citalopram in pervasive developmental disorders. *J. Dev. Behav. Pediatr.* **24**, 104–108.

Ollendick, T.H., Oswald, D.P. & Ollendick, D.G. (1993): Anxiety disorders in mentally retarded persons. In: *Psychopathology in the mentally retarded*, eds. J.L. Matson & R.P. Barret, pp. 123-143. Boston, MA: Allyn & Bacon Inc.

Posey, D.J., Guenin, K.D., Kohn, A.E. & McDougle, C.J. (2001): A naturalistic open-label study of mirtazapine in autistic and other pervasive developmental disorders. *J. Child Adolesc. Psychopharmacol.* **11**, 267–277.

Potter, H.W. (1971): Mental retardation: the Cinderella of psychiatry. In: *Psychiatric aspects of diagnosis and treatment of mental retardation*, ed. F.J. Menolascino, pp. 9-23. Seattle: Special Child Publications.

Reiss, S., Levitan, G.W. & Szyso, J. (1982): Emotional disturbance and mental retardation: diagnostic overshadowing. *Am. J. Ment. Defic.* **86**, 567–574.

Research Units on Pediatric Psychopharmacology (RUPP) Autism Network (2002): Risperidone in children with autism and serious behavioral problems. *N. Engl. J. Med.* **347,** 314–321.

Rutter, M., Graham, P. & Yule, W. (1970): A neuropsychiatric study in childhood. *Clin. Dev. Med.* **35/36**. London: Heinemann/Spastics Society.

Snyder, R., Turgay, A., Aman, M., Binder, C., Fisman, S., Carroll, A. & The Risperidone Conduct Study Group (2002): Effects of risperidone on conduct and disruptive behavior disorders in children with subaverage IQs. *J. Am. Acad. Child Adolesc. Psychiatry* **41,** 1026–1036.

Steingard, R.J., Zimnitzky, B., De Maso, D.R., Bauman, M.L. & Bucci, J.P. (1997): Sertraline treatment of transition-associated anxiety and agitation in children with autistic disorder. *J. Child Adolesc. Psychopharmacol.* **7,** 9–15.

Venstraelen, M. & Tyrer, S.P. (1999): Rapid cycling bipolar affective disorder in people with intellectual disability: a systematic review. *J. Intellect. Disabil. Res.* **43,** 349–359.

Vitiello, B., Behar, D. & Spreat, S. (1989): Obsessive-compulsive disorder in mentally retarded patients. *J. Nerv. Ment. Dis.* **177,** 232–236.

Williams, H., Clarke, R., Bouras, N., Martin, J. & Holt, G. (2000): Use of atypical antipsychotics olanzapine and risperidone in adults with intellectual disability. *J. Intellect. Dis. Res.* **44,** 164–169.

Chapter 14

Neuropsychological rehabilitation in children with cognitive impairment

Chiara Gagliardi, Sara Martelli and Renato Borgatti

Neurorehabilitation Unit, IRCCS 'E. Medea', via Don Luigi Monza 20, 23842 Bosisio Parini (Lc), Italy
renato.borgatti@bp.lnf.it

Summary

In general, the study of a growing organism implies a peculiar viewpoint and specific standards for analysis. This is far more evident if there is substantial plasticity involved – as in the developing nervous system. In case of neural malformations, the development of cognitive functions is both a result of and a starting point for the current and future profile. The category of adaptation, or re-adaptation, must be applied to developmental neuropsychology, which thus needs to find its own specificity and be differentiated from adult neuropsychology. The underlying variables and theories are so complex that a suitable method is still to be defined.

In order to apply adequate environmental stimulation, which is essential for cognitive improvement, developmental neuropsychology is involved at the level of both evaluation and therapy.

Rehabilitation is a complex process, aimed at promoting the best possible quality of life for the child and the family. This is put into practice by formulating a rehabilitation plan and a combination of active therapeutic programmes in the three fields of re-education, assistance, and education. Rehabilitation therapy is the medical intervention phase which therefore proves to be discontinuous and limited in time. The main field of intervention is the improvement in the adaptive resources and functional adaptations in clinical situations.

In this chapter we will discuss the three themes of evaluation, intervention (variables, planning, end), and environment empowerment.

Introduction

Developmental neuropsychology has differentiated from adult neuropsychology, thanks to a progressive identification and emphasis on its specificity. This specificity is linked to the growing organism, both for the presence of particular processes of organization and rearrangement, and for the impact that a congenital lesion or a lesion acquired early in life can have on functions still to be formed. This is a fascinating field, the enormous expansion of which also reflects concurrent developments in genetics, neurobiology, pharmacology and new technologies. It is also a complex field, continuously at risk of mistakes and simplifications, as Annette Karmiloff-Smith has emphasized: in their excitement at using the human genome project to uncover the functions of specific genes, researchers have often ignored one fundamental factor – the gradual process of ontogenetic development. The *developing* brain is very different from the adult brain. It starts out highly interconnected across regions and is neither localized nor specialized at birth, allowing interaction with the environment to play an important role in gene expression and the ultimate cognitive phenotype. From a neuroconstructivist perspective we can argue that domain-specific end states can stem from more domain-general start states, that associations may turn out to be as informative as dissociations, and that genetic mutations that alter the trajectory of ontogenetic development can inform nature/nurture debates. (Karmiloff-Smith & Thomas, 2003; Karmiloff-Smith, 2006).

Cognitive modules are the outcome of development, not its starting point

In the developmental period, pathogenic damage occurring during foetal life (as produced by congenital malformations) causes anatomical and functional re-adaptations, while at the same time directly influencing and limiting many opportunities for development; early functional impairment can cause extreme limitation of functional organization and jeopardize the possible later organization of connected functions (cascade effect).

Furthermore, phenotypes are more complex than what could be assumed based on the linear sequence of genetic codification, and proteins can interact with more than one structure and modify more than one function (Weiss, 1995). Moreover, the micro- and macro-malformational aspects, which are often multisystemic, can be the most obvious modification – though not necessarily the only one – and may involve several structures. The cognitive phenotype will thus depend on the rearrangement processes, on the malformation, and on the involvement of other structures or functions (correlated or linked by common final routes or by mediators) in a dynamic process.

Neuropsychological rehabilitation is a therapeutic process with complex methodological problems still unsolved. This lack of a general definition is due to subtle differences between schools, thoughts, and theories, with aims that range over the different functions or summarize them. Studies in neuropsychological rehabilitation have thus proceeded rather slowly in a field full of variables, aiming at a better definition of methods, objectives and verification, and combining clinical medicine/therapy and scientific approaches, thereby ensuring appropriate interventions.

Nervous system plasticity – which is especially high during the developmental period – is responsible for the production of new cells in the hippocampus (Gould *et al.*, 1999) and experience-related changes in the adult brain (Recanzone *et al.*, 1993; Robertson & Murre, 1999). Not all the experiences involve advantageous changes: some types of experience or stimulation can highlight, sometimes dramatically, deficits in vulnerable circuits because of the activation of a competitor network, involving further inhibition in an already malfunctioning module (Kapur, 1996). The rehabilitation process, with interactive stimulation and procedural organization, is based on opportunities provided by nervous system plasticity. Recent research shows that the neuroscientists' complete rejection of such untapped potential is misplaced (Robertson & Murre, 1999; Robertson, 2000), and there is considerable potential for the strengthening of connected neural networks. Lack of use and lack of stimulation should lead to atrophy of neural circuits with consequent loss of function, while the effects of environmental enrichment have now been described (see, for instance, Cancedda *et al.*, 2004, for visual system development).

The importance of adequate environmental stimulation is well known. It has been demonstrated in recent years – in humans as well as in animal models – that an environment rich in stimuli can lead to an increase in cortical synapses. In clinical examples of acquired damage (Duffau,

2006; Kelly et al., 2006) it has been shown that the type and amount of treatment can influence cortical reconnections, and that the type of experience can guide synaptic reorganization after cerebral damage.

'Cognitive impairment' is only a descriptive definition, aimed at providing an overall view and codifying a wide range of clinical pictures that are characterized by various relatively well-preserved abilities alongside other markedly compromised ones. The diagnosis of mental retardation based on standardized scale scores (World Health Organisation) in fact uses a general functioning indicator referred to the overall population. The performance on general tasks (based on scale criteria) does not provide any information on single functions or strategies/expedients. Moreover, especially in cases of difficult task solutions, an inadequate response is poorly informative from a qualitative point of view, both for any hypothesis of structure/function correlation and at a clinical/rehabilitation level. These problems are far more evident in the developmental period. Therefore it is more important to identify tools and methods leading to a deeper understanding and so intervene adequately and as early as possible.

The neuropsychological rehabilitation intervention

The rehabilitation process and neuropsychological rehabilitation

Rehabilitation is a complex process aimed at promoting the best possible quality of life for the child and the family. This process is concerned with the physical, mental, affective, communicative and relational skills of the individual, developed through direct and indirect actions in a familiar social and environmental context (ecological prerogative). This is put into practice by formulating a rehabilitation plan and a combination of active therapeutic programmes in the three fields of re-education, assistance, and education.

Rehabilitation, which could be called rehabilitation therapy, is a medical intervention phase which is discontinuous and limited in time. Like all therapies, its definition in terms of duration, intensity, and frequency is referred to guidelines and the latest knowledge about the biological processes involved in recovery; like all therapies, it must also define its conditions, methods, and characteristics and respond to the criteria of verification and effectiveness; and like all therapies it has an end point which identifies the end of the therapeutic phase but which does not coincide with the end of the rehabilitation process.

Neuropsychological rehabilitation therapy is placed within this framework. Its main field of intervention is the improvement of adaptive resources and functional adaptations in clinical situations. In the latter, the presence of damage (congenital or acquired) to the central nervous system implies a structural and functional change. This is often complex and is determined by multidimensional factors that can lead to an impoverishment of expression and potential. Neuropsychological rehabilitation does not therefore involve a single pathological picture. Knowledge of basic characteristics and of the impairment and involvement of structures instead constitute the fundamental components.

To date, it has not been possible to define a specific, exclusive approach to neuropsychological rehabilitation for the condition of 'cognitive impairment' because of the multidimensional nature of the impairment, and the inter- and intra-phenotype variability. The final aim of any therapeutic intervention can be identified as the improvement in the patients' wellbeing, enabling them to express their potential and, if possible, removing the unfavourable factors, or alternatively, reducing their impact to a minimum. By acquiring operative autonomies, each child will be able to follow their own evolutionary pathway, coping with limits and restrictions, but hopefully conscious that the presence of obstacles on the pathway does not in itself prevent anyone from reaching their destination (Gagliardi, 2002). The neuropsychological rehabilitation intervention thus constitutes a phase of an organized rehabilitation path, especially when mental retardation is involved. As it is not the only therapeutic/rehabilitation resource available, activation of this specific re-educational route is not necessarily required, even though better adaptation and an expansion of learning are to be hoped for in most patients. Furthermore it is not necessarily the only intervention (even where indicated). It should rather be coordinated with other re-educational or educational fields.

Neuropsychological rehabilitation: qualitative or quantitative evaluation?

Neuropsychological evaluation is an excellent tool in detecting specific deficits caused by a mosaic of several cortical functional deficits. The evaluation must be tailored to the level of functioning and adapted, in order to obtain reliable data and to avoid a floor effect (Jakab, 1990).

The level of cognitive impairment, and thus the level of general functioning, and the harmony (or lack of it) between the impairments across cognitive domains, can be very diverse. There are now several studies about typical characteristics in the cognitive profile of specific clinical pictures (for instance Williams syndrome, see elsewhere in this volume). Increasing knowledge and increasing specificity lead to a better identification of areas and domains to be investigated within the different clinical pictures.

Every neuropsychological evaluation must include an evaluation of general intellectual competence, thus providing a reference picture of the average competence level. However, this variable in itself is not very informative for the interpretation of the data collected because of the construction procedures of the tests, the complexity of the processes analysed, and the methodological problems involved in obtaining a control or reference group (Aylward, 2002).

Specific tests are used (see examples elsewhere in this volume) to define more precisely the specific characteristics of the different functions and their integration systems. The contribution of these tests to the evaluation of the patient enables a reference frame to be established. Thus, undertaking these tests requires the activation of many competences, either simultaneously or in sequence; lack of success on one subtest does not necessarily define a specific problem but is indicative of a complex process, with dysfunction at one or more levels yet to be defined. Analysis of results allows the identification of strengths, which will prove fundamental in the organization of rehabilitation treatment and in identifying the strategies to be facilitated. Specific tests and items targeting different functions enable us to explore and document individual functions on a quantitative level. The definition of mental retardation, however, covers a vast range of organization (or impairment) levels; the results are often non-significant quantitatively and sometimes it is not possible to administer (or interpret) specific tests to examine a particular function more thoroughly because of the presence of significant attention, cooperation, or activation deficits. Therefore, alongside the quantitative evaluation, it is essential to carry out a qualitative evaluation of the data collected, as this is often decisive in determining the therapy route; qualitative information is often neglected in comparison with the numerical data of the scores, but it is valuable and very informative. The qualitative components to evaluate could, for example, be the strategies and the compensations used, the type of error and how modifiable it is, the tendency to fatigue and therefore the ability to remain attentive to the task, the ability to take advantage of facilitations, and so on. The degree of motivation and the possibility of mobilizing both personal and environmental resources on the one hand, and low self-esteem, repeated failure, or the tendency to evade frustrating or unfulfilling tasks on the other, constitute some of the many variables that can influence the rehabilitation process (Gagliardi, 1999; 2002).

In theory, neuropsychological evaluation is possible in all situations; in reality, it proves difficult to obtain reliable data without a floor effect, particularly at a quantitative level, when there is significant impairment at the level of organization, especially across different domains. In our opinion, this limitation does not mean that the evaluation should be foregone; it should instead lead to careful consideration of the route to rehabilitation, using any available resource to enable residual potential to be expressed.

Neuropsychological evaluation, in its complexity, enables us to achieve two complementary but definitely not coincident aims: on the one hand, it allows a better definition of the characteristics of the cognitive profile (at its different levels and paying attention to its individual functions); on the other hand, it allows us to express a valid judgment on the modifiability of the clinical picture and on the timing and way in which the adaptive changes may be induced.

Neuropsychological rehabilitation: adaptation in cognitive impairment

Neuropsychological rehabilitation therapy is based on the data included in the subject's individual functional profile, though the general picture of what is known about the basic syndrome or pathology is available as a reference. As in any other clinical situation, the strategies and routes to follow, as well as the hierarchical order of the objectives (including diachronic ones), are indissolubly tied to the characteristics and needs of that individual. Also, as a general rule, the earlier the action is taken, the more effective it is, within the limits of the basic biological framework. In our experience, competences are best harmonized and procedures stabilized only if the interventions are flexible and are carried out over time (Gagliardi, 1999).

Rehabilitation therapy can act by attempting to recover lost functions through rebuilding connections in the damaged area, with stimuli and objectives established on the basis of the competence hierarchy (restoration therapy); or by seeking a substitute for the functions (reintegration therapy). In the latter case, the improvement is the result of the functional reorganization of the system. Once the retained abilities and strategies are identified – as well as those that are ineffective or latent – and the individual potential for learning new strategies is determined, compensatory strategies and alternative approaches to the problem are taught, using the preserved functions. Neuropsychological rehabilitation therapy can then be adjusted to help the subject adapt to the disability rather than rehabilitating the damaged function. Stimulation of cognitive processing, functional adaptation, and specific process stimulation can be a direct cognitive rehabilitation method.

The therapeutic plan, its content, methods (type of treatment, frequency), and duration can be formulated once the strong points, the existing strategies to be reinforced, and the types of stimuli have been identified, along with the route whereby the strategies are to be facilitated and the level of cooperation to be expected.

The criteria and methods of treatment planning differ according to age; the possibility of achieving significant results is also linked to the 'echo effect' – that is, to the possibility that facilitating and strengthening strategies are adopted synergistically in the different existential contexts. Moreover, whatever has been established during the course of treatment must of course be applicable in the different existential contexts, in order that the child does not to remain either activity-dependent or bound to the rehabilitation setting. The strategy for connecting and interfacing the various existential contexts (family, school, and other significant contexts) is therefore strictly part of the rehabilitation plan.

The clinical condition of 'cognitive impairment' is heterogeneous and the structure/function correlation is complex. During the developmental period in particular, the structural limitation connected with the presence of biological damage (which can rarely be pinpointed with precision, even though our knowledge of genotype/phenotype correlations has expanded) interacts in a complex way with the environment, the individual (clinical and existential) history and with the level of stimulation received. Clinical expression can vary and this necessarily requires a high degree of individualization in the clinical and rehabilitation approach; for this reason, any generalization of the intervention methods tends to be limiting and inevitably imprecise. By recognizing this limitation, however, we can try to identify valid clues to the different situations in which cognitive impairment is the central component.

INDIVIDUAL VARIABLES

• Age group
• Presence/absence of multisystemic impairment (e.g. sensory neural deficit; neuromotor deficit and/or limitation; significant, considerably limiting internal problems)
• Presence/absence of behavioural problems
• Level of attention and activation
• Possibility of voluntary control activation
• Adjustability

ENVIRONMENTAL VARIABLES

• Family compliance
• Type of settling and compliance at school

A rehabilitation approach method that takes the neuropsychological viewpoint into account can be put into practice very early on; however, a specific neuropsychological therapy intervention requires greater levels of cooperation and the ability at least to share the awareness of working together towards a common goal (an adapted version of the 'adult's rehabilitation contract'). Providing stimulation for improved functional adaptation means that adaptive methods and strategies can be activated, even early on. This stimulation may be provided by facilitating the behaviour and calibrating the stimuli, so that the environment can offer available situations for small children and motivate them to act and interact. Furthermore if the overall characteristics expected in the basic picture are already known, facilitations for establishing an expedient – even in the presence of structural limitations – may be introduced. At older ages, the plans can become more specific, always bearing in mind that the integration of all the different functions is interconnected and interdependent.

The concomitant presence of behavioural problems – which are sometimes the most obvious clinical component in a clinical picture of cognitive retardation – limits the real effectiveness of a traditional neuropsychological intervention. Aside from the pharmacological therapeutic resources (see elsewhere in this volume) and from the proposals for targeted routes (see, for example, the cognitive behavioural approach), it is still possible to individualize a route that takes into account the elements that come to light during the neuropsychological evaluation. Furthermore, behavioural and emotional aspects are sometimes constituent parts typical of the syndromic picture – as for example in Williams syndrome (Gagliardi, 2002; Frigerio et al., 2006) – and of the specific rehabilitation route.

Adaptations to the types of stimuli (for example, their size, localization, and intensity, and the scanning methods) are required because of the concurrent presence of neuromotor and sensory neural deficits, thus enabling one to decide whether it is appropriate to use one or more afferent methods at the same time or in sequence (such as the use or avoidance of auditory stimuli to recall visual attention, feedback, feed forward). Adjustments in both fields of facilitation (grip, technological adaptation, interface) and posture allow the planning of specific interventions, even in presence of neuromotor damage.

Aside from specific objectives, other more 'functional' objectives may be identified, which can turn out to be less process-specific and to involve overall cognitive functioning to a higher degree. Other competences besides those at which the treatment is specifically directed will also be activated, both in the rehabilitation field and in various existential contexts. The ability of both the children and their environment to use what is planned for them in a functional way and to apply it flexibly can lead to empowerment. In this sense, it is possible to reverse the tendency through an increase in attention span, a greater ability to structure activities within time and space, and the opportunity to obtain results more in line with those expected by the child and recognizable by others. Repeated experience of failure tends sometimes to cause stagnation, whereas the possibility of experiencing successful situations can lead to a greater willingness to try.

Neuropsychological rehabilitation: the length of a specific rehabilitative intervention

The choice of when to end treatment poses complex problems, especially in a pathological picture characterized by chronicity, or more specifically by the absence of definite recovery, as in *restitutio ad integrum*. A process of assistance – variable over time but nevertheless continuous – entails the involvement of many implied components and the presence of different problems occurring in the various stages of life. The different stages of life are accompanied by changes in the environment, stimulation, and educational input, all of which sustain and direct the process of change implied by learning. Rehabilitation therapy has, on the other hand, a beginning and an end, often with alternation between moments of therapeutic intervention and times when intervention is suspended. The expression of a rehabilitation prognosis, together with the expectation of possible change – albeit with inevitable uncertainty – is therefore necessary.

Thus discharge from rehabilitation therapy does not coincide with the end of rehabilitation, nor with the end of the child's development and learning. A cycle of therapy comes to an end either because the stated objectives have been achieved or because no significant effect or change can be achieved within a reasonable period of time. Discharge is already planned at the start of the cycle, even if this is often not explicit.

This general concept is even more relevant in clinical pictures of a congenital nature which are often characterized by chronicity rather than evolution. Chronicity subsumes situations with a different aetiopathogenesis. Expansion of knowledge and learning – more or less marked, more or less continuous, and more or less ubiquitous in multisystem problems which are in turn stable or unstable – is destined to continue in some way throughout life under favourable environmental conditions, while rehabilitative intervention must be targeted and limited to specific periods of life.

The active involvement of the family through the process of communicating the diagnosis and the prognosis, the definition of aims and the choice of tools, the allocation of tasks, and the adaptation of the physical, psychological, and social contexts are always fundamental.

Conclusions

The route to neuropsychological rehabilitation in mental retardation constitutes a significant resource to be included within the therapeutic possibilities in these conditions, and the earlier it is begun, the greater its effectiveness. Neuropsychological rehabilitation cannot solve the problem by itself, it does not cancel the difficulties, and it must not promise impossible changes; but it works towards an improvement in adaptation, an understanding of the present potential, and an upgrading of the quality of life. The tools are improving thanks to the expansion of research and knowledge. This is a road to be travelled by researchers, therapists and patients together – a road in which children with cognitive retardation can teach us how to help them to learn.

References

Aylward, G.P. (2002): Cognitive and neuropsychological outcomes: more than IQ scores. *Ment. Retard. Dev. Disabil. Res. Rev.* **8,** 234–240.

Cancedda, L., Putignano, E., Sale, A., Viegi, A., Berardi, N. & Maffei, L. (2004): Acceleration of visual system development by environmental enrichment. *J. Neurosci.* **24,** 4840–4848.

Duffau, H.J. (2006): Brain plasticity: from pathophysiological mechanisms to therapeutic applications. *Clin. Neurosci.* **13,** 885–897.

Frigerio, E., Burt, D.M., Gagliardi, C., Ciuffi, G., Martelli, S., Perrett, D.I. & Borgatti, R. (2006): Is everybody always my friend? Perception of approachability in Williams syndrome. *Neuropsychologia* **44,** 254–259.

Gagliardi, C. (1999): Aspetti visuospaziali e visuocostruttivi. In: *La sindrome di Williams*, eds. S.Vicari & A. Gianotti. Milan: FrancoAngeli.

Gagliardi, C. (2002): La compromissione delle competenze visuospaziali e visuocostruttive in età evolutiva. In: *I disturbi dello sviluppo*, eds. S. Vicari & M.C. Caselli. Bologna: Il Mulino.

Gould, E., Beylin, A., Tanapat, P., Reeves, A. & Shors, T.J. (1999): Learning enhances adult neurogenesis in the hippocampal formation. *Nat. Neurosci.* **2,** 260–265.

Jakab, I. (1990): Neuropsychological evaluation and rehabilitation in mental retardation. *Neuropsychol. Rev.* **1,** 137–164.

Kapur, N. (1996): Paradoxical functional facilitation in brain behaviour research: a critical review. *Brain* **119,** 775–790.

Karmiloff-Smith, A. (2006): The tortuous route from genes to behaviour: a neuroconstructivist approach. *Cogn. Affect. Behav. Neurosci.* **6,** 9–17.

Karmiloff-Smith, A. & Thomas, M. (2003): What can developmental disorders tell us about the neurocomputational constraints that shape development? The case of Williams syndrome. *Dev. Psychopathol.* **15,** 969–990.

Kelly, C., Foxe, J.J. & Garavan, H. (2006): Patterns of normal human brain plasticity after practice and their implications for neurorehabilitation. *Arch. Phys. Med. Rehabil.* **87** (Suppl. 12), 20–29.

Recanzone, G.H., Schreiner, C.E. & Merzenich, M.M. (1993): Plasticity in the frequency representation of primary auditory cortex. *J. Neurosci.* **13,** 87–103.

Robertson, I. & Murre, J.M. (1999): Rehabilitation of brain damage: brain plasticity and principles of guided recovery. *Psychol. Bull.* **125,** 544–575.

Robertson, I. (2000): Compensation for brain deficits. *Br. J. Psychiatry* **174,** 412–413.

Weiss, V. (1995): The advent of a molecular genetics of general intelligence. *Intelligence* **20,** 115–124.

Chapter 15

An educational approach in mental retardation: how to build an individualized education plan (IEP)

Stefania Bargagna, Margherita Bozza, Francesca Liboni and Anastasia Dressler

Department of Developmental Neuroscience, Stella Maris Scientific Institute, University of Pisa, viale del Tirreno 331, 56018 Calambrone, Pisa, Italy
sbargagna@inpe.unipi.it

Summary

Mental retardation is a disability characterized by significant limitations in both intellectual functioning and adaptive behaviour, as expressed in conceptual, social, and practical skills. Every person, even the most severely disabled, needs to be educated before undergoing a rehabilitation programme. The Individualized Education Plan (IEP) outlines in detail the objectives for improving the child's skills and may include activities focused on the family or a parent. Health care services and educational programmes may include special education provided by a certified teacher and focused on the needs of the child.
Normal needs are often forgotten in disabled children because their special needs predominate. The diagnosis forms a mask covering the real child beneath, and everything is interpreted in the light of the syndrome or disorder. Assessment of the child should define a diagnosis that is not aetiological or nosographic but functional. This means that it not only concerns the syndrome, but also describes points of weakness and strength in the affected child. The functional diagnosis must be updated on a regular basis, because needs and strengths may change over time. In the assessment, all areas of normal development, cognition, language, motor skills, school learning, and affective and social attitudes must be evaluated. A functional diagnosis helps to define the main current needs. School provides many opportunities for a child to learn and have new experiences. One of the main points of this chapter is to describe the role of academic learning in developing adaptive skills. School can contribute to cognitive empowerment and to social development. Academic achievements only have real meaning if they are linked to adaptive skills. Adaptive behaviour is defined as the performance of daily activities required for personal and social sufficiency and is an essential component in the evaluation of intellectual disability, as it allows us to assess how well individuals function in their own environment. This provides important clues for therapeutic and occupational interventions in childhood and adult life.

Normal and abnormal development in children with mental retardation

According to the American Association of Intellectual and Developmental Disabilities (AAIDD, formerly the AAMR), mental retardation is a disability characterized by significant limitations in both intellectual functioning and adaptive behaviour, as expressed in conceptual, social, and practical skills. This disability must show an onset before the age of 18 years.

There are five essential features of the definition: (1) limitations in present functioning must be considered in the context of the community environment typical of the individual's age and culture; (2) valid assessment needs to consider cultural and linguistic diversity as well as differences in communication, sensory, motor, and behavioural factors; (3) within one individual, limitations often coexist with strengths; (4) an important purpose of describing limitations is to develop a profile of the support required; (5) with appropriate personalized support over a sustained period, the functioning of people with mental retardation will generally improve (American Association on Mental Retardation, 2002).

While the medical and psychosocial communities were developing an acceptable definition and classification system, the educational community adopted its own system of classification. Their three-level system separated school-aged children with mental retardation into three groups, based on their predicted ability to learn (Kirk *et al.*, 1955). Children who were *educable* could learn simple academic skills but could not progress above fourth grade level. Children who were believed to be *trainable* could learn to care for their daily needs but had very few academic skills. Children who appeared to be *untrainable* or totally dependent were considered in need of long-term care, possibly in a residential setting.

Human development in both typically-developing and disabled children is determined not only by genetics and cognition, but also by the interaction with the environment, and by stimuli coming from environment itself. The progression of developmental stages is the same as in normal children, though much slower; children with mental retardation have many difficulties in progression from the sensory-motor stage to the representative stage – that is, from preoperative to operative. Progression may be enhanced by appropriate activities.

Because children with mental retardation often present with several problems, it is necessary to involve a team of practitioners from different areas (child psychiatrist, social worker, child psychologist, special education teacher, speech and language specialist, community agencies) to make a comprehensive diagnosis. This type of interdisciplinary team approach is relatively new, but is considered to be imperative for comprehensive assessment, treatment and management of children with mental retardation (Lubetsky *et al.*, 1995).

Medical, developmental and psychiatric histories are obtained. Behavioural analysis and psychoeducational, speech and language testing are completed. Medical and neurological assessments are carried out. Because of the complexity of mental retardation syndrome, an integrated programme is needed, with varied approaches. In 1980, Krebs wrote 'At the present time mental handicap has become a multidimensional polydisciplinary task. A structurally static consideration of the pathological anatomic data as an unalterable situation due to cerebral organic deficiency or classifying the handicap as a disease is no longer tenable. Therefore training programs with a joint medical and medical pedagogic approach are becoming increasingly important.' (Krebs, 1980).

The overall plan is a set of proposals for goals, activities and instruments that can be applied over a certain period of time and must be updated every 6 to 9 months. Several kinds of specialists contribute to the plan on the basis of their own knowledge and expertise regulated by national Italian Law (Law n. 4, August 1977, n. 517, art. 2;7). A diagnosis of function is necessary to achieve correct planning of the rehabilitation programme. This plan, the Individualized Education Plan (IEP), outlines in detail the objectives for improving the child's skills and may include activities focused on the family or a parent. Health care services and educational programmes may include special education provided by a certified teacher and focused on the needs of the child, such as child counselling, occupational therapy, physical therapy, speech therapy, recreational activities, school health services, transportation services, and parent training or counselling. Thus IEP in school is a substantial responsibility. It is required by law and is operated throughout Italy wherever a group of specialists can be assembled to undertake the programme.

The programme is composed of two parts: the first is the 'normal' educational approach and the second depends on the clinical features of the individual case. What is a normal educational approach? This signifies any common educational intervention that parents and caregivers initiate towards a child. Every individual, even the most severely disabled, needs to be educated before undergoing a rehabilitation programme.

Normal needs are often forgotten in disabled children, because their special needs predominate. The diagnosis forms a mask that covers the real child beneath, and everything is interpreted in the light of the syndrome or disorder.

The will to learn

The will to learn is a basic function in all children, but is generally forgotten in normal childhood because normal children succeed in whatever their surroundings propose. This is not true for children with mental retardation, because they lack motivation and cognitive strategies. This is a consequence not only of poor intelligence – a quantitative intelligence deficit – but also of the lack of strategies for using their skills. These abilities are also called metacognitive factors; they are particularly poor in several domains in children with mental retardation, as they exhibit no planning or self-monitoring, no personal theory of mental functioning, and poor affective motivation with low self-esteem.

A comprehensive assessment must be undertaken to obtain sufficient knowledge of the child. Such an assessment is necessary to make a diagnosis that is not aetiological or nosographic but functional. This means that it does not concern only the features of the child's syndrome, but also the areas of weakness and strength. The functional diagnosis must be updated, because needs and strengths may change over time. All areas of normal development must be evaluated: cognition, language, motor skills, school learning, and affective and social attitudes. The team members contribute to the assessments by their clinical impressions, written or oral records, and by tests, checklists and interviews.

The assessments involve clinical and school tests and free observations collected from parents, teachers and any other persons having a role in the child's life. Intelligence tests are the most common tools used in evaluating people with mental retardation (for instance, WISC-R, Leiter scale, Raven Matrices) to obtain a quantitative measure of intelligence. They must be used in conjunction with qualitative assessments of intelligence and adaptive function scales (adaptive behaviour is an important and necessary part of the definition and diagnosis of mental retardation). Assessment of adaptive behaviour focuses on how well an individual can function and maintain independence and how well they meet the personal and social demands imposed on them by their cultures. The most common scale is the Vineland Adaptive Behaviour Scale (VABS) (Sparrow *et al.*, 1984). The VABS – a revision of the Vineland Social Maturity Scale – assesses the social competence of individuals with and without disabilities from birth to 19 years. The VABS measures four domains: communication, daily living skills, socialization, and motor skills. A combination of the scores from the four domains gives an Adaptive Behaviour Composite.

Achievement tests (such as reading and mathematics) are heavily dependent on formal learning, are more culturally specific, and tend to sample more specific skills than intelligence tests do.

From this assessment we can obtain a personalized picture of strengths and weaknesses, integrating temperament, behaviour, and affect. The observational setting needs to be enlarged to cover the individual and group setting. The assessment must be global and integrated, but specific to an individual and adjusted for that individual's age.

Social and interpersonal interventions can be both preventive and therapeutic. As noted above, children with mental retardation are at increased risk of behavioural disorders. Thus, a variety of social and recreational activities in a group should be included in the child's educational programme. These activities should include non-disabled peers and may involve participation at parties, attending recreational activities such as ball games and movies, participating in youth sports, and visiting community sites such as the zoo. The goal of these activities should be to teach appropriate social skills relevant to group participation and the building of self-esteem.

From observational assessments, the interdisciplinary team formulates a functional diagnosis that identifies the main current needs. 'Need' is different from the general target or objective of therapy; it is determined by crucial and urgent difficulties due to external and internal factors; great importance is attributed to subjective suggestions for defining these needs.

The appropriate choice of therapeutic goals and strategies of intervention involves defining partial objectives, necessary activities, and the tools to be used. Every treatment plan must be reevaluated after a certain period of application. Educational, therapeutic, and scholastic goals together define a personalized programme which forms the IEP; families, schools and rehabilitation staff need to agree on the subjects, while at the same time differentiating their own intervention.

Aetiology and the pedagogic approach

A thorough knowledge of the causes of mental retardation can help in establishing a rehabilitation programme, but it should not obscure the individual needs of a child. Information about the clinical features of any given syndrome certainly helps in assessing the individual patient, because of the known risk factors in a particular disorder. However, the areas of weakness and strength defined by known genetic syndromes or imaging abnormalities are not sufficient to plan a rehabilitation programme. At the individual level, we are concerned with a person and not a syndrome. A plan suitable for all mentally retarded people is not feasible; on the contrary, treatments and educational courses need to be established for each child on a regular basis during development. The programme for every child must be individualized as far as possible, in a global assessment as described above (see Fig. 1 for a summary).

OBSERVATION	NEEDS
Cognitive (I.Q., strategies and use)	
Language	
Visual-perceptual abilities	
Motor skills	
Social and affective skills (Adaptive functions)	

⟹ **INTERVENTION**

Fig. 1. Pre-treatment evaluations.

Schooling and autonomy

Autonomy is often considered only secondary compared to school achievements. Nevertheless, adaptive functions are strictly linked to autonomy and have great impact on the quality of life. To be 'adapted' means to be able to do something autonomously and in a conscious way. Real autonomy in daily living skills may increase coping and self-monitoring strategies. In this way the main goal of an educational rehabilitative approach is to develop self-organizing abilities rather than conditioned skills. The acquisition of everyday skills is not sufficiently fostered by formal education, but rather by planning, thinking, and applying strategies of modelling and monitoring. School learning is important in our world, but writing, reading, and arithmetic are useful skills for life rather than primary goals.

In academic learning and in daily personal experience, everybody uses criteria of classification, exploration and memory. Typically-developing children learn without any apparent effort and their parents tend to forget about the importance of their learning strategies. Parents of children with mental retardation are generally more concerned about results than about strategies. They may find it difficult to support cognitive progression.

From a developmental perspective the gradual progression of thought needs to be encouraged and applied to problem solving: cognitive strategies can be supported in an educational approach.

In our clinical practice we support families in developing their children's autonomy as a necessary goal for an adequate quality of life. We attach importance to explaining the dual goal of achieving results, and applying learning strategies.

How and when should families be included in decision-making? Families must always be involved and are of crucial importance in the child's development. The family, especially the parents, have to be supported in their normal and enhanced educational role.

Health and education professionals who participate as team members must actively pursue a parent-professional partnership in the decision-making process. The logical first step is to acknowledge the value of the parent-professional relationship. Parents should be viewed as equal partners who can make important and necessary contributions to planning and decision-making. The family must be helped to find their own resources in these endeavours.

As a consequence of a recent diagnosis, parents may often be unable to see 'normal' parts in their 'ill' child. They often are depressed and have to be helped in seeing through the mask of the illness to recreate a good bond with their baby. Parent-child interactions must be addressed before motor and language skills are taught. To restore the affective balance is the first level of any 'prise en charge'.

In children with mental retardation, play is generally forgotten as a need. Play is an excellent way of exploring intellectual and relational skills and social competencies in children. It is a window into a child's mind and enriches many areas of development. There is a strong correlation between play and cognitive development. Thus, in children with mental retardation, play may be poorer. The quality of play ameliorates cognitive development, and mother-child interactions may be enriched through play activities (Bargagna et al., 1997).

Parent counselling should support the reinforcement of affective relationships and also provide an educational approach, with suggestions for activities, changes to the environment, and modifications of attitudes. It is quite common to see adolescents with mental retardation playing with inappropriate kinds of toys. Parents must be supported in choosing new steps towards autonomy for their child. The environment needs to be modified and enriched to offer new stimuli appropriate for the child's age and present needs.

Because meetings generally take place in school, it is quite easy to make the common mistake of assuming that IEP is meant to decide only what the teachers need to do in school for a particular pupil. This simplified view has to be expanded to involve all parts of the child's life – home, friends, sports, hobbies, and health.

School can provide opportunities for both the child and the family to learn and have new experiences. One of the main purposes of this chapter is to emphasize the way in which school achievement can be oriented towards adaptive functioning.

School can certainly contribute to cognitive empowerment and to improving social life, as it provides a unique occasion to socialize. Academic achievements only have real meaning if they help in developing adaptive skills. Even simplified participation in classes leads to a subjective sense of satisfaction. Moreover, the achievement of learning something increases self-esteem. School achievements are means rather than goals. No subject should be neglected, though a 'mechanical' approach should be avoided. Lessons in history, mathematics, and languages can enhance social competencies. Academic skills are not the main goal but they are part of an overall educational plan to develop social competence.

Adaptive function and quality of life

Adaptive behaviour is defined as the performance of daily activities required for personal and social sufficiency. It is an essential part of the evaluation of intellectual disability as it permits us to assess how well individuals function in their own environment. This provides important clues for therapeutic and occupational interventions. Adolescents with mental retardation show adaptive abilities that are generally greater than expected when compared to the level of retardation. Moreover, there are suggestions that people with mental retardation can improve their abilities even in adult life. It is therefore very important that individuals with mental retardation are provided with work or with some kind of occupation to avoid loss of performance. Down syndrome represents a typical condition in which neuropsychiatric assessment and rehabilitative treatment are required (for a review see Bargagna *et al.*, 2001; 2005). Because of its characteristics it can also be used as a model for other groups of children with mental retardation. Research has demonstrated a slowing down of adaptive behaviour and cognitive abilities in Down syndrome with increasing age, but opinions diverge about the age at which this starts. Adaptive behaviour in Down syndrome is described as increasing until middle childhood and then beginning to decline in adolescence. Studies have focused on adaptive skills in adulthood as an early sign of decline. Zigman *et al.*, in a cross-sectional study, found an increasing decline in adaptive behaviour in subjects with Down syndrome over 50 years of age compared with younger adults, and a greater decline in Down syndrome than in intellectual disability of other aetiology (Zigman *et al.*, 1987). Particularly affected areas were gross motor functioning, working, dressing/grooming, eating, and independent living. To avoid the onset of dementia, a training programme to reinforce daily skills may be useful. In recent research from our group, we found that in childhood and adolescence, areas of strength in adaptive behaviour were communication and daily living skills, whereas in young and middle adult life, performance in socialization and daily living skills were better (Bargagna *et al.*, 2004). Mental functioning can be improved by operative strategies in persons with mental retardation, leading to increased independence and adaptive abilities. Daily skills are often acquired in mentally retarded people by conditioning activities and have a limited association with mental cognitive ability. Our suggestion is that an integrated approach to patients with mental retardation involves not only *doing* things, but also *planning* to do them. Training that starts with daily activities may, through monitoring, analysis of strategies, and problem solving empower skills and cognition. We suggest a rehabilitative approach where cognitive development is strictly linked to adaptive skills. Thus, the main defective areas in mental retardation can sustain one another. In a sample of 10 patients with mild mental retardation (five male, five female, age range 23 to 34 years) a follow-up study over 18 months showed improvement in cognitive functioning as well as in adaptive functions. The subjects lived independently, attending to household work, shopping, and organising their leisure time. Their perception of satisfaction improved.

The great interest of this approach is the increase in quality of life for people with mental retardation. Self-determination is generally poor in individuals with mental retardation because of poor strategies and lack of opportunities to make choices. Studies by Lachapelle and Nota (Lachapelle *et al.*, 2005; Nota *et al.*, 2006) have explored work self-determination, autonomy, and life choices in people with mental retardation before and after they moved from a more restrictive to a less restrictive type of work. This change resulted in improvement in skills, enhancing self-determination and quality of life.

References

American Association on Mental Retardation (2002): *Mental retardation: definition, classification, and systems of supports*. Washington, DC: American Association on Mental Retardation.

Bargagna, S. (2001): *Il ritardo mentale in età evolutiva: indicazioni per un percorso educativo e riabilitativo*. Pisa Edizioni del Cerro.

Bargagna, S. (2005): *La sindrome di Down: proposte per un percorso educativo e riabilitativo*. Pisa: Edizioni del Cerro.

Bargagna, S., Millepiedi, S., Marcheschi, M. & Battaglia, A. (1997): Play development and mother-child interaction in DS. In: Sixth World Congress on Down Syndrome, Madrid 23–26 October, 1997.

Bargagna, S., Perelli, V., Dressler, A., Pinsuti, M., Colleoni, A., Rafanelli, V. & Chilosi, A.M. (2004): Rapporti fra abilità linguistiche, cognitive e profili di sviluppo adattivo in giovani adulti con sindrome di Down. *Psicologia Clinica dello Sviluppo* **3,** 459–484.

Cicchetti, D.V. & Beeghly, M. (1990) *Children with Down Syndrome*. Cambridge: Cambridge University Press.

Krebs, H. (1980): Present problems in the mentally handicapped. *MMW Münch. Med. Wochenschr.* **122,** 1849–1854.

Kirk, S.A., Karnes, M.B. & Kirk, W.D. (1955): *You and your retarded child*. New York: Macmillan.

Lachapelle, Y., Wehmeyer, M.L., Haelewyck, M.C., Courbois, Y., Keith, K.D., Schalock, R., Verdugo, M.A. & Walsh, P.N. (2005): The relationship between quality of life and self-determination: an international study. *J. Intellect. Disabil. Res.* **49,** 740–744.

Lubetsky, M.J., Mueller, L., Madden, K., Walker, R. & Len, D. (1995): Family-centered/interdisciplinary team approach to working with families of children who have mental retardation. *Ment. Retard.* **33,** 251–256.

Nota, L., Soresi, S. & Perry, J. (2006): Quality of life in adults with an intellectual disability: the evaluation of Quality of Life Instrument. *J. Intellect. Disabil. Res.* **50,** 371–385.

Sparrow, S.S., Balla, D.A. & Cicchetti, D.V. (1984): *The Vineland Adaptive Behaviour Scales*. Circle Pines, MN: America Guidance Service.

Zigman, W.B., Schupf, N., Lubin, R.A. & Silverman, W.P. (1987): Premature regression in adults with Down syndrome. *Am. J. Ment. Defic.* **92,** 161–168.

Chapter 16

Medical treatments for mental retardation: the neurobiological bases for new therapeutic approaches

Alessandro Zuddas, Nicoletta Adamo, Cristina Peddis, Giulia Congia and Tatiana Usala

Centre for Pharmacological Therapies in Child and Adolescent Neuropsychiatry, Department of Neuroscience, University of Cagliari, via Ospedale 119, 09124 Cagliari, Italy
azuddas@unica.it

Summary

In the past few years, several pharmacological agents used to improve syndromes that are not categorized primarily as cognitive disorders have been shown to enhance learning and memory, providing important insights into specific neurobiological processes regulating the mechanisms of cognition. New compounds specifically designed to improve learning and memory have been investigated. Although at its initial stage, the very concept of cognitive enhancement in normal people is controversial, giving rise to important ethical issues which, in turn, may be slowing the development of new pharmacological tools for people with mental retardation.

Introduction

The medical approach to mental retardation is founded on the prevention of possible aetiological factors (for example, genetic syndromes or hereditary metabolic diseases), and on the treatment of concomitant medical or psychiatric disorders (comorbidities). In individuals with developmental disabilities, however, the behavioural resultants of comorbidities are often severe enough to require integrated behavioural and psychopharmacological treatment to stabilize the patient's condition and enhance their quality of life (Chen *et al.*, 2006).

In the past few years, several lines of evidence have elucidated how specific neurobiological processes may regulate the abilities of information capturing, maintenance, and processing, as well as modulating cognitive and behavioural responses to external stimuli. Impaired attention, problems in information processing, and difficulties with working memory characterize subjects with mental retardation and patients with psychiatric disorders.

Subjects with mental retardation usually consult mental health care specialists because of impairment of adaptive function rather than for cognitive deficit. Nevertheless, improvement in attention, visuospatial skills, time and space perception, and memory is crucial for rehabilitation in mental retardation. Thus the enhancement of these features could be useful for improving autonomy and social integration skills, such as reading, writing, computation, money management, using the phone, household skills, interpersonal skills, and occupational abilities. Cognitive improvement has great importance in facilitating the development and reinforcement of skills that have not been developed and consolidated spontaneously.

Neurobiology of cognition

Behind an apparently straightforward action, there is an enormous complexity of processes which the brain faces in perceiving the scene, deciding on a course of action, and then executing it. Choosing a toy from a toy box, like innumerable actions carried out every day, involves a surprising array of cognitive functions. First, the visual system reconstructs an accurate representation of the scene, and a higher level decision processes must evaluate the perceptual information and select one toy in particular. More specifically, the brain must categorize the toys (the specific kind, colour, and so on), assign appropriate affective associations to them (likes or dislikes), deploy spatial attention to salient objects in the scene, and discriminate fine differences in colour, size, and shape to select the best. Thus the decision is shaped by immediate sensory information, by previously learned categories drawn from visual memory, and by likes and dislikes based on accumulated experience. Other elements in the scene that are irrelevant to the decision must be ignored. Finally, once the brain reconstructs the scene and makes a decision, voluntary movement systems must plan and execute the appropriate behavioural response (Nichols & Newsome, 1999).

The recent positron emission tomography (PET) and functional magnetic resonance imaging (fMRI) studies have provided many insights into the localization of mental functions (Posner & Raichle, 1998; Rueda *et al.*, 2004). Cognitive functions involve complex cellular and circuit interactions centred in the prefrontal cortex (Robbins, 2000). Both procedural learning (that is, the process of learning either a cognitive or a motor procedure in which the strategy of execution cannot be explicitly described, such as learning by doing) and memory also require intact basal ganglia to operate properly. In addition, emotions have powerful influences on learning and memory: they involve multiple brain systems engaged at different stages of information processing. Studies of declarative emotional memory show how fronto-temporal brain regions act jointly to promote the retention of emotionally arousing events and retrieve them from long-term storage. Memory-enhancing effects of emotional arousal involve interactions between subcortical and cortical structures and the engagement of central and peripheral neurohormonal systems that are coordinated by the amygdala. The contributions of the amygdala, prefrontal cortex, and medial temporal lobe to the memory system extend beyond the initial period of memory consolidation, and involve the retrieval of emotional memories, including those from the personal past (LaBar & Cabeza, 2006).

The role of executive functions in cognition

Definitions of executive function hinge on the classic distinction between automatic and effortful processing – while the former provides an efficient means of responding to routine situations, the latter is required for adaptive responses to novel or complex situations. Executive functions involve a range of higher order cognitive processes (for example, set shifting, inhibition of prepotent responses, self-monitoring, and planning), associated with the functions of the prefrontal cortex (Pennington & Ozonoff, 1996; Ozonoff et al., 2004). Executive functions are commonly described as a set of mental control processes that enable self-control (Denckla, 1996; Pennington & Ozonoff, 1996) and are necessary to maintain an appropriate problem-solving set for the attainment of a future goal and to optimize performance in complex tasks (Welsh & Pennington, 1988). Executive functions include different metacognitive domains such as response inhibition, working memory, cognitive flexibility (set shifting), allocation of attention, planning, and fluency (Pennington & Ozonoff, 1996; Fuster, 1999). Working memory, in particular, serves to maintain temporary active representations of information for further processing or recall (Baddeley, 1996). It plays an important role in reducing distraction and controlling attention during complex cognitive activities such as mental calculation and language comprehension (Baddeley, 1996; Miyake & Shaw, 1999; de Fockert et al., 2001).

Two of the most studied developmental disorders – attention deficit hyperactivity disorder (ADHD) and autism – have been associated with executive function deficits (Pennington & Ozonoff, 1996; Barkley, 1997; Russell, 1997; Geurts et al., 2004). Subjects with paediatric bipolar disorder, regardless of the type of drug treatment, show impairments in the domains of attention, executive functioning, working memory, and verbal learning, compared with healthy controls. The cognitive deficits found in these individuals suggest significant involvement of frontal lobe (neocortical) systems, supporting working memory, and mesial temporal lobe systems, supporting verbal memory (Fuster, 1999; Cabeza & Nyberg, 2000; Pavuluri et al., 2006).

The prefrontal cortex modulates the ability to form internal representation of the external world for planning, organizing, and guiding forthcoming response sequences, based on ideas and thoughts instead of immediate external stimulation (Goldman-Rakic, 1995). Findings from recent studies suggest a role of prefrontal neurons in the representation of multiple attributes of sensory stimuli, including their associated motor connotations. The prefrontal cortex is crucial in motor preparation and in the cross-temporal mediation of sensory-motor contingencies, and therefore in the temporal organization of behaviour (Quintana et al., 1988; D'Esposito et al., 2000).

Neurochemical aspects of cognition

Attention is crucial for the initiation and modulation of cognition. The attentional system is characterized by three distinct neural networks processing. The *alerting network* suppress background neural noise to establish readiness to react and inhibit ongoing activity. It is linked to frontal lobe brain regions. The *orienting network* mobilizes neural resources to prepare for expected input, facilitating one type and inhibiting the others; it is centred on the posterior parietal cortex. The *executive control system* coordinates multiple specific neural process to direct behaviour, detecting the presence of a target, starting and stopping mental operations, and ordering multiple responses. It is centred in the prefrontal cortex and anterior cingulate gyrus and includes basal ganglia (Posner & Peterson, 1990).

Catecholamines modulate neuronal function in all these three networks. Both dopamine and noradrenaline depress the spontaneous activity of prefrontal cortical neurons and the responsiveness of cortical neurons to new inputs, enhancing their response to specific inputs. Dopamine also interacts with other systems such as the serotonin (5-HT) systems, which are components of the multiple attentional networks. The noradrenergic system is considered intimately associated with the modulation of higher cortical functions including attention, alertness, and vigilance. Dysregulation of the noradrenergic neurons in the locus coeruleus causes functional disruption to the cortical posterior attention system (Pliska et al., 1996). Electrophysiological and neurosurgical lesion studies on experimental animals have implicated the ascending dorsal noradrenergic bundle of the locus coeruleus system in cognitive processes such as memory, learning, and selective attention. Within the frontal lobes, noradrenaline is also crucial in the prevention of distractibility by irrelevant stimuli (Coull, 1994).

A crucial role for dopamine in regulating prefrontal cortex function has also been described. Dopamine neurons originating in the ventral tegmental area innervate the prefrontal cortex or septum and the nucleus accumbens (the mesocortical and mesolimbic dopamine systems, respectively). Mesocortical dopamine projections mediate cognitive functions such as verbal fluency, serial learning, vigilance for executive functioning, sustaining and focusing attention, prioritizing behaviour, and modulating behaviour based upon social cues (Solanto, 1998; Nieoullon, 2002). Decreased dopamine function at prefrontal synapses leads to deficits in inhibitory control and working memory. Negative and cognitive symptoms of schizophrenia have been shown to be related to a deficit of dopamine in the mesocortical pathway, such as the dorsolateral prefrontal cortex (Lewis & Gonzalez-Burgos, 2006; Tanaka, 2006). α_2-adrenoceptors have been found on a substantial number of dopamine cells in the substantia nigra and ventral tegmental area (Lee *et al.*, 1998) and may control both noradrenaline and dopamine release in the prefrontal cortex. It has been shown that in the prefrontal regions but not in the nucleus accumbens or in other limbic regions, blockade of α_2-adrenoceptors increases both dopamine and noradrenaline output (Devoto *et al.*, 2004; Devoto *et al.*, 2005).

Brain regions related to social cognition (amygdala, hippocampus, and other specific parieto-temporal regions) are modulated by prefrontal executive functions. Impairment of the modulating activity of the prefrontal cortex on the activity of the amygdala and the hippocampus has been observed in schizophrenia, obsessive-compulsive disorder, and ADHD. The brain regions for both executive function and social cognition are modulated by a dense serotoninergic innervation from the raphé nuclei of the brain stem. A deficit in serotoninergic function has been associated with worsened sleep, depressed mood, altered arousal, increased aggression, greater impulsivity, and reduced social behaviours. The actions of 5-HT are complex and depend greatly upon the specific location and class of receptor stimulated – depending on brain regions, a marked increase in extracellular 5-HT release can reduce appetite and aggression but also lead to a syndrome of distinctive repetitive behaviours. Serotonin also plays an important role in prenatal and postnatal brain development, regulating cell division, differentiation, neurite outgrowth, and synaptogenesis (Anderson *et al.*, 2002). More recently, several lines of evidence strongly suggest that specific 5-HT receptors (the $5-HT_6$ receptors, see below) can modulate long-term memory.

Hippocampal processes of neuroplasticity, such as long-term potentiation, have been proposed as a neurophysiological correlate of learning and memory (Bliss & Collingridge, 1993; Malenka & Nicoll, 1999; Morris *et al.*, 2003). In the hippocampus, excitatory transmission is mediated by glutamate acting on ionotropic NMDA and non-NMDA receptors, as well as on metabotropic receptors (Hollmann & Heinemann, 1994). The best understood form of long-term potentiation is induced by the activation of the N-methyl-D-aspartate receptor complex. This subtype of glutamate receptor endows long-term potentiation and allows electrical events at the postsynaptic membrane to be transduced into chemical signals; these activate both pre- and postsynaptic mechanisms to generate a persistent increase in synaptic strength (Williams *et al.*, 2003). Glutamatergic neurotransmision modulates physiological and pathological conditions such as neuronal plasticity, memory, and learning (Lynch, 2004). Agents that indirectly enhance NMDA-receptor function through the glycine modulatory site reduce negative symptoms and variably improve cognitive functioning in schizophrenic subjects receiving typical antipsychotic agents (Goff & Coyle, 2001; Coyle & Tsai, 2004).

Finally, diminished cholinergic activity has been associated with memory impairment. Acetylcholine is directly involved in anxiety, arousal, attention, fatigue, and sleep, as well as in several memory processes such as acquisition and consolidation (Karson et al., 1996).

Pharmacological modulation of cognition

Several lines of evidence indicate that drugs effective at ameliorating behavioural symptoms or thought disturbances in patients affected by different psychiatric disorders may also improve specific cognitive deficits in the same individuals. These observations have provided significant insight in the current knowledge the biology of cognition, leading to the characterization of new compounds specifically designed to improve learning and memory.

Second-generation antipsychotics as cognitive enhancers

Second-generation antipsychotic agents (clozapine, risperidone, olanzapine, and quetiapine) interact with serotonin and dopamine neurotransmission by blocking both 5-HT$_{2a}$ and D$_2$ receptors (Kapur et al., 1999). Some also show a more rapid dissociation from the dopamine D$_2$ receptor than the classic neuroleptics (Kapur & Remington, 2001). By modulating α_2-adrenoreceptors, these drugs also increase both dopamine and noradrenaline output in the prefrontal cortex but not in the limbic regions (Devoto et al., 2004).

The antipsychotic effect becomes evident only at doses at which their D$_2$ dopamine receptor occupancy in the limbic regions exceeds 65 per cent – a threshold of efficacy no different from that of haloperidol (a typical antipsychotic agent). This confirm the crucial role of the D$_2$ receptors in the modulation of the salience of the external stimulus (Kapur et al., 1999). In the prefrontal cortex the combined blockade of the 5-HT$_{2a}$ receptors and α_2-adrenoreceptors promotes dopamine release; this effect allows the redundant dopamine to stimulate D$_1$ receptors and to compete with the drug in the contrasting D$_2$ receptor blockade (Kapur et al., 2000). Some of these drugs, such as clozapine, have also shown a higher dissociation constant – they attach to and dissociate from the receptors 100 times in the time it takes haloperidol to do so once. As the concentration of endogenous dopamine increases in response to physiological stimuli, drugs such as clozapine decrease their occupancy much faster, providing greater access to surges of dopamine and promoting more effective stimulus acquisition and manipulation (Seeman & Tallerico, 1999; Kapur & Remington, 2001).

Risperidone is the second-generation antipsychotic agent that has been most extensively studied in childhood and adolescence. A few studies have been designed specifically to investigate its effects on cognitive function (Pandina et al., 2007). In trials assessing the efficacy and safety of this drug, not only was there no evidence of any deterioration in cognitive variables during its use (Aman et al., 2002; Snyder et al., 2002), but marked improvements in cognitive function were observed in specific tests of verbal learning and memory tasks (Turgay et al., 2002; Reyes et al., 2006). Although in some studies risperidone treatment has exacerbated deficits in the maintenance of spatial information in working memory, perhaps by impairing the encoding of information (Purdon et al., 2000; Reilly et al., 2006), several studies on adult schizophrenic patients have shown an improvement in episodic memory, verbal fluency, vigilance, executive functioning, and visuo-motor speed in patients treated with risperidone, olanzapine, clozapine, ziprasidone, and quetiapine, but not with haloperidol (Purdon et al., 2000; Harvey et al., 2003a;

Harvey *et al.*, 2003b). These effects appear independent of changes in clinical symptoms or movement disorders, suggesting a direct effect of atypical antipsychotic drugs on cognitive deficits in schizophrenia.

Stimulants

Psychostimulant drugs such as methylphenidate are the primary treatment for ADHD (Taylor *et al.*, 2004; Banaschewski *et al.*, 2006). Several randomized controlled studies conducted in children and adolescents have confirmed the effects of psychostimulants in improving impulsivity, inattention, and hyperactivity – the core symptoms of ADHD – in a consistent, rapid, and lasting way. Stimulants have been also reported to enhance social skills, reduce anger and aggressive behaviours, and improve cooperation with interventions (Santosh & Taylor, 2000; Taylor *et al.*, 2004).

In ADHD, accumulating evidence of structural and functional abnormalities in prefrontal and striatal brain regions, which are modulated by catecholaminergic neurotransmitters, provides the theoretical basis for the pharmacological treatment of this disorder (Volkow *et al.*, 2001). Significant differences in the neurophysiology of frontal-striatal brain regions important for inhibitory control have been reported between ADHD subjects and normal controls. Brain structures involved in working memory and modulated by catecholamines (Braver *et al.*, 2001, Giedd *et al.*, 2001), have been found to be impaired in ADHD (Bush *et al.*, 2005; Volkow *et al.*, 2005). ADHD has been shown to be characterized by atypical fronto-striatal function, and methylphenidate affects striatal activation differently in ADHD than in healthy children (Vaidya *et al.*, 1998). A methylphenidate-induced increase in dopamine levels in the synaptic clefts of these structures enhances several aspects of cognitive processing, including working memory (Mehta *et al.*, 2000). In children with ADHD, methylphenidate significantly and selectively improves performance on a visual-spatial working memory task and on the maintenance of visual-spatial information. On the other hand, this drug appears to have no effects on measures of visual-spatial planning ability or recognition memory, suggesting a selective effect on visual-spatial memory (Bedard *et al.*, 2004). Recently, the administration of a single-dose of methylphenidate has been found to restore performance on a visual memory task, but this restorative effect diminished with repeated administration, showing that this drug restores visual memory but not working memory in ADHD (Rhodes *et al.*, 2004).

Because most clinical trials in child psychiatry exclude children with subaverage IQs to avoid heterogeneity within samples, few pharmacological studies have been conducted to assess the effects of stimulants in individuals presenting with both ADHD and mental retardation (Pearson *et al.*, 2004). Reports from these studies suggest that the use of stimulants in this population improves ADHD symptoms, although the effect is inversely proportional to the degree of mental retardation. In a pilot study assessing the safety and efficacy of an acute single-dose methylphenidate test and the effects of the subsequent ongoing therapy in children with pervasive developmental disorder (PDD) and moderate to severe hyperactivity/impulsivity, we have shown that methylphenidate is effective at improving measures of hyperactivity and impulsivity, while core symptom measures of autism were unaffected (Di Martino *et al.*, 2004). Two large studies have confirmed the long-term effects of methylphenidate on symptoms of hyperactivity, impulsivity, inattention, oppositionality, aggression, and intermittent explosive rage in PDD subjects (RUPP Autism Network, 2005).

Baseline cognitive measures may be predictive of drug response (Buitelaar *et al.*, 1995). In a group of normal adult volunteers, a single dose of methylphenidate improved self-ordered spatial working memory performance: the drug-induced changes in performance measures were related to individual differences at baseline (Mehta *et al.*, 2000). In healthy adult volunteers, stimulants have been also found to enhance performance in visual-spatial working memory and planning, with less activation of prefrontal cortex. The biggest benefit has been found in subjects with poor executive function (Elliott *et al.*, 1997; Mattay *et al.*, 2000).

Modulating memory to improve cognition: the new cognitive enhancers

Ampakines

'Ampakines' are a family of benzamide compounds that act as positive modulators at the glutamatergic amino-3-hydroxy-5-methylisoxazole-4-propionic acid (AMPA) receptor complex by increasing the peak and duration of glutamate-induced AMPA-receptor-gated currents and reducing the amount of afferent activity needed to induce long-term potentiation (Staubli *et al.*, 1994a; Arai *et al.*, 1996). This effect may boost the activity of glutamate-promoting plasticity at the synapse, which could translate into better cognitive performance and also enhance attention span and alertness. Unlike earlier stimulants (for example, caffeine, methylphenidate, and amphetamines), because of their short half-life (hours) ampakines do not induce unpleasant long-lasting side effects such as sleeplessness. Ampakines are currently being investigated as a potential treatment for a range of conditions involving mental disability including Alzheimer's disease, Parkinson's disease, schizophrenia, and neurological disorders such as ADHD. Prototypical compounds of the ampakines family are CX-516, CX-546, CX-614, and CX-717.

Several studies on rats suggest that ampakines cause a cumulative enhancement of performance in a spatial short-term memory task during behavioural training (Hampson *et al.*, 1998). Ampakines have also been shown to facilitate long-term potentiation and cognition in spatial tasks (Staubli *et al.*, 1994b), to promote the acquisition of a conditioned response (Shors *et al.*, 1995), and to reduce the number of trials needed to form stable olfactory memory (Larson *et al.*, 1995). In healthy volunteers, ampakines have shown a positive effect on the delayed recall of nonsense syllables as well as on several common memory tasks (Lynch, 2004). Performance steadily improved and the improvement persisted after completion of drug treatment in both animal and human trials (Goff *et al.*, 2001). In a recent study conducted in non-human primates, CX717 given to sleep-deprived monkeys produced a striking removal of the behavioural impairment and returned performance to above-normal levels. The AMPA receptor modulator CX717, given to monkeys engaged in cognitive processing and short-term memory tasks, improved performance under normal alert conditions and under effects of sleep deprivation (Porrino *et al.*, 2005).

The glutamatergic neurons are the major excitatory pathways linking the cortex, limbic system, and thalamus, three regions believed to be involved in schizophrenia. Blockade of the glutamate NMDA receptor can induce behavioural and cognitive deficits in normal subjects, mimicking schizophrenia. In a recent placebo-controlled pilot study involving 18 people with schizophrenia, the ampakine CX516 was added to clozapine and when compared with placebo was associated with moderate to large effect sizes, improving several measures of attention and memory (Goff *et al.*, 2001).

Consistent with clinical observations that depression is commonly associated with cognitive dysfunction in learning and memory tasks (Grasby *et al.*, 1993; Mineka *et al.*, 1998), it has been suggested that long-term antidepressant therapy improves cognitive function in parallel with the remission of depression in depressed human subjects (Sternberg & Jarvik, 1976;

O'Brien et al., 1993). In a behavioural task linked to depression, Knapp and colleagues designed a trial to test the activity of nootropic drugs: both antidepressants and cognitive enhancers improved depression and cognitive dysfunction, suggesting that ampakines may have antidepressant activity (Knapp et al., 2002).

5-HT$_6$ receptor antagonists

Over the past decade, there has been increasing interest in the role of the serotonin 6 (5-HT$_6$) receptor in higher cognitive processes. This appears to influence long-term memory more than anxiety (Roth et al., 2004). The 5-HT$_6$ receptor is one of the most recently discovered serotonin receptor subtypes among the 14 identified; it is expressed relatively early in brain development (in the rat diencephalon on E12, in the caudate by E17). It is positively coupled to the Gs protein and activates adenylate cyclase (cAMP), following the protein kinase A transduction cascade (Monsma et al., 1993; Plassat et al., 1993; Ruat et al., 1993). During development, these receptors are involved in axonal growth and guidance (Grimaldi et al., 1998). Immunohistochemical studies have demonstrated the highest receptor expression in the striatum, nucleus accumbens, olfactory tubercle, and cortex, with moderate expression in the amygdala, hypothalamus, thalamus, cerebellum, and hippocampus (Gerard et al., 1997; Boess et al., 1998). 5-HT$_6$ receptors are localized in dopamine-rich areas such as the striatum and nucleus accumbens (Gerard et al., 1997), on aminobutyric acid (GABA)ergic interneurons (Ward & Dorsa, 1996), and mostly on hippocampal glutamatergic neurons (Gerard et al., 1997), where they decrease glutamate release (Gerard et al., 1997). *In vivo*, 5-HT$_6$ blockade potentiates dopamine transmission induced by stimulants drugs such as amphetamine (Pullagurla et al., 2004), affecting dopamine through the modulation of acetylcholine rather than by a direct pathway.

In several studies, 5-HT$_6$ receptor antagonists reversed the anticholinergic-mediated deficits in memory performance during a learning task (Meneses, 2001; Woolley et al., 2003; Hirst et al., 2006), suggesting that acetylcholine release may be modulated by 5-HT$_6$ inhibition. Some researchers have investigated the possibility that 5-HT$_6$ blockade modulates learning, memory, and passive avoidance through increased cholinergic transmission, showing that 5-HT$_6$ antagonists may aid memory and fear-memory consolidation. In animal models, the administration of selective 5-HT$_6$ antagonists improves spatial memory, both alone and in combination with acetylcholinesterase inhibitors (Woolley et al., 2001). Recent studies have shown the 5-HT$_6$ antagonists Ro 04-6790 and SB 21076 enhance memory consolidation (King et al., 2004).

Phosphodiesterase-4 inhibitors

Classical cognitive enhancers interact with single neurotransmitter systems involved in the complex mechanisms that underlie cognition. An alternative approach would be to target second messenger systems that are used by multiple neurotransmitters.

The regulation of memory consolidation occurs in the CA1 subregion of the hippocampus, through biochemical processes in which a second messenger, cyclic adenosine monophosphate (cAMP), plays a key role. The postsynaptic cAMP/protein kinase A (PKA)/cAMP responsive element binding protein (CREB) pathway is involved in long-term potentiation, in part by activating CREB-dependent gene expression (Slack & Walsh, 1995; Lu & Hawkins, 2002). Thus cAMP is implicated in the synaptic plasticity necessary for learning and memory. Prolongation of cAMP signals can be accomplished by inhibiting phosphodiesterases. Phosphodiesterase enzymes, components of NMDA receptor-mediated cAMP signalling, are responsible for the degradation of neuronal cAMP. Inhibitors of phosphodiesterases – drugs that modulate

CREB function by enhancing cAMP signalling – enhance CREB-dependent gene expression and facilitate long-term memory (Bourtchouladze et al., 2003).

In rats, two selective type IV phosphodiesterase inhibitors (PDE-4), quinoline and rolipram, have been reported to have pharmacological effects on the locus coeruleus, habenula, the paraventricular nucleus of the thalamus, the amygdala, and the nucleus accumbens, all structures with strong limbic connectivity implicated in arousal, memory, and the affective aspects of behaviour (Bureau et al., 2006). Rolipram increases both the intensity and duration of cAMP-mediated signalling (Scuvee-Moreau et al., 1987), enhancing hippocampus-dependent memory and long-term potentiation (Barad et al., 1998; Bourtchouladze et al., 2003). Furthermore, it has been shown to reverse rat memory impairment caused by scopolamine (Rutten et al., 2006), or by serotonin deficit resulting from acute tryptophan depletion, improving the performance of object recognition tasks (Rutten et al., 2007). There is growing evidence that PDE-4 inhibitors have positive effects on learning and memory in animal models, suggesting their potential use for improving symptoms of cognitive decline associated with neurodegenerative and psychiatric diseases (Rose et al., 2005; Zhang et al., 2005). MEM 1414 is a new PDE-4 inhibitor that has been developed for the treatment of Alzheimer's disease. Phase I trials of this experimental drug have been completed in humans (Memory Pharmaceuticals). MEM 1414 may also be applicable for other indications, including mild cognitive impairment, a disorder characterized by a decline in long-term memory capabilities.

Ethical issues in cognitive enhancement

For the most part, psychotropic drugs are used to treat neurological and psychiatric illnesses, and there is relatively little controversy about their use for this purpose. Many aspects of psychological function, however, can be potential targets for pharmacological enhancement – including memory, executive function, mood, appetite, libido, and sleep – in individuals who are not ill (Farah, 2002; Farah et al., 2004). Although in its initial stage, the concept of cognitive enhancement in normal people raises important ethical issues which may have slowed the development of new pharmacological agents for people with mental retardation (Farah, 2004).

In comparison with other elective treatments, such as cosmetic surgery and the chemical modulation of sexual and reproductive function, neurocognitive enhancement involves an extremely complex system, with a greater risk of unanticipated problems. Safety is a concern with all drugs and procedures, but common tolerance for risk is smallest when the treatment is purely elective, without clear therapeutic effects on specific disorders. The potential for subtle, rare, or long-term side effects cannot be excluded, so is important to assess what side effects are an acceptable trade-off for the drug's benefits. This prudent approach needs to be applied to agents developed for neurocognitive enhancement.

While safety concerns can be readily managed, 'coercion' is a more debatable issue – with the development of agents for neurocognitive enhancement, there will inevitably be situations in which people are pressured into enhancing their cognitive abilities. Employers will recognize the benefits of a more attentive and less forgetful workforce. Competing against enhanced co-workers or students may provide an incentive to use neurocognitive enhancement, and it is a harder to identify any existing legal framework for protecting people against such incentives to compete. A straightforward legislative approach of outlawing or restricting the use of neurocognitive enhancement in the workplace or in school, as for 'doping' in the sporting world, is itself also coercive by denying people the freedom to practise safe means of self-improvement (Farah et al., 2004).

Moreover, it is likely that neurocognitive enhancement – like almost everything else – will not be fairly distributed. Methylphenidate use by normal healthy people is greatest among college students, an overwhelmingly middle class and privileged segment of the population. There will undoubtedly be cost barriers to new legal neurocognitive enhancement and possibly social barriers as well for certain groups. Such barriers could compound the disadvantages that are already faced by people of low socioeconomic status in education and employment. Nevertheless, in comparison with other forms of enhancement that contribute to gaps in socioeconomic achievement – from good nutrition to high quality schools – neurocognitive enhancement could prove easier to distribute equitably.

The main ethical issues encompass the many ways in which neurocognitive enhancement intersects with our understanding of what it means to be a person, to be healthy and whole, to do meaningful work, and to value human life in all its imperfection. Although cognitive enhancement is a desirable goal for neuroscience and clinical practice, especially for people with mental retardation, these ethical concerns must always be considered so as to avoid these drugs becoming the trigger for unpredicted problems.

References

Anderson, G.M., Gutknecht, L., Cohen, D.J., Brailly-Tabard, S., Cohen, J.H., Ferrari, P., Roubertoux, P.L. & Tordjman, S. (2002): Serotonin transporter promoter variants in autism: functional effects and relationship to platelet hyperserotonemia. *Mol. Psychiatry* **7**, 831–836.

Aman, M.G., De Smedt, G., Derivan, A., Lyons, B., Findling, R.L. & the Risperidone Disruptive Behavior Study Group (2002): Double-blind, placebo-controlled study of risperidone for the treatment of disruptive behaviours in children with subaverage intelligence. *Am. J. Psychiatry* **159**, 1337–1346.

Arai, A., Kessler, M., Rogers, G. & Lynch, G. (1996): Effects of a memory-enhancing drug on DL-alpha-amino-3-hydroxy-5-methyl-4-isoxazolepropionic acid receptor currents and synaptic transmission in hippocampus. *J. Pharmacol. Exp. Ther.* **278**, 1–12.

Baddeley, A.D. (1996): *Human memory: theory and practice* [revised edition]. New York: Allyn & Bacon.

Banaschewski, T., Coghill, D., Santosh, P., Zuddas, A., Asherson, P., Buitelaar, J., Dankaerts, M., Dopfner, M., Faraone, S.V., Rothenberger, A., Sergeant, J., Steinhausen, H.C., Sonuga-Barke, E.J. & Taylor, E. (2006): Long-acting medications for the hyperkinetic disorders. A systematic review and European treatment guideline. *Eur. Child Adolesc. Psychiatry* **15**, 476–495.

Barad, M., Bourtchouladze, R., Winder, D.G., Golan, H. & Kandel, E. (1998): Rolipram, a type IV-specific phosphodiesterase inhibitor, facilitates the establishment of long-lasting long-term potentiation and improves memory. *Proc. Natl. Acad. Sci. USA* **95**, 15020–15025.

Barkley, R.A. (1997): Behavioural inhibition, sustained attention, and executive functions: constructing a unifying theory of AD/HD. *Psychol. Bull.* **121**, 65–94.

Bedard, A.C., Martinussen, R., Ickowicz, A. & Tannock, R. (2004): Methylphenidate improves visual-spatial memory in children with attention-deficit/hyperactivity disorder. *J. Am. Acad. Child Adolesc. Psychiatry* **43**, 260–268.

Bliss, T.V. & Collingridge, G.L. (1993): A synaptic model of memory: long-term potentiation in the hippocampus. *Nature* **361**, 31–39.

Boess, F.G., Riemer, C., Bos, M., Bentley, J., Bourson, A. & Sleight, A.J. (1998): The 5-hydroxytryptamine 6 receptor-selective radioligand [3H]Ro 63-0563 labels 5-hydroxytryptamine receptor binding sites in rat and porcine striatum. *Mol. Pharmacol.* **54**, 577–583.

Bourtchouladze, R., Lidge, R., Catapano, R., Stanley, J., Gossweiler, S., Romashko, D., Scott, R. & Tully, T. (2003): A mouse model of Rubinstein-Taybi syndrome: defective long-term memory is ameliorated by inhibitors of phosphodiesterase 4. *Proc. Natl. Acad. Sci. USA* **100**, 10518–10522.

Braver, T.S., Barch, D.M., Kelley, W.M., Buckner, R.L., Cohen, N.J., Miezin, F.M., Snyder, A.Z., Ollinger, J.M., Akbudak, E., Conturo, T.E. & Petersen, S.E. (2001): Direct comparison of prefrontal cortex regions engaged by working and long-term memory tasks. *Neuroimage* **14**, 48–59.

Buitelaar, J.K., Van der Gaag, R.J., Swaab-Barneveld, H. & Kuiper, M. (1995): Prediction of clinical response to methylphenidate in children with attention-deficit hyperactivity disorder. *J. Am. Acad. Child Adolesc. Psychiatry* **34**, 1025–1032.

Bureau, Y., Handa, M., Zhu, Y., Laliberte, F., Moore, C.S., Liu, S., Huang, Z., MacDonald, D., Xu, D.G. & Robertson, G.S. (2006): Neuroanatomical and pharmacological assessment of Fos expression induced in the rat brain by the phosphodiesterase-4 inhibitor 6-(4-pyridylmethyl)-8-(3-nitrophenyl) quinoline. *Neuropharmacology* **51**, 974–985.

Bush, G., Valera, E.M. & Seidman, L.J. (2005): Functional neuroimaging of attentiondeficit/hyperactivity disorder: a review and suggested future directions. *Biol. Psychiatry* **57**, 1273–1284.

Cabeza, R. & Nyberg, L. (2000): Imaging cognition II: an empirical review of 275 PET and fMRI studies. *J. Cogn. Neurosci.* **12**, 1–47.

Chen, C.Y., Lawlor, J.P., Duggan, A.K., Hardy, J.B. & Eaton, W.W. (2006): Mild cognitive impairment in early life and mental health problems in adulthood. *Am. J. Public Health* **96**, 1772–1778.

Coull, J.T. (1994): Pharmacological manipulations of the alpha 2-noradrenergic system. Effects on cognition. *Drugs Aging* **5**, 116–126.

Coyle, J.T. & Tsai, G. (2004): The NMDA receptor glycine modulatory site: a therapeutic target for improving cognition and reducing negative symptoms in schizophrenia. *Psychopharmacology (Berl.)* **174**, 32–38.

de Fockert, J., Rees, G., Frith, C.D. & Lavie, N. (2001): The role of working memory in visual selective attention. *Science* **291**, 1803–1806.

D'Esposito, M., Ballard, D., Zarahn, E. & Aguirre, G.K. (2000): The role of prefrontal cortex in sensory memory and motor preparation: an event-related fMRI study. *Neuroimage* **11**, 400–408

Denckla, M.B. (1996): A theory and model of executive function: a neuropsychological perspective. In: *Attention, memory, and executive function*, eds. G.R. Lyon & N.A. Krasnegor, pp. 263–277. Baltimore: Paul H. Brookes.

Devoto, P., Flore, G., Pira, L., Longu, G. & Gessa, G.L. (2004): Alpha2-adrenoceptor mediated co-release of dopamine and noradrenaline from noradrenergic neurons in the cerebral cortex. *J. Neurochem.* **88**, 1003–1009.

Devoto, P., Flore, G., Saba, P., Fa, M. & Gessa, G.L. (2005): Stimulation of the locus coeruleus elicits noradrenaline and dopamine release in the medial prefrontal and parietal cortex. *J. Neurochem.* **92**, 368–374.

Di Martino, A., Melis, G., Cianchetti, C. & Zuddas, A. (2004): Methylphenidate for pervasive developmental disorders: safety and efficacy of acute single dose test and ongoing therapy: an open-pilot study. *J. Child Adolesc. Psychopharmacol.* **14**, 207–218.

Elliott, R., Sahakian, B.J., Matthews, K., Bannerjea, A., Rimmer, J. & Robbins, T. (1997): Effects of methylphenidate on spatial working memory and planning in healthy young adults. *Psychopharmacology (Berl.)* **131**, 196–206.

Farah, M.J. (2002): Emerging ethical issues in neuroscience. *Nat. Neurosci.* **5**, 1123–1129.

Farah, M.J., Illes, J., Cook-Deegan, R., Gardner, H., Kandel, E., King, P., Parens, E., Sahakian, B. & Wolpe, P.R. (2004): Neurocognitive enhancement: what can we do and what should we do? *Nat. Rev. Neurosci.* **5**, 421–425.

Fuster, J.M. (1999): Synopsis of function and dysfunction of the frontal lobe. *Acta Psychiatr. Scand. Suppl.* **395**, 51–57.

Gerard, C., Martres, M.P., Lefevre, K., Miquel, M.C., Verge, D. & Lanfumey, L. (1997): Immunolocalization of serotonin 5-HT6 receptor-like material in the rat central nervous system. *Brain Res.* **746**, 207–219.

Geurts, H.M., Verté, S., Oosterlaan, J., Roeyers, H. & Sergeant, J.A. (2004): How specific are executive functioning deficits in attention deficit hyperactivity disorder and autism? *J. Child Psychol. Psychiatry* **45**, 836–854.

Giedd, J.N., Blumenthal, J., Molloy, E. & Castellanos, F.X. (2001): Brain imaging of attention deficit/hyperactivity disorder. *Ann. N.Y. Acad. Sci.* **931**, 33–49.

Goff, D.C. & Coyle, J.T. (2001): The emerging role of glutamate in the pathophysiology and treatment of schizophrenia. *Am. J. Psychiatry* **158**, 1367–1377.

Goff, D.C., Leahy, L., Berman, I., Posever, T., Herz, L., Leon, A.C., Johnson, S.A. & Lynch, G. (2001): A placebo-controlled pilot study of the ampakine CX516 added to clozapine in schizophrenia. *J. Clin. Psychopharmacol.* **21**, 484–487.

Goldman-Rakic, P.C. (1995): Cellular basis of working memory. *Neuron* **14**, 477–485.

Grasby, P.M., Friston, K.J., Bench, C.J., Cowen, P.J., Frith, C.D., Liddle, P.F., Frackowiak, R.S. & Dolan, R.J. (1993): The effect of the dopamine agonist, apomorphine, on regional cerebral blood flow in normal volunteers. *Psychol. Med.* **23**, 605–612.

Grimaldi, B., Bonnin, A., Ruat, M., Traiffort, E. & Fillion, G. (1998): Characterization of 5-HT6 receptor and expression of 5-HT6 mRNA in the rat brain during ontogenetic development. *Naunyn-Schmiedebergs Arch. Pharmacol.* **357**, 393–400.

Hampson, R.E., Rogers, G., Lynch, G. & Deadwyler, S.A. (1998): Facilitative effects of the ampakine CX516 on short-term memory in rats: correlations with hippocampal neuronal activity. *J. Neurosci.* **18**, 2748–1763.

Harvey, P.D., Green, M.F., McGurk, S.R. & Meltzer, H.Y. (2003a): Changes in cognitive functioning with risperidone and olanzapine treatment: a large-scale, double-blind, randomized study. *Psychopharmacology (Berl.)* **169**, 404–411.

Harvey, P.D., Napolitano, J.A., Mao, L. & Gharabawi, G. (2003b): Comparative effects of risperidone and olanzapine on cognition in elderly patients with schizophrenia or schizoaffective disorder. *Int. J. Geriatr. Psychiatry* **18**, 820–829.

Hirst, W.D., Stean, T.O., Rogers, D.C., Sunter, D., Pugh, P., Moss, S.F., Bromidge, S.M., Riley, G., Smith, D.R., Bartlett, S., Heidbreder, C.A., Atkins, A.R., Lacroix, L.P., Dawson, L.A., Foley, A.G., Regan, C.M. & Upton, N. (2006): SB-399885 is a potent, selective 5-HT6 receptor antagonist with cognitive enhancing properties in aged rat water maze and novel object recognition models. *Eur. J. Pharmacol.* **553**, 109–119.

Hollmann, M. & Heinemann, S. (1994): Cloned glutamate receptors. *Annu. Rev. Neurosci.* **17**, 31–108.

Kapur, S. & Remington, G. (2001): Atypical antipsychotics: new directions and new challenges in the treatment of schizophrenia. *Annu. Rev. Med.* **52**, 503–517.

Kapur, S., Zipursky, R.B. & Remington, G. (1999): Clinical and theoretical implications of 5-HT2 and D2 receptor occupancy of clozapine, risperidone, and olanzapine in schizophrenia. *Am. J. Psychiatry* **156**, 286–293.

Kapur, S., Zipursky, R., Jones, C., Remington, G. & Houle, S. (2000): Relationship between dopamine D2 occupancy, clinical response, and side effects: a double-blind PET study of first-episode schizophrenia. *Am. J. Psychiatry* **157**, 514–520.

Karson, C.N., Mrak, R.E., Husain, M.M. & Griffin, W.S. (1996): Decreased mesopontine choline acetyltransferase levels in schizophrenia. *Mol. Chem. Neuropathol.* **29**, 181–191.

King, M.V., Sleight, A.J., Woolley, M.L., Topham, I.A., Marsden, C.A. & Fone, K.C. (2004): 5-HT6 receptor antagonists reverse delay-dependent deficits in novel object discrimination by enhancing consolidation – an effect sensitive to NMDA receptor antagonism. *Neuropharmacology* **47**, 195–204.

Knapp, R.J., Goldenberg, R., Shuck, C., Cecil, A., Watkins, J., Miller, C., Crites, G. & Malatynska, E. (2002): Antidepressant activity of memory-enhancing drugs in the reduction of submissive behaviour model. *Eur. J. Pharmacol.* **440**, 27–35.

LaBar, K.S. & Cabeza, R. (2006). Cognitive neuroscience of emotional memory. *Nat. Rev. Neurosci.* **7**, 54–64.

Larson, J., Lieu, T., Petchpradub, V., LeDuc, B., Ngo, H., Rogers, G.A. & Lynch, G. (1995): Facilitation of olfactory learning by a modulator of AMPA receptors. *J. Neurosci.* **15**, 8023–8030.

Lee, A., Wissekerke, A.E., Rosin, D.L. & Lynch, K.R. (1998): Localization of (2c adrenergic receptor immunoreactivity in catecholaminergic neurons in the rat central nervous system. *Neuroscience* **84**, 1085–1096.

Lewis, D.A. & Gonzalez-Burgos, G. (2006): Pathophysiologically based treatment interventions in schizophrenia. *Nat. Med.* **12**, 1016–1022.

Lu, Y.F. & Hawkins, R.D. (2002): Ryanodine receptors contribute to cGMP-induced latephase LTP and CREB phosphorylation in the hippocampus. *J. Neurophysiol.* **88**, 1270–1278.

Lynch, M.A. (2004): Long-term potentiation and memory. *Physiol. Rev.* **84**, 87–136.

Malenka, R.C. & Nicoll, R.A. (1999): Long-term potentiation – a decade of progress? *Science* **285**, 1870–1874.

Mattay, V.S., Callicott, J.H., Bertolino, A., Heaton, I., Frank, J.A., Coppola, R., Berman, K.F., Goldberg, T.E. & Weinberger, D.R. (2000): Effects of dextroamphetamine on cognitive performance and cortical activation. *Neuroimage* **12**, 268–275.

Mehta, M.A., Owen, A.M., Sahakian, B.J., Mavaddat, N., Pickard, J.D. & Robbins, T.W. (2000): Methylphenidate enhances working memory by modulating discrete frontal and parietal lobe regions in the human brain. *J. Neurosci.* **20**, RC65.

Meneses, A. (2001): Effects of the 5-HT(6) receptor antagonist Ro 04-6790 on learning consolidation. *Behav. Brain Res.* **118**, 107–110.

Mineka, S., Watson, D. & Clark, L.A. (1998): Comorbidity of anxiety and unipolar mood disorders. *Annu. Rev. Psychol.* **49**, 377–412.

Miyake, A. & Shaw, P. (1999): *Models of working memory: mechanisms of active maintenance and executive control.* New York: Cambridge University Press.

Monsma, F.J., Shen, Y., Ward, R.P., Hamblin, M.W. & Sibley, D.R. (1993): Cloning and expression of a novel serotonin receptor with high affinity for tricyclic psychotropic drugs. *Mol. Pharmacol.* **43**, 320–327.

Morris, R.G., Moser, E.I., Riedel, G., Martin, S.J., Sandin, J., Day, M. & O'Carroll, C. (2003): Elements of a neurobiological theory of the hippocampus: the role of activity-dependent synaptic plasticity in memory. *Philos. Trans. R Soc. Lond. B Biol. Sci.* **358**, 773–786.

Nichols, M.J. & Newsome, W.T. (1999): The neurobiology of cognition. *Nature* **402**, C35-C38.

Nieoullon, A. (2002): Dopamine and the regulation of cognition and attention. *Prog. Neurobiol.* **67**, 53–83.

O'Brien, J.T., Sahakian, B.J. & Checkley, S.A. (1993): Cognitive impairments in patients with seasonal affective disorder. *Br. J. Psychiatry* **163**, 338–343.

Ozonoff, S., Cook, I., Coon, H., Dawson, G., Joseph, R.M. & Klin, A. (2004): Performance on Cambridge Neuropsychological Test Automated Battery subtests sensitive to frontal lobe function in people with autistic disorder: evidence from the Collaborative Programs of Excellence in Autism Network. *J. Autism Dev. Disord.* **34**, 139–150.

Pandina, G.J., Bilder, R., Harvey, P.D., Keefe, R.S., Aman, M.G. & Gharabawi, G. (2007): Risperidone and cognitive function in children with disruptive behavour disorders. *Biol. Psychiatry* [E-pub ahead of print].

Pavuluri, M.N., Schenkel, L.S., Aryal, S., Harral, E.M., Hill, S.K., Herbener, E.S. & Sweeney, J.A. (2006): Neurocognitive function in unmedicated manic and medicated euthymic paediatric bipolar patients. *Am. J. Psychiatry* **163**, 286–293.

Pearson, D.A., Lane, D.M., Santos, C.W., Casat, C.D., Jerger, S.W., Loveland, K.A., Faria, L.P., Mansour, R., Henderson, J.A., Payne, C.D., Roache, J.D., Lachar, D. & Cleveland, L.A. (2004): Effects of methylphenidate treatment in children with mental retardation and ADHD: individual variation in medication response. *J. Am. Acad. Child Adolesc. Psychiatry* **43**, 686–698.

Pennington, B.F. & Ozonoff, S. (1996): Executive functions and developmental psychopathology. *J. Child Psychol. Psychiatry* **37**, 51–87.

Plassat, J.L., Amlaiky, N. & Hen, R. (1993): Molecular cloning of a mammalian serotonin receptor that activates adenylate cyclase. *Mol. Pharmacol.* **44**, 229–236.

Pliszka, S.R., McCracken, J.T. & Maas, J.W. (1996): Catecholamines in attention-deficit hyperactivity disorder: current perspectives. *J. Am. Acad. Child Adolesc. Psychiatry* **35**, 264–272.

Porrino, L.J., Daunais, J.B., Rogers, G.A., Hampson, R.E. & Deadwyler, S.A. (2005): Facilitation of task performance and removal of the effects of sleep deprivation by an ampakine (CX717) in nonhuman primates. *PLoS Biol.* **3**, e299

Posner, M.I. & Raichle, M.E. (1998): The neuroimaging of human brain function. *Proc. Natl. Acad. Sci. USA* **95** 763–764.

Posner, M.I. & Peterson, S.E. (1990): The attention system of the human brain. *Annu. Rev. Neurosci.* **13**, 25–42.

Pullagurla, M., Bondareva, T., Young, R. & Glennon, R.A. (2004): Modulation of the stimulus effects of (+)amphetamine by the 5-HT6 antagonist MS-245. *Pharmacol. Biochem. Behav.* **78**, 263–268.

Purdon, S.E., Jones, B.D., Stip, E., Labelle, A., Addington, D., David, S.R., Breier, A. & Tollefson, G.D. (2000) Neuropsychological change in early phase schizophrenia during 12 months of treatment with olanzapine, risperidone or haloperidol. The Canadian Collaborative Group for research in schizophrenia. *Arch. Gen. Psychiatry* **57**, 249–258

Quintana, J., Yajeya, J. & Fuster, J.M. (1988): Prefrontal representation of stimulus attributes during delay tasks. I Unit activity in cross-temporal integration of sensory and sensorymotor information. *Brain Res.* **474**, 211–221.

Reilly, J.L., Harris, M.S., Keshavan, M.S. & Sweeney, J.A. (2006): Adverse effects of risperidone on spatial working memory in first-episode schizophrenia. *Arch. Gen. Psychiatry* **63**, 1189–1197.

Reyes, M., Croonenberghs, J., Augustyns, I. & Eerdekens, M. (2006): Long-term use of risperidone in children with disruptive behavior disorders and subaverage intelligence: efficacy, safety, and tolerability. *J. Child Adolesc. Psychopharmacol.* **16**, 260–272.

Rhodes, S.M., Coghill, D.R. & Matthews, K. (2004): Methylphenidate restores visual memory, but not working memory function in attention deficit-hyperkinetic disorder. *Psychopharmacology (Berl.)* **175**, 319–330.

Robbins, T.W. (2000): Chemical neuromodulation of frontal-executive functions in humans and other animals. *Exp Brain Res.* **133**, 130–138.

Rose, G.M., Hopper, A., De Vivo, M. & Tehim, A. (2005): Phosphodiesterase inhibitors for cognitive enhancement *Curr. Pharm. Des.* **11**, 3329–3334.

Roth, B.L., Hanizavareh, S.M. & Blum, A.E. (2004): Serotonin receptors represent highly favorable molecular targets for cognitive enhancement in schizophrenia and other disorders. *Psychopharmacology (Berl.)* **174**, 17–24.

Ruat, M., Traiffort, E., Arrang, J.M., Tardivel-Lacombe, J., Diaz, J., Leurs, R. & Schwartz, J.C. (1993): A novel rat serotonin (5-HT6) receptor: molecular cloning, localization and stimulation of cAMP accumulation. *Biochem. Biophys Res. Commun.* **193**, 268–276.

Rueda, M.R., Fan, J., McCandliss, B.D., Halparin, J.D., Gruber, D.B., Lercari, L.P. & Posner, M.I. (2004): Development of attentional networks in childhood. *Neuropsychologia* **42**, 1029–1040.

RUPP, Research Units on Paediatric Psychopharmacology Autism Network (2005): A randomized controlled crossover trial of methylphenidate in pervasive developmental disorders with hyperactivity. *Arch. Gen. Psychiatry* **62**, 1266–1274.

Russell, J. (1997): *Autism as an executive disorder.* Oxford: Oxford University Press.

Rutten, K., Prickaerts, J. & Blokland, A. (2006): Rolipram reverses scopolamine-induced and time-dependent memory deficits in object recognition by different mechanisms of action. *Neurobiol. Learn. Mem.* **85**, 132–138.

Rutten, K., Lieben, C., Smits, L. & Blokland, A. (2007): The PDE$_4$ inhibitor rolipram reverses object memory impairment induced by acute tryptophan depletion in the rat. *Psychopharmacology (Berl.)* **192**, 275–282.

Santosh, P.J. & Taylor, E. (2000): Stimulant drugs. *Eur. Child Adolesc. Psychiatry* **9**, 127–143.

Scuvee-Moreau, J., Giesbers, I. & Dresse, A. (1987): Effect of rolipram, a phosphodiesterase inhibitor and potential antidepressant, on the firing rate of central monoaminergic neurons in the rat. *Arch. Int. Pharmacodyn. Ther.* **288**, 43–49.

Seeman, P. & Tallerico, T. (1999): Rapid release of antipsychotic drugs from dopamine D2 receptors: an explanation for low receptor occupancy and early clinical relapse upon withdrawal of clozapine or quetiapine. *Am. J. Psychiatry* **156**, 876–884.

Shors, T.J., Servatius, R.J., Thompson, R.F., Rogers, G. & Lynch, G. (1995): Enhanced glutamatergic neurotransmission facilitates classical conditioning in the freely moving rat. *Neurosci Lett.* **186**, 153–156.

Slack, J.R. & Walsh, C. (1995): Effects of a cAMP analogue simulate the distinct components of long-term potentiation in CA1 region of rat hippocampus. *Neurosci Lett.* **201**, 25-28.

Snyder, R., Turgay, A., Aman, M., Binder, C., Fisman, S., Carroll, A. & the Risperidone Conduct Study Group (2002): Effects of risperidone on conduct and disruptive behaviour disorders in children with subaverage IQs. *J. Am. Acad. Child Adolesc. Psychiatry* **41**, 1026–1036.

Solanto, M.V. (1998): Neuropsychopharmacological mechanisms of stimulant drug action in attention-deficit hyperactivity disorder: a review and integration. *Behav. Brain Res.* **94**, 127–152.

Staubli, U., Perez, Y., Xu, F.-B., Rogers, G., Ingvar, M., Stone-Elander, S. & Lynch, G. (1994a): Centrally active modulators of glutamate receptors facilitate the induction of long-term potentiation in vivo. *Proc. Natl. Acad. Sci. USA* **91**, 11158–11162.

Staubli, U., Rogers, G. & Lynch, G. (1994b): Facilitation of glutamate receptors enhances memory. *Proc. Natl. Acad. Sci. USA* **91**, 777–781.

Sternberg, D.E. & Jarvik, M.E. (1976): Memory functions in depression. *Arch. Gen. Psychiatry* **33**, 219–224.

Tanaka, S. (2006): Dopaminergic control of working memory and its relevance to schizophrenia: a circuit dynamics perspective. *Neuroscience* **139**, 153–171.

Taylor, E., Sergeant, J., Doepfner, J., Buitelaar, J., Rothenberger, A., Zuddas, A., Danckaerts, M., Banaschewski, T., Setinhausen, H.C., Asherson, P., Sonuga Barke, E. & Coghill, D. (2004): Clinical guidelines for hyperkinetic disorder. *Eur. Child Adolesc. Psychiatry* **7**, 184–200.

Turgay, A., Binder, C., Snyder, R. & Fisman, S. (2002): Long-term safety and efficacy of risperidone for the treatment of disruptive behaviour disorders in children with subaverage IQs. *Pediatrics* **110**, e34.

Vaidya, C.J., Austin, G., Kirkorian, G., Ridlehuber, H.W., Desmond, J.E., Glover, G.H. & Gabrieli, J.D. (1998): Selective effects of methylphenidate in attention deficit hyperactivity disorder: a functional magnetic resonance study. *Proc. Natl. Acad. Sci. USA* **95**, 14494–14499.

Volkow, N.D., Wang, G., Fowler, J.S., Logan, J., Gerasimov, M., Maynard, L., Ding, Y., Gatley, S.J., Gifford, A. & Franceschi, D. (2001): Therapeutic doses of oral methylphenidate significantly increase extracellular dopamine in the human brain. *J. Neurosci.* **21**, RC121.

Volkow, N.D., Wang, G.J., Fowler, J.S. & Ding, Y.S. (2005): Imaging the effects of methylphenidate on brain dopamine: new model on its therapeutic actions for attention deficit/hyperactivity disorder. *Biol. Psychiatry* **57**, 1410–1415.

Ward, R.P. & Dorsa, D.M. (1996): Colocalization of serotonin receptor subtypes 5-HT2A, 5-HT2C, and 5-HT6 with neuropeptides in rat striatum. *J. Comp. Neurol.* **370**, 405–414.

Welsh, M.C. & Pennington, B.F. (1988): Assessing frontal lobe functioning in children: views from developmental psychology. *Dev. Neuropsychol.* **4**, 199–230.

Williams, J.M., Guevremont, D., Kennard, J.T., Mason-Parker, S.E., Tate, W.P. & Abraham, W.C. (2003): Long-term regulation of N-methyl-D-aspartate receptor subunits and associated synaptic proteins following hippocampal synaptic plasticity. *Neuroscience* **118**, 1003–1013.

Woolley, M.L., Bentley, J.C., Sleight, A.J., Marsden, C.A. & Fone, K.C. (2001): A role for 5-ht6 receptors in retention of spatial learning in the Morris water maze. *Neuropharmacology* **41** (Suppl. 2), 210–219.

Woolley, M.L., Marsden, C.A., Sleight, A.J. & Fone, K.C. (2003): Reversal of a cholinergic induced deficit in a rodent model of recognition memory by the selective 5-HT6 receptor antagonist, Ro 04-6790. *Psychopharmacology (Berl.)* **170**, 358–367.

Zhang, H.T., Huang, Y., Suvarna, N.U., Deng, C., Crissman, A.M., Hopper, A.T., De Vivo, M., Rose, G.M. & O'Donnell, J.M. (2005): Effects of the novel PDE4 inhibitors MEM1018 and MEM1091 on memory in the radial-arm maze and inhibitory avoidance tests in rats. *Psychopharmacology (Berl.)* **179**, 613–619.

Chapter 17

The Feuerstein method: an effective tool for rehabilitation in mental retardation

Antonia Madella Noja

AIAS (Associazione Italiana Assistenza Spastici), via Paolo Mantegazza 10, 20156 Milan, Italy
antoniamadellanoja@tiscali.it

Summary

The Feuerstein method is of increasing interest for clinicians who assess and treat people with neurological disorders and genetic syndromes associated with mental retardation. In this chapter, the method is reviewed and the cultural framework underlying the method is outlined. Relative points of strength and weakness of the method are discussed.

Between the 1970's and the end of the 1990's, Reuven Feuerstein's method developed and applied mainly in the educational field as rehabilitative intervention for general learning disabilities. However, in the recent years there has been much interest in applying the method in the clinical field, in the rehabilitation of patients with neurological disorders and genetic syndromes associated with mental retardation.

Reuven Feuerstein was born in Romania. He studied psychology in Paris at the Sorbonne University. For a long time he worked in Geneva with Jean Piaget and André Rey, whose philosophical and pedagogic theories he studied in depth. Later he expanded the studies of Lev Vygotski, the great Russian pedagogist connected with the Neuropsychological Circle in Moscow, who died young and only became well known in Western countries much later than Piaget.

These two great thinkers were the most important influences on Feuerstein, and provided the inspiration for his Theory of Structural Cognitive Modifiability and Theory of Mediated Learning Experience.

Like Piaget, Feuerstein is a member of the cognitive school which characterized the last century in this field. Indeed his approach is more than 'cognitive' – it is 'metacognitive' as it considers 'elaboration and insight' the most particular characteristics of human thought. The cognitive and metacognitive perspective emphasizes the phase of elaboration of strategies for solving problems during the learning process. In addition, Feuerstein followed Vygotsky in his interpretation of the sociocultural nature of human learning.

From the start, the cognitive and psychological activities of the child have to do with the influences exercised by other humans. While for Piaget the human is an isolated discoverer of rules, for Vygotsky and Feuerstein human beings are individuals who can learn only by relating their personal context to the instruments offered them by their own 'culture' (from latin 'colere': to cultivate, to grow).

From this dichotomy there arise different ways of assessing learning ability. According to Piaget, the best way of assessing the child's learning process is to have the child deal with an unfamiliar task, so that performance can be tested without any contamination arising from the adult's logic. On the other hand, for Feuerstein – as for Vygotsky – what really counts is not the overt level of performance but the learning potential and propensity, which is better emphasized by a task that is both difficult and familiar at the same time, but which is solved through an adult's mediation. In such a cooperative situation, an individual can express his own 'zone of proximal development' (ZPD, elaborated by Vygotsky in 1927), which is evaluated by dynamic and interactive assessment aimed at showing the child's intellectual evolution and ability to change rather than a static level of performance. The ZPD contains functions that are currently in a state of being formed, and the situation of collaborative or assisted problem-solving creates conditions for the development of new psychological functions.

This concept permitted to Feuerstein to organize a system of assessment which he called the 'learning propensity assessment device' (LPAD), which provides an ongoing evaluation of discrepancies in quality and quantity between current functioning and modifiability, in order to suggest an appropriate intervention.

The theoretical basis of Feuersteins's method has two components. The first is the concept of *structural cognitive modifiability*, which is based on the possibility that cognitive functions can be modified irrespective of the aetiology of the problem and the degree of impairment. To be effective, the changes in cognitive functioning should be structural, permanent, pervasive, and generalizable. This assumption is strictly related to the second concept of the theory, which is that much of a person's modifiability is directly linked to the *amount and quality of mediated learning experiences* – defined by Feuerstein as 'the interactional process between the developing human organism and an experienced adult who, by interposing himself between the child and external sources of stimulation, mediates the world to him by framing, selecting, focusing, and feeding back environmental experience in such a way as to create appropriate learning sets.' (Feuerstein, 1968: The learning potential assessment device. Unpublished manuscript).

In the light of these two fundamental concepts, Feuerstein and the ICELP team (International Centre for Enhancement of Learning Potential) in Jerusalem have organized several systems of assessment and intervention between 1968 and the present day. The first of these, and also the most tested throughout the world over many years, is the LPAD (Learning Propensity Assessment Device) 'Classic' – a series of tests and activities that evaluate how a person learns, what kinds of teaching are required to obtain an improved response, and how much of the observed learning is retained. The LPAD differs from traditional educational and psychological evaluations in that we gain information not from scores or single responses, but from observations of the cognitive modifiability of the individual, and from helping the individual to solve problems through mediation.

An LPAD assessment consists of a battery of instruments, chosen to allow the assessor to observe how the learner responds in as many ways as possible. As the learner responds, the evaluator gathers information, develops ideas about the learner's needs and functions, and uses these insights to analyse the subject's performance in subsequent tasks: '...the LPAD produces processes of change *in vitro* during the assessment procedure and, rather than to establish an inventory of existing functions that the individual can mobilize efficiently, it assesses general learning modifiability, the extent of modifiability itself and the probability of transfer of new learning to other areas.' (Feuerstein & Shalom, 1968).

Because the process rather than the product is the main assessment target of LPAD, it offers a wide variety of possibilities for direct, specific, and systematic intervention, and this is perhaps the most important novel feature of the dynamic approach.

The LPAD – with its major goal of evaluating the degree of modifiability of a person with cognitive impairment above and beyond his low manifest level of functioning – cannot be of real significance unless it is accompanied by strategies of intervention to modify the subject's profile. With this in mind, Feuerstein elaborated the 'Instrumental Enrichment Programme. Classic' (IE Classic) in 1980: 'Instrumental enrichment is defined as a direct and focused attack on those intellectual functions diagnostically determined as being responsible, because of their weakness or nonexistence, for poor intellectual performance.' (Feuerstein *et al.*, 1980).

The IE Classic consists of more than 500 pages of paper-and-pencil 'content-free' exercises, divided into 14 instruments. The programme is presented for two to five hours weekly, at spaced intervals, over a period of two years, and its primary target population is children from 8 years old. Each instrument focuses on a specific cognitive deficiency, but also addresses itself to the acquisition of many other prerequisites of learning. Unlike other general enrichment programmes, which deal with cognitive deficits in terms of a gap to be compensated for by adding a certain amount of experience of contents, in the IE programme the emphasis is placed on the creation of awareness – in both the mediator and the pupil – of the significance of cognitive functioning implied in the activity particular to the task, and also in its generalization to other situations.

The instruments have different modalities (graphic, verbal, pictorial) to stimulate the child to produce structural cognitive changes in different areas and with different tasks. In the battery of the classic IE programme, there are the following:

Three non-verbal instruments: (1) Organization of dots; (2) Analytic perception; (3) Illustrations.

Six instruments with a limited vocabulary which require directions to be read: (1) Orientation in space-1; (2) Orientation in space-2; (3) Comparisons; (4) Family relations; (5) Numerical progressions; (6) Stencil design.

Five instruments that require independent reading and comprehension skills: (1) Categorization; (2) Instructions; (3) Temporal relations; (4) Transitive relations; (5) Syllogisms.

Except for 'Illustrations' and 'Temporal relations', exercises in each instrument are graded in difficulty and complexity, with later learning based on the mastery of earlier tasks. Two different instruments are taught in alternate lessons. This prevents the frustration that would accompany the use of only one instrument in which either the predominant modality or the deficient function emphasized by the instrument poses too much of a problem for a subject with specific difficulties. In this way we can provide the child with a balance between the kinds of functions addressed, the modality of presentation, and the subject's needs.

The programme's purpose is to enhance the individual's ability to benefit from direct exposure to new experiences in both formal and informal situations.

Instrumental enrichment achieves its purpose through six goals.

• *Goal 1:* The first goal is the correction of deficient cognitive functions in the three phases – input, elaboration, and output – provided for the intellectual framework of the method. Compared with the mental operations of Piaget, the cognitive functions in the IE programme are simpler portions of the mental process. For this reason when they are deficient they are more approachable by rehabilitation and more changeable in a positive way.

Correction of deficient cognitive functions is conditional on further modifiability and enhancement of individual capacities, and is the ultimate target for both assessment and intervention. The tasks of the IE programme provide a generalized approach to a wide range of cognitive deficiencies so as to correct and compensate them.

• *Goal 2:* The second goal of the programme is to help the subject acquire the concepts, vocabulary, strategies, and skills necessary to complete the task.

• *Goal 3:* The third goal is the production of intrinsic motivation through the formation of habits and the consolidation and internalization of new strategies, principles, and skills. Internalization is very important so that the subject can apply the acquired concepts, operations, and strategies spontaneously and without effort in different fields of learning and everyday experience.

• *Goal 4:* The fourth goal is the creation of insight so that the subjects can understand the reasons for their success or failure, the nature and value of their cognitive processes, and the possibility of transferring and generalizing their mental activities in different areas (the famous 'bridging activity' highlighted by Feuerstein).

• *Goal 5:* The fifth goal is the creation of task-intrinsic motivation: the tasks of the programme are intrinsically interesting, challenging, and complex, thus stimulating the motivation of child *per se*.

• *Goal 6:* The sixth goal is to change the state of the subject from a passive recipient of information to an active generator of new information.

Each instrument is structured with an internal coherence so that more complex tasks are based on learning acquired following the mastery of earlier tasks and instruments. A typical session of the IE programme includes an introduction, independent work, a discussion (which is the core of work), and a summary statement.

The programme involves a change in both mediator and mediatee: the attitude of both participants changes from passive acceptance to an active modification approach. The insight, generalization, use of errors as a source of further learning, capacity to plan from page to page, expansion of the mental field, and increasing flexibility represent the real content of the IE programme. In all the instruments the subject learns to encode and decode, to select the relevant items in the available data, and to reflect and delay the provision of an answer. The emphasis is on the abstract rather than the concrete; on representation rather than manipulation, and on becoming aware of the process whereby the solution is reached.

From 2000 to the present, Feuerstein and his team at ICELP have developed two further large 'chapters' of the method: LPAD Basic and IE Basic.

Alongside LPAD Classic, they have designed and systematized a new organic body of dynamic tests to assess the basic cognitive functions that precede those functions that are already structured and the mental operations that ensue. In fact, the term 'basic' refers to situations where the fundamental cognitive functions are deficient or latent, or have been insufficiently organized. The LPAD Basic is very useful in preschool children and also in other subjects affected by severe cognitive deficiencies resulting from neurological disorders (such as cerebral palsy) or genetic syndromes with mental retardation. As in LPAD Classic, the nature of the assessment is qualitative, not quantitative, and the goal is the analysis of the process whereby the learner finds the answer, rather than the answer itself. The aim of LPAD Basic is to show us whether, during the assessment, any small changes have arisen which prove the possibility of cognitive modifiability and the achievement of the zone of proximal development. The batteries of intervention linked with LPAD Basic are included in IE Basic.

The Feuerstein Instrumental Enrichment Programme-Basic (FIEB) is an extension and elaboration of the IE Classic and is based on the same theories of cognitive modifiability and mediated learning experience as the classic programme. The initial battery of instruments was presented for the first time in Guildford (England) and in Chicago (Illinois) in 2003 and includes seven instruments; the second battery was presented in Paris in 2005 and includes four instruments. Compared with IE Classic, the particular feature of IE Basic is that it is addresses younger children (preschool age children) or older individuals with very impaired mental functioning and needing a more systematic and developmentally based approach. Because these populations have significant cognitive and developmental disabilities or delay, they are unable to use and learn IE Classic.

The IE Basic can be considered to lay the foundation for later learning and to establish the cognitive and specific skills required for the use of the IE Classic programme. Like IE Classic, IE Basic is also organized in a systematic and clear way, with a focus on developmental and cognitive objectives. It not only facilitates the development of children, but ensures that further development will take place. With IE Basic it is possible to create a systematic and focused enhancement and acceleration of the natural process of cognitive functioning, not only in early childhood but also in situations of severe attention deficit disorder, neurological deficiencies, genetic syndromes with mental retardation, and so on. Compared with IE Classic, the content of Basic is much more than a pretext for the establishment of operations, it is a goal in itself. Indeed for the younger child and for low-functioning older learners, the content must be more expressly and systematically taught and linked to specific aspects of experience at the outset of the teaching. For these populations cognitive function is in a state of emergence, and the mediator must be ready to assess and build on the basic concepts so that the blend of content and process within the instruments can be utilized for the child's maximal development.

The 11 instruments comprising the IE Basic are as follows:

- Two instruments that serve as a preparation for the same at a higher level: *Organization of dots B*; *Orientation in space B*.

- Five instruments that strengthen the relation between emotional states and their cognitive correlates (a novelty in the method): *Identifying the emotions*; *From empathy to action*; *Absurd-1*; *Absurd-2*; *Prevention of violence*.

- One instrument that helps the learner to use and consolidate the cognitive operations necessary to build mathematical skills: *From unit to group*.

- One instrument organized to prevent and remedy a variety of difficulties and/or deficiencies in the attentional and perceptual fields: *Tri-channel attentional learning*.

- One instrument that trains the ability to categorize and prepare the skills necessary for playing with the instrument 'Categorization' in IE Classic: *Know, use and classify*.

- One instrument that provides the skills necessary for reading: *Reading comprehension*.

An important element in the presentation and teaching of the instruments of the IE Basic is the systematic, persistent, and structured creation of conditions that encourage the child to ask and answer questions, to be engaged in some active cognitive activities, and to define and solve problems.

Despite the early age and the low level of functioning, the subject is required to work in an abstract manner in IE Basic, as in IE Classic – the setting is not a psychomotor one but a purely cognitive one, and the experiences of work are not sensorimotor but formal and representative thinking.

In addition to LPAD Classic and Basic and IE Classic and Basic, Feuerstein has given us three other powerful tools for the rehabilitation of people with mental retardation. These three instruments are: (1) analysis of deficient cognitive function, (2) analysis of the characteristics of the stimulus (cognitive map), and (3) analysis of the quality of mediation (mediation criteria).

The first instrument is the analysis of *deficient cognitive function*, which lies at the core of inadequate cognitive performance and is the ultimate target for both assessment and intervention. Correction of deficient cognitive function is the most important condition for further modifiability and enhancement of the individual adaptable capacities. A list of deficient cognitive functions in the three phases of the mental act (input – elaboration – output) helps towards a better understanding of both the assessment procedures and the methods of intervention. The integrative model of the function itself includes four basic components: capacity, need, orientation, and operation. Obviously the existing list of the deficient cognitive functions is far from exhaustive, and this integrative model cannot encompass all possible factors which play a determining role in eliciting the appropriate cognitive behaviour. However, the analysis of deficient cognitive function is useful in drawing up a realistic profile of the capacities and deficiencies of the child.

Another consideration in constructing programmes for low-functioning individuals is to decide the areas on which to place the greatest emphasis. Because the goal of the intervention programme is to create a greater facility for benefiting from the learning processes, any decision about which dimensions to choose for greater investment must be guided by a conceptual framework.

This involves the second of Feuerstein's three additional instruments, the *cognitive map*. This, in contrast to the list of deficient cognitive functions, does not describe the individual but instead describes the tasks and their requisites. Each cognitive task can be analysed in terms of the following seven dimensions: (1) overall content; (2) language of presentation; (3) phase of the mental act (input – elaboration – output); (4) type of operation; (5) level of abstraction; (6) level of complexity; (7) degree of efficiency.

Feuerstein's third instrument for organizing the best programme for low-functioning individuals is the *analysis of quality of mediation*. So that the teacher or therapist acts as a mediator and not merely as dispenser of information, they need to follow certain criteria and categories of mediation. Mediated learning, in contrast to learning by direct exposure to stimuli, creates a relationship between a human mediator, a mediated stimulus, and a response. The quality of mediation and all mediational interactions are characterized by several criteria and categories. In particular there are three features that are universal and apply to every experience of cognitive interaction. These are:

- *Intentionality and reciprocity*, which refer to the fact that the mediator is motivated by an intention to modify the mediatee, and also that mediatee responds to the mediator. A unilateral effort to mediate is doomed to failure, or at least to limited meaning.
- *Transcendence*, defined as the widening of the interaction beyond its immediate goals to others that are more remote in time and space.
- *Meaning*, being the emotional, affective, energetic component of the interaction.

These three features are always present when a person wishes to have a cognitive interaction with someone else; the other criteria are situation-specific and are implemented by the mediator as a function of special needs of the individual and of the specific conditions of their life.

Conclusions

In our 15-year experience, we have identified three relative points of weakness and three points of strength in Feuerstein's method.

The points of weakness are as follows: (1) The method has attracted few external references. (2) Relating to this, there is a lack of clinical validation of the method. Feuerstein's method developed mainly in the educational field. Application of the method in the clinical field is more recent and it is very complex to harmonize the strict quantitative rules of scientific research in order to validate the system for application in pathological states such as cerebral palsy or genetic syndromes with mental retardation. (3) The third point of weakness relates to the setting necessary for cognitive intervention with instrumental enrichment – that is, a paper and pencil setting. The child must be able to cope with the situation, and children with severe behavioural and relational disturbance cannot be exposed successfully to this kind of setting. In our experience, with such patients it is better to start with a psychomotor rehabilitation system and only later to use instrumental enrichment.

Despite these areas of weakness, Feuerstein's method has three important strengths. These are as follows: (1) There is a very large 'repertoire' of interventions (either for assessment or for rehabilitation tools); reviewing other methods of cognitive rehabilitation, it is not possible to find a system that is so complete, rich, and differentiated as Feuerstein's. (2) The method is capable of generating changes in individuals with very low levels of cognitive functioning. From this point of view there is no limit to the application of the method, because even children with very inadequate cognitive performance can achieve important 'microchanges'. (3) The third advantage is related to the abstract nature of the tasks used in the method. The tasks in LPAD and IE are always representational and abstract, despite the young age of children who can be tested and their very low mental age. These characteristics activate the child's propensity to generalize, to self-reflect, and to internalize. The concept of internalization is an integral part of Feuerstein's theory, originating from Vygotskian thought. The process is gradual, proceeding developmentally from other-regulation to self-regulation, until the individual achieves independence.

In conclusion, despite the points of weakness still needing to be overcome, Feuerstein's method is an effective and powerful system of rehabilitation in mental retardation.

References

Feuerstein, R. & Shalom, H. (1968): The learning potential assessment device. In: *Proceedings of the First Congress of the International Association for the Scientific Study of Mental Deficiency*. ed. B.W. Richards. Reigate, UK: Michael Jackson.

Feuerstein, R., Rand, Y., Hoffman, M. & Miller, R. (1980): *Instrumental enrichment: an intervention program for cognitive modifiability*. Baltimore: University Park Press.

Additional bibliography

Feuerstein, R. (1969): *The instrumental enrichment method: an outline of theory and technique*. Jerusalem: Hadassah-WIZO-Canada Research Institute.

Feuerstein, R. (1977): Mediated learning experience: a theoretical basis for cognitive modifiability during adolescence. In: *Research to practice in mental retardation*, Vol. 2, ed. P. Mittler. Baltimore: University Park Press.

Feuerstein, R. (1980): *Instrumental enrichment*. Baltimore: University Park Press.

Feuerstein, R. (1990): The theory of structural cognitive modifiability. In: *Learning and thinking styles: classroom interaction*, ed. B. Presseisen. Washington DC: National Education Association.

Feuerstein, R. & Krasilowsky, D. (1967): The treatment group technique. *Israeli Annals of Psychiatry and Related Disciplines* **5,** 61–90.

Feuerstein, R., Rand, Y. & Hoffman, M. (1979): The dynamic assessment of retarded performers. In: *The learning potential assessment device (LPAD): theory, instruments and techniques*. Baltimore: University Park Press. [New revised edition: Feuerstein, R. *et al.* (2003): *The dynamic assessment of cognitive modifiability*. Jerusalem: ICELP Press].

Feuerstein, R., Klein, P.S. & Tannenbaum, A. (1991): *Mediated learning experience: theoretical, psychosocial and learning implications*. Tel Aviv: Freund.

Feuerstein, R., Rand, Y., Haywood, C., Kyram, L. & Hoffman, M. (1995): *Revised LPAD examiner's manual*. Jerusalem: ICELP.

Feuerstein, R., Falik, L.H. & Feuerstein, R.S. (1998): *Definition of essential concepts and terms. A working glossary*. Jerusalem: ICELP Press.

Kozulin, A. (1990): *Vygotsky's psychology: a biography of ideas*. Cambridge, MA: Harvard University Press.

Kozulin, A. (1998): *Psychological tools: a sociocultural approach to education*. Cambridge, MA: Harvard University Press.

Mecacci, L. (1983): *Lezioni di psicologia: Vygotsky*. Bologna: Il Mulino.

Mecacci, L. (1992): *Vygotsky: antologia di scritti*, pp. 7–40. Bologna: Il Mulino.

Piaget, J. (1952): *The origins of intelligence in children*. New York: Norton.

Piaget, J. (1954): *The construction of reality in the child*. New York: Ballantine.

Piaget, J. (1966): *La psychologie de l'enfant*. Paris: PUF.

Piaget, J. & Inhelder, B. (1947): *La représentation de l'espace chez l'enfant*. Paris: PUF.

Vygotsky, L. (1978): *Mind in society*. Cambridge, MA: Harvard University Press.

Vygotsky, L. (1986): *Thought and language*. Cambridge, MA: MIT Press.

Chapter 18

Understanding alterations during human brain development with molecular imaging: a guide to new treatment approaches for mental retardation

Diane C. Chugani

Carman and Ann Adams Department of Paediatrics and Department of Radiology, Children's Hospital of Michigan, Wayne State University School of Medicine, 3901 Beaubien Blvd., Detroit, Michigan 48201, USA.
dchugani@pet.wayne.edu

Summary

Molecular imaging studies using positron emission tomography (PET) can provide information on time course differences in the ontogeny of various neurochemical processes in children with developmental disabilities, and can therefore aid in designing treatment strategies. Developmental changes in brain glucose metabolism, serotonin synthesis, and $GABA_A$ receptor binding in children, measured with PET, are described. Studies using PET tracer to estimate serotonin synthesis show that humans undergo a period of high brain serotonin synthesis capacity during childhood, and that this developmental process is disrupted in autistic children. As serotonin is known to be an important factor involved in postnatal synaptogenesis, one therapeutic treatment for autism could be the use of serotonergic agents in children less than 6 years of age, when serotonin synthesis capacity is *lower* in autistic children than in non-autistic controls. The goal of treatment would be to provide a more normal modulation of synaptic plasticity for a finite period of brain development. In this chapter we explore strategies for defining critical periods of brain development using molecular imaging, as well as for exploiting critical periods for therapeutic alteration of brain development in children with mental retardation.

Introduction

Brain development involves a series of overlapping processes, occurring with distinct time courses, during which brain structure and function are established. Normal development depends upon the execution of genetically coded developmental programmes under optimal environmental conditions. Mental retardation occurs when there is disruption of normal brain development because of genetic mutations or adverse environmental events. Each developmental process may be considered a window in time in which pharmacological or behavioural interventions may have a distinct effect owing to the interactions of the interventions with that particular process at that point in development (Andersen, 2003). Measures of biochemical processes by positron emission tomography (PET) can be used to delineate normal biochemical patterns of brain maturation. The identification of deviations in the evolution of biochemical processes in developmental disorders can provide a rationale for a time-limited pharmacological or behavioural intervention to influence that particular process.

Studies of brain development with PET

At present, the time courses of relatively few molecular processes have been studied in humans *in vivo*. PET studies in humans have shown significant changes in glucose metabolism during normal brain development (Chugani *et al.*, 1987). Similarly, PET studies of neurotransmitter synthesis (Chugani *et al.*, 1999) and receptor binding (Chugani *et al.*, 2001) have also demonstrated significant changes during human brain development. A summary of these studies is presented below.

Glucose metabolism

Studies of regional cerebral glucose metabolism in human infants using PET with the tracer 2-deoxy-2[^{18}F]-fluoro-D-glucose (FDG) have shown that the pattern of glucose utilization undergoes dramatic changes in the first postnatal year. A consistent pattern is seen in the newborn, with the highest glucose metabolic activity in primary sensorimotor cortex, thalamus, brain stem, and cerebellar vermis (Chugani & Phelps, 1986; Chugani *et al.*, 1987; Chugani, 1994; Kinnala *et al.*, 1996). Intermediate levels of glucose metabolism are present in the cingulate cortex, amygdala, hippocampus, and occasionally the basal ganglia (Chugani, 1996; Chugani, 1998). The major portion of the cerebral cortex shows the lowest glucose metabolism. This neonatal pattern of glucose metabolism, largely confined to subcortical structures, is consistent with the less complex behaviour of neonates compared with infants. Subsequently, the ontogeny of regional brain glucose metabolism appears to follow a phylogenetic order, with functional maturation of older anatomical structures preceding that of newer areas (Chugani & Phelps, 1986; Chugani *et al.*, 1987; Chugani, 1994; Kinnala *et al.*, 1996; Chugani, 1996; Chugani, 1998). Moreover, functional maturation of various brain regions, as depicted by a rise in regional glucose metabolism, correlates well with the maturation of behavioural, neurophysiological, and neuroanatomical events in the infant. As visuo-spatial and visuo-sensorimotor integrative functions are acquired in the second and third months of life, and primitive reflexes become reorganized (André-Thomas *et al.*, 1960; Parmelee & Sigman, 1983), increases in glucose metabolism are observed in parietal, temporal, and primary visual cortical regions, frontal eye fields (Brodmann area 8), basal ganglia, and cerebellar hemispheres. Increasing glucose metabolism in the cerebral cortex during the second and third months of life presumably reflects maturation of the cortex and is consistent with the dramatic maturation of the electroencephalogram seen during the same period (Kellaway, 1979). Between 6 and 8 months, the remaining frontal cortex begins to show a maturational rise in glucose metabolism, which continues until one year of age. Functional maturation of the frontal cortex begins in the lateral and inferior portions, and later proceeds to include the medial and lastly the dorsal prefrontal areas. Functional maturation of these frontal cortical regions coincides with the emergence of higher cortical and cognitive abilities. By 1 year of age, the overall pattern of brain glucose metabolism is similar to that seen in adults. Measurement of the local cerebral metabolic rates of glucose utilization (LCMRglc) in children using PET show that they undergo a period during development when brain energy demand exceeds that of adults (Chugani *et al.*, 1987). The typically low neonatal values of LCMRglc, which are about 30 per cent lower than adult rates, increase rapidly from birth and reach adult values by about the second year. Thereafter, LCMRglc values continue to increase and begin to exceed adult values during the third postnatal year. By about 3 years, a plateau is reached which extends until about 9 to 10 years; following this, there is a gradual decline in LCMRglc to reach adult values again by about 16 to 18 years (Chugani et al., 1987; Chugani, 1994; Chugani, 1998). The relative increase in LCMRglc over adult values, which is most pronounced in neocortical regions between 3 and 10 years, reaches a peak value of over twice the LCMRglc levels seen in adults.

Serotonin synthesis

As with the developmental changes shown for cerebral glucose metabolism, ontogeny studies in non-human primates also demonstrate changes in neurotransmitter content and receptor binding (Goldman-Rakic & Brown, 1982; Lidow et al., 1991). For example, in the macaque there is a steep rise in cortical serotonin content beginning before birth and reaching a peak at 2 months of age, followed by a slow decline until about 3 years of age, when puberty occurs (Goldman-Rakic & Brown, 1982). The same group of investigators has reported a similar time course for expression of serotonin receptors (Lidow et al, 1991). We (Chugani et al., 1999) measured whole brain serotonin synthesis capacity at different ages using the tryptophan analogue $\alpha[^{11}C]$methyl-L-tryptophan (AMT) and PET in autistic children and a comparison group comprising eight healthy non-autistic siblings of autistic children (six male, two female, aged 2 to 14 years), as well as 16 children with epilepsy who were developing normally (nine male, seven female, aged 3 months to 13 years). We obtained permission to study healthy siblings of children with autism in order to examine the broader phenotype of autism present in many autism family members, thus providing potential benefit to the healthy siblings who participated. For this group of 'control' children, serotonin synthesis capacity was > 200 per cent of adult values until the age of 5 years and then declined towards adult values. Serotonin synthesis capacity values declined at an earlier age in girls than in boys. These data suggest that humans undergo a period of high brain serotonin synthesis capacity during childhood followed by a decline towards adult values, and that there are sex differences.

$GABA_A$ receptors

An understanding of human $GABA_A$ receptor ontogeny is highly relevant in elucidating the pathophysiology of neurodevelopmental disorders in which GABAergic mechanisms play a role, as well as in understanding age-related differences in the pharmacology of drugs acting on this system. We have measured age-related changes in the brain distribution of the $GABA_A$ receptor complex in vivo using PET in children with epilepsy under evaluation for surgical treatment (Chugani et al., 2001). PET imaging was undertaken using the tracer $[^{11}C]$flumazenil (FMZ), a ligand which binds to α subunits of the $GABA_A$ receptor. FMZ binding was quantified using a two-compartment model yielding values for the volume of distribution (VD) of the tracer in tissue. All brain regions studied showed the highest value for FMZ VD at the youngest age measured (2 years), and the values then decreased exponentially with age. Medial temporal lobe structures, primary visual cortex, and thalamus showed larger differences between age 2 years and adulthood (approximately a 50 per cent decrease) as compared with basal ganglia, cerebellum, and other cortical regions (which showed 25 to 40 per cent decreases from 2 years to adulthood). Furthermore, subcortical regions reached adult values earlier (14 to 17.5 years) than cortical regions (18 to 22 years).

Alterations of a biochemical developmental programme in a developmental disorder

Autism is a neurodevelopmental disorder characterized by deficits in social interaction and communication (verbal and non-verbal), and associated with restricted, repetitive, or stereotyped behaviours. It is associated with mental retardation in approximately 75 per cent of cases. In order to determine whether there are brain serotonergic abnormalities in children with autism, we have evaluated serotonin synthesis capacity *in vivo* with PET, using AMT as the tracer. Our results show two fundamentally different types of serotonergic abnormality in children with autism (Chugani *et al.*, 1997; Chugani *et al.*, 1999; Chandana *et al.*, 2005). The first is a difference in whole brain serotonin synthesis capacity in autistic children compared with age-matched non-autistic children. As described above, serotonin synthesis capacity was > 200 per cent of adult values until the age of 5 years and then declined toward adult values in non-autistic children. In contrast, serotonin synthesis capacity in autistic children increased gradually between the ages of 2 years and 15 years to values 1.5 times the adult normal values (Chugani *et al.*, 1999). These data suggest that humans undergo a period of high brain serotonin synthetic capacity during early childhood, and that this developmental process is disrupted in autistic children.

The second type of abnormality we have reported relates to focal abnormalities in brain serotonin synthesis. Asymmetries of AMT uptake in the frontal cortex, thalamus, and cerebellum were visualized in children with autism (Chugani *et al.*, 1997). In addition, we measured brain serotonin synthesis in a large group of autistic children (n = 117) with AMT PET, and related these data to handedness and language function (Chandana *et al.*, 2005). Cortical AMT uptake abnormalities were objectively derived from small homotopic cortical regions using a predefined cut-off asymmetry threshold (> 2 SD of normal asymmetry). Autistic children showed several patterns of abnormal cortical involvement, including right cortical, left cortical, and absence of abnormal asymmetry. Groups of autistic children defined by the presence or absence and side of cortical asymmetry differed on a measure of language as well as on handedness. Autistic children with left cortical AMT decreases showed a higher prevalence of severe language impairment, whereas those with right cortical decreases showed a higher prevalence of left and mixed handedness. These results suggest that global as well as focal abnormally asymmetrical development in the serotonergic system could lead to miswiring of the neural circuits specifying hemispheric specialization.

Pharmacological intervention in autism to restore the developmental pattern for serotonin

Pharmacological interventions in autism have been carried out predominantly in older children and adults (for reviews, see Posey & McDougle, 2001 and Palmero & Curatolo, 2004). The primary goal of these studies was to target certain disruptive behaviours such as aggression, self-injurious behaviour, and sleep problems, or specific behaviours characteristic of autism, such as stereotyped behaviours (reviewed in Aman, 2004 and Bostic & King, 2005). Here we propose pharmacological intervention to restore the normal pattern of brain biochemical development based upon our finding of an altered pattern of serotonin synthesis in autistic children, together with a large animal literature showing changes in synaptic connectivity at a time when there were alterations in serotonin during critical periods of brain development.

Evidence from both pharmacological and gene knock-out experiments (for a review, see Gaspar *et al.*, 2003) show that serotonin plays a role in modulation of synaptogenesis.

Immunocytochemistry for serotonin and [^{3}H]citalopram binding to serotonin uptake sites have both demonstrated a transient serotonergic innervation of primary sensory cortex between postnatal days 2 and 14 during the period of synaptogenesis in rat cortex (D'Amato et al., 1987; Cases et al., 1995). Two early studies (Bennett-Clarke et al., 1996; Lebrand et al., 1996) reported that this transient innervation actually represented transient expression of the high-affinity serotonin transporter and vesicular monoamine transporter by glutamatergic thalamo-cortical neurons. The serotonin transporter is transiently expressed by glutamatergic thalamo-cortical afferents (Bennett-Clarke et al., 1996; Lebrand et al., 1996) during the first two postnatal weeks in rats. During this period, these thalamocortical neurons take up and store serotonin although they do not synthesize serotonin. While the role of serotonin in glutamatergic neurons with cell bodies located in the sensory nuclei of the thalamus is not yet known, there is evidence that the serotonin concentration must be neither too high nor too low during this period. Thus depletion of serotonin delays the development of the barrel fields of the rat somatosensory cortex (Blue et al., 1991; Osterheld-Haas & Hornung, 1996) and decreases their size (Bennett-Clarke et al., 1994). Conversely, increased serotonin during this critical period – as in the MAO-A knock-out mouse – results in increased tangential arborization of these axons, with blurring of the boundaries of the cortical barrels (Cases et al., 1996). Decreased or increased brain serotonin during this period of development causes disruption of synaptic connectivity in sensory cortices (Cases et al., 1995; Bennett-Clarke et al., 1994; Cases et al., 1996). Furthermore, disruption of serotonin transporter functions impairs the cerebral glucose metabolic response to whisker stimulation (Esaki et al., 2005). The effect of serotonin on synaptogenesis and synaptic function is not limited to the sensory cortices. For example, Yan et al. (1997) have reported that depletion of serotonin with p-chloroamphetamine (PCA) or 5,7-dihydroxytryptamine in neonatal rat pups resulted in large decreases in the numbers of dendritic spines in hippocampus.

Mechanisms of serotonin effects on synaptic plasticity

The changes in serotonin receptor density, serotonergic innervation, and serotonin synthesis with age suggest that serotonin plays an important role in brain development. Indeed, there is a body of evidence indicating that serotonin regulates several aspects of brain development including cell division, differentiation, neurite outgrowth, and synaptogenesis. These effects have been observed on serotonergic neurons as well as in the tissues innervated by serotonergic terminals. There are several different mechanisms by which serotonin influences brain development. These include the regulation of trophic factors and direct regulation of activity-dependent plasticity. There is evidence that one mechanism by which serotonin exerts trophic effects during brain development may be through the regulation of trophic factors such as the $5HT_{1A}$-mediated release of S100β (Nishi et al., 1996) and brain-derived neurotrophic factor (BDNF) (Galter & Unsicker, 2000). One study has reported evidence that serotonin, the $5HT_{1A}$ receptor, BDNF, and its receptor trkB form an autoparacrine loop which regulates the differentiation of serotonergic neurons (Galter & Unsicker, 2000). This study reported that serotonin and the $5HT_{1A}$ agonists BP-554 and 8-OH-DPAT (but not $5HT_{1B}$ and $5HT_{1D}$ agonists) increased the numbers of cultured raphé neurons expressing serotonergic markers and BDNF rRNA. Treatment with the $5HT_{1A}$ antagonist WAY-100635 or trkB-IgG fusions protein blocked the induction of serotonergic markers in the cultures.

During brain development, activity-dependent processes may also play a role in the refinement of synaptic connections. Axons are thought to compete for post-synaptic targets during critical periods when synapses are stabilized or lost depending upon synaptic activity (Goodman & Shatz, 1993). One mechanism by which synapses are believed to be stabilized is by long-term potentiation (LTP). Interestingly, serotonin and its alterations during development have effects on LTP. These effects have been documented in several brain regions, including the somatosensory cortex (Isaac et al., 1997), visual cortex (Edagawa et al., 1998a; Edagawa et al., 1998b; Edagawa et al., 1999; Kojic et al., 2000; Edagawa et al., 2001), spinal cord (Li & Zhuo, 1998), and hippocampus (Tecott et al., 1998). In addition, evidence for serotonergic modulation of synaptic development has been demonstrated for the lateral superior olive in developing gerbils (Fitzgerald & Sanes, 1999) and for segregation of retinal projections in MAO-A knock-out mice (Upton et al., 1999). In summary, it is now clear that serotonin influences postnatal synaptogenesis in multiple brain regions.

Designing pharmacological studies for developmental disabilities

The design of pharmacological studies aimed at altering brain development in autism requires various critical decisions to be made (Scahill et al., 2001; Hollander et al., 2004) – including choice of pharmacological agent, subject inclusion and exclusion criteria, timing (age) and duration of treatment, combination with behavioural intervention, and assessment of efficacy and adverse outcomes. There are several classes of pharmacological agents for modifying brain development. One class of compounds includes trophic or regulatory hormones that are developmentally regulated and are pivotal in certain aspects of brain development for discrete periods of time. There appears to be an abundance of evidence that serotonergic agents may be logical first choices in employing this approach in modifying brain developmental processes in autism, as described above.

In order to determine the optimal time to treat an autistic child, both the normal developmental process and deviation from normal development need to be considered. In the case of serotonin synthesis and autism, there is a rationale for targeting the period of 2 to 6 years, when serotonin synthesis is lower in autistic children than in typically developing children. We have reported preliminary results of a trial of the serotonin partial agonist buspirone in 2–6 year old autistic children (Rothermel et al., 2006). This pilot study showed buspirone treatment resulted in significant improvements in social and stereotyped behaviours, as well as in anxiety and sensory problems. A larger trial based upon these results is ongoing.

It is likely that some interventions will only work in autistic children during a certain age range or during a certain period of brain development. In general, one would hypothesize that the earlier the intervention and the closer in time to the actual disorder-driven deviation in brain development, the better the chance of recovery of function. However, one can also imagine that the side effects of a treatment – that is, the actions of the pharmacological agent at sites where its expression may be normal – may be less if the intervention occurs after that normal process is complete. In other words, timing of an intervention may be one means of having some specificity when administering compounds that have actions in widespread areas of the brain, but the target areas are somewhat discrete. The question of how long to treat an autistic child is similar to that of when to treat. Again, specific insight of the normal developmental time course of the process being targeted and deviation in autism from the process must first be achieved. However, it is conceivable that treatment for a period longer than the normal time course could be beneficial for various reasons. For example, treatment may lengthen the critical period, thus providing a longer period of time for sensory interventions to affect synaptic plasticity. Length of treatment might also be determined empirically by ascertaining when the side effects of the treatment begin to surpass the perceived benefits.

Combining pharmacological and behavioural interventions

The combination of particular behavioural interventions during critical period targeted pharmacotherapy could also be considered. For example, it is well demonstrated that GABA mechanisms are involved in the refinement of ocular dominance columns. Treatment with GABAergic drugs during a critical period alters the time course of this development (Hensch et al., 1998). There is abundant evidence that developmental changes in GABA neurotransmission are related to critical periods of activity-dependent synaptic plasticity in response to sensory experience in animals (Wolf et al., 1986; Ramoa et al., 1988; Reiter & Stryker, 1988). Furthermore, there are dramatic changes in $GABA_A$ receptor subunit composition in the developing brain – for example, in the visual cortex (Huntsman et al., 1994; Huang et al., 1999) somatosensory cortex (Golshani et al., 1997; Huntsman et al., 1995), and cerebellum (Carlson et al., 1998). A specific role for benzodiazepine-sensitive $GABA_A$ receptors in the critical period for establishing ocular dominance has been suggested by investigators who have demonstrated that infusion of diazepam can restore visual cortex plasticity in mice with gene-targeted disruption of the 65 kDa isoform of the GABA synthetic enzyme glutamic acid decarboxylase (GAD_{65}) (Hensch et al., 1998). GAD_{65} knock-out mice showed no shift in ocular dominance with eye closure during the critical period. However, ocular dominance shift in response to eye closure *did* occur in these mice if diazepam was infused in the visual cortex during the critical period. We suggested that the high ^{11}C-flumazenil volume of distribution (VD) in early childhood, as demonstrated by PET scanning (Chugani et al., 2001), may be related to a specific role of benzodiazepine-sensitive $GABA_A$ receptors in critical periods of synaptic plasticity during human brain development. Pairing of visual sensory experience with the lengthening of the critical period may be a powerful way to provide a therapeutic intervention in this system. Similarly, serotonergic drugs have been shown to alter the thalamocortical connectivity of the somatosensory cortex as described above. Pairing of various sensory interventions with pharmacological treatment affecting serotonergic tone may improve the efficacy of this type of intervention.

The possibility of reopening critical periods

As mentioned above, treatment with benzodiazepines can lengthen the critical period for establishment of the ocular dominance columns. Therefore, it is not inconceivable that pharmacological agents might also be employed in children with developmental disorders to reopen critical periods for therapeutic intervention. For example, the length of time for the expression of serotonin transporters on thalamocortical afferents was shown to be prolonged by decreasing thyroid hormone (Auso et al., 2001). Thus, manipulation of thyroid hormone may be a strategy for altering the critical period for thalamocortical synaptogenesis. The purpose of lengthening or reopening a critical period might allow more time for acquisition of certain skills – for example, language skills. Pairing of this opening with intensive behavioural interventions might lead to improved efficacy of experience-dependent plasticity. This approach may also be useful for 'correcting' sensory problems such as hypersensitivity to sound, light, touch, and smell.

Practical and ethical considerations

There is much need for the development of tools to assess therapeutic change for clinical trials in autism (Scahill et al., 2001; Hollander et al., 2004) and other developmental disorders. The assessment of a treatment that is designed to change brain development is even more problematic. The improvement in behaviour may require a rather protracted period during which there may be apparent adverse effects on behaviour. In any case, the assessment of change in a chronic treatment requires tools for assessing the targeted behaviours and adverse events, and these tools must be amenable to periodic repeated use over the course of the treatment.

One must be cautious in designing interventions during development, as there is the possibility of adversely affecting brain development. For example, lack of expression of the $5HT_{1A}$ receptor (Gross et al., 2002) and blockade of the serotonin transporter (Ansorge et al., 2004) during early brain development is linked to anxiety in adult rodents (for a review, see Gross & Hen, 2004). It is difficult to know precisely which timing and which dose one must use to achieve beneficial effects, and it is possible that only a certain dose at a certain time will be beneficial, whereas other doses or the appropriate dose at other time points may be detrimental. Furthermore, as discussed above, drugs act at many locations in the brain, and the beneficial action may occur in one specific area of the brain whereas a detrimental effect may occur by the action of the drug in another part of the brain.

Conclusions

A new era of pharmacological interventions in developmental disorders is possible owing to increasing understanding of the molecular events regulating critical periods of brain development. In addition, the ability to ascertain the genetic variations in individuals with developmental disorders to determine which developmental process may be affected might guide rational strategies for intervention. The use of pharmacological strategies, paired with behavioural interventions, holds promise for influencing brain function in children with developmental disorders.

Acknowledgments: This work was supported in part by U01 HD37261-04S2, one of the NICHD funded Pediatric Pharmacology Research Units, and R01 HD34942.

References

Aman, M.G. (2004): Management of hyperactivity and other acting-out problems in patients with autism spectrum disorder. *Semin. Pediatr. Neurol.* **11**, 225–228.

Andersen, S.L. (2003): Trajectories of brain development: point of vulnerability or window of opportunity? *Neurosci. Biobehav. Rev.* **27**, 3–18.

André-Thomas, C.Y. & Saint-Anne Dargassies, S. (1960): *The neurological examination of the infant.* London: Medical Advisory Committee of the National Spastics Society.

Ansorge, M.S., Zhou, M., Lira, A., Hen, R. & Gingrich, J.A. (2004): Early-life blockage of the 5-HT transporter alters emotion behaviour in adult mice. *Science* **29**, 879–881.

Auso, E., Cases, O., Fouquet, C., Camacho, M., Garcia-Velasco, J.V., Gaspar, P. & Berbel, P. (2001): Protracted expression of serotonin transporter and altered thalamocortical projections in the barrelfield of hypothyroid rats. *Eur. J. Neurosci.* **14**, 1968–1980.

Bennett-Clarke, C.A., Leslie, M.J., Lane, R.D. & Rhoades, R.W. (1994): Effect of serotonin depletion on vibrissae-related patterns in the rat's somatosensory cortex. *J. Neurosci.* **14**, 7594–7607.

Bennett-Clarke, C.A., Chiaia, N.L. & Rhoades, R.W. (1996): Thalamocortical afferents in rat transiently express high-affinity serotonin uptake sites. *Brain Res.* **733**, 301–306.

Blue, M.E., Erzurumlu, R.S. & Jhaveri, S. (1991): A comparison of pattern formation by thalamocortical and serotonergic afferents in the rat barrel field cortex. *Cereb. Cortex* **1**, 380–389.

Bostic, J.Q. & King, B.H. (2005): Autism spectrum disorders: emerging pharmacotherapy. *Expert Opin. Emerg. Drugs* **10**, 521–536.

Carlson, B.X., Elster, L. & Schousboe, A. (1998): Pharmacological and functional implications of developmentally-regulated changes in GABA(A) receptor subunit expression in the cerebellum. *Eur. J. Pharmacol.* **352**, 1–14.

Cases, O., Seif, I., Grimsby, J., Gaspar, P., Chen, K., Pournin, S., Müller, U., Aguet, M., Babinet, C., Shih, J.C. & De Maeyer, E. (1995): Aggressive behaviour and altered amounts of brain serotonin and norepinephrine in mice lacking MAOA. *Science* **268**, 1763–1766.

Cases, O., Vitalis, T., Seif, I., De Maeyer, E., Sotelo, C. & Gaspar, P. (1996): Lack of barrels in the somatosensory cortex of monoamine oxidase A-deficient mice; role of a serotonin excess during the critical period. *Neuron* **16**, 297–307.

Chandana, S.R., Behen, M.E., Juhasz, C., Muzik, O., Rothermel, R.D., Mangner, T.J., Chakraborty, P.K., Chugani, H.T. & Chugani, D.C. (2005): Significance of abnormalities in developmental trajectory and asymmetry of cortical serotonin synthesis in autism. *Int. J. Dev. Neurosci.* **23**, 171–182.

Chugani, H.T. (1994): Development of regional brain glucose metabolism in relation to behaviour and plasticity. In: *Human behaviour and the developing brain*, eds. G. Dawson & K.W. Fischer, pp. 153–175. New York: Guilford Publications.

Chugani, H.T. (1996): Neuroimaging of developmental nonlinearity and developmental pathologies. In: *Developmental neuroimaging: mapping the development of brain and behavior*, eds. R.W. Thatcher, G.R. Lyon, J. Rumsey & N. Krasnegor, pp. 187–195. San Diego: Academic Press.

Chugani, H.T. (1998): The ontogeny of cerebral metabolism. In: *Neuroimaging in child neuropsychiatric disorders*, ed. B. Garreau, pp. 89–96. Berlin: Springer-Verlag.

Chugani, H.T. & Phelps, M.E. (1986): Maturational changes in cerebral function in infants determined by 18FDG positron emission tomography. *Science* **231**, 840–843.

Chugani, H.T., Phelps, M.E. & Mazziotta, J.C. (1987): Positron emission tomography study of human brain functional development. *Ann. Neurol.* **22**, 487–497.

Chugani, D.C., Muzik, O., Rothermel, R., Behen, M., Chakraborty, P., Mangner, T., da Silva, E.A. & Chugani, H.T. (1997): Altered serotonin synthesis in the dentato-thalamo-cortical pathway in autistic boys. *Ann. Neurol.* **42**, 666–669.

Chugani, D.C., Muzik, O., Behen, M.E., Rothermel, R.D., Lee, J. & Chugani, H.T. (1999): Developmental changes in brain serotonin synthesis capacity in autistic and non-autistic children. *Ann. Neurol.* **45**, 287–295.

Chugani, D.C., Muzik, O., Juhasz, C., Janisse, J.J., Ager, J. & Chugani, H.T. (2001): Postnatal maturation of human GABAA receptors measured with positron emission tomography. *Ann. Neurol.* **49**, 618–626.

Cook, E.H., Courchesne, R.Y., Cox, N.J., Lord, C., Gonen, D., Guter, S.J., Lincoln, A., Nix, K., Haas, R., Leventhal, B.L. & Courchesne, E. (1998): Linkage-disequilibrium mapping of autistic disorder, with 15q11-13 markers. *Am. J. Hum. Genet.* **62**, 1077–1083.

D'Amato, R.J., Blue, M.E., Largent, B.L., Lynch, D.R., Ledbetter, D.J., Molliver, M.E. & Snyder, S.H. (1987): Ontogeny of the serotonergic projection to rat neocortex, transient expression of a dense innervation to primary sensory areas. *Proc. Natl Acad Sci USA* **84**, 4322–4326.

Edagawa, Y., Saito, H. & Abe, K. (1998a): Serotonin inhibits the induction of long-term potentiation in rat primary visual cortex. *Prog. Neuropsychopharmacol. Biol. Psychiatry* **22**, 983–997.

Edagawa, Y., Saito, H. & Abe, K. (1998b): $5HT_{1A}$ receptor-mediated inhibition of long-term potentiation in rat visual cortex. *Eur. J. Pharmacol.* **349**, 221–224.

Edagawa, Y., Saito, H. & Abe, K. (1999) Stimulation of the $5HT_{1A}$ receptor selectively suppresses NMDA receptor-mediated synaptic excitation in the rat visual cortex. *Brain Res.* **827**, 225–228.

Edagawa, Y., Saito, H. & Abe, K. (2001): Endogenous serotonin contributes to a developmental decrease in long-term potentiation in the rat visual cortex. *J. Neurosci.* **21**, 1532–1537.

Esaki, T., Cook, M., Shimoji, K., Murphy, D.L., Sokoloff, L. & Holmes, A. (2005): Developmental disruption of serotonin transporter function impairs cerebral responses to whisker stimulation in mice. *Proc. Natl. Acad. Sci. USA* **102**, 5582–5587.

Fitzgerald, K.K. & Sanes, D.H. (1999): Serotonergic modulation of synapses in the developing gerbil lateral superior olive. *J. Neurophysiol.* **81**, 2743–2752.

Galter, D. & Unsicker, K. (2000): Sequential activation of the 5HT1A serotonin receptor and TrkB induces the serotonergic neuronal phenotype. *Mol. Cell. Neurosci.* **15**, 446–455.

Gaspar, P., Cases, O. & Maroteaux, L. (2003): The developmental role of serotonin: news from mouse molecular genetics. *Nat. Rev. Neurosci.* **4**, 1002–1012.

Goldman-Rakic, P.S. & Brown, R.M. (1982): Postnatal development of monoamine content and synthesis in the cerebral cortex of rhesus monkeys. *Dev. Brain Res.* **4**, 339–349.

Golshani, P., Truong, H. & Jones, E.G. (1997): Developmental expression of $GABA_A$ receptor subunit and GAD genes in mouse somatosensory barrel cortex. *J. Comp. Neurol.* **383**, 199–219.

Goodman, C. & Shatz, C. (1993): Developmental mechanisms that generate precise patterns of neuronal connectivity. *Cell* **72** (Suppl. 10), 77–98.

Gross, C. & Hen, R. (2004): The developmental origins of anxiety. *Nat. Rev. Neurosci.* **5**, 545–552.

Gross, C., Zhuang, X., Stark, K., Ramboz, S., Oosting, R., Kirby, L., Santarelli, L., Beck, S. & Hen, R (2002): Serotonin 1A receptor acts during development to establish normal anxiety-like behaviour in the adult. *Nature* **416**, 396–400.

Hensch, T.K., Fagiolini, M., Mataga, N., Stryker, M.P., Baekkeskov, S. & Kash, S.F. (1998): Local GABA circuit control of experience-dependent plasticity in developing visual cortex. *Science* **282**, 1504–1508.

Hollander, E., Phillips, A., King, B.H., Guthrie, D., Aman, M.G., Law, P., Owley, T. & Robinson, R. (2004): Impact of recent findings on study design of future autism clinical trials. *CNS Spectrums* **9**, 49–56.

Huang, Z.J., Kirkwood, A., Pizzorusso, T., Porciatti, V., Morales, B., Bear, M.F., Maffei, L. & Tonegawa, S. (1999): BDNF regulates the maturation of inhibition and the critical period of plasticity in mouse visual cortex. *Cell* **98**, 739–755.

Huntsman, M.M., Isackson, P.J. & Jones, E.G. (1994): Lamina-specific expression and activity-dependent regulation of seven $GABA_A$ receptor mRNAs in monkey visual cortex. *J. Neurosci.* **14**, 2236–2259.

Huntsman, M.M., Woods, T.M. & Jones, E.G. (1995): Laminar patterns of expression of $GABA_A$ receptor subunit mRNAs in monkey sensory motor cortex. *J. Comp. Neurol.* **362**, 565–582.

Isaac, J.T.R., Crair, M.C., Nicoll, R.A. & Malenka, R.C. (1997): Silent synapses during development of thalamocortical inputs. *Neuron* **18**, 269–280.

Kellaway, P. (1979): An orderly approach to visual analysis: parameters of the normal EEG in adults and children. In: *Current practice of clinical electroencephalography*, eds. D.W. Klass & D.D Daly, pp. 69–147. New York: Raven Press.

Kinnala, A., Suhonen-Polvi, H., Äärimaa, T., Kero, P., Korvenranta, H., Ruotsalainen, U., Bergman, J., Haaparanta, M., Solin, O., Nuutila, P. & Wegelius, U. (1996): Cerebral metabolic rate for glucose during the first six months of life: an FDG positron emission tomography study. *Arch. Dis. Child.* **74**, F153-F157.

Kojic, L., Dyck, R., Gu, Q., Douglas, R.M., Matsubara, J. & Cynader, M.S. (2000): Columnar distribution of serotonin-dependent plasticity within kitten striate cortex. *Proc. Natl. Acad. Sci. USA* **97**, 1841–1844.

Lebrand, C., Cases, O., Adelbrecht, C., Doye, A., Alvarez, C., Mestikawy, S.E., Seif, I. & Gaspar, P. (1996): Transient uptake and storage of serotonin in developing thalamic neurons. *Neuron* **17**, 823–835.

Li, P. & Zhou, M. (1998): Silent glutamatergic synapses and nociception in mammalian spinal cord. *Nature* **393**, 695–698.

Lidow, M.S., Goldman-Rakic, P.S. & Pakic, P. (1991): Synchronized overproduction of neurotransmitter receptors in diverse regions of the primate cerebral cortex. *Proc. Natl. Acad. Sci. USA* **88**, 10218–10221.

Nishi, M., Whitaker-Azmitia, P.M. & Azmitia, E.C. (1996): Enhanced synaptophysin immunoreactivity in rat hippocampal culture by 5-HT 1A agonist, S100b, and corticosteroid receptor agonists. *Synapse* **23**, 1–9.

Osterheld-Haas, M.C. & Hornung, J.P. (1996): Laminar development of the mouse barrel cortex, effects of neurotoxins against monoamines. *Exp. Brain Res.* **110**, 183–195.

Palermo, M.T. & Curatolo, P. (2004): Pharmacologic treatment of autism. *J. Child Neurol.* **19**, 155–164.

Parmelee, A.H. & Sigman, M.D. (1983): Perinatal brain development and behaviour. In: *Biology and infancy*, vol. II, eds. M. Haith & J. Campos, pp. 95–155. New York: John Wiley.

Phelps, M.E., Barrio, J.R., Huang, S.C., Keen, R.E., Chugani, H. & Mazziotta, J.C. (1984): Criteria for the tracer kinetic measurement of cerebral protein synthesis in humans with positron emission tomography. *Ann. Neurol.* **15**, S192-S202.

Posey, D.J. & McDougle, C.J. (2001): Pharmacotherapeutic management of autism. *Expert Opin. Pharmacother.* **2**, 587–600.

Ramoa, A.S., Paradiso, M.A. & Freeman, R.D. (1988): Blockade of intracortical inhibition in kitten striate cortex: effects on receptive field properties and associated loss of ocular dominance plasticity. *Exp. Brain Res.* **73**, 285–298.

Reiter, H.O. & Stryker, M.P. (1988): Neural plasticity without postsynaptic action potentials, less active inputs become dominant when kitten visual cortical cells are pharmacologically inhibited. *Proc. Natl. Acad. Sci. USA* **85**, 3623–3627.

Rothermel, R.R., Behen, M.E., Geenen, E., Fish, A., Chugani, H.T. & Chugani, D.C. (2006): Pilot efficacy of treatment with buspirone in autistic children: a randomized double blind study in children 2 to 6 years of age. International Meeting for Autism Research, Montreal, Canada, June 1–3.

Scahill, L., McCracken, J., McDougle, C.J., Aman, M., Arnold, L.E., Tierney, E., Cronin, P., Davies, M., Ghuman, J., Gonzalez, N., Koenig, K., Lindsay, R., Martin, A., McGough, J., Posey, D.J., Swiezy, N., Volkmar, F., Ritz, L. &

Vitiello, B. (2001): Methodological issues in designing a multisite trial of risperidone in children and adolescents with autism. *J. Child Adolesc. Psychopharmacol.* **11,** 377–388.

Tecott, L.H., Logue, S.F., Wehner, J.M. & Kauer, J.A. (1998): Perturbed dentate gyrus function in serotonin 5-HT2C receptor mutant mice. *Proc. Natl. Acad. Sci. USA* **95,** 15026–15031.

Upton, A.L., Salichon, N., Lebrand, C., Ravary, A., Blakely, R., Seif, I. & Gaspar, P. (1999): Excess of serotonin (5-HT) alters the segregation of ipsilateral and contralateral retinal projections in monoamine oxidase A knock-out mice: possible role of 5-HT uptake in retinal ganglion cells during development. *J. Neurosci.* **19,** 7007–7024.

Wolf, W., Hicks, T.P. & Albus, K. (1986): The contribution of GABA-mediated inhibitory mechanisms to visual response properties of neurons in the kitten's striate cortex. *J. Neurosci.* **6,** 2779–2796.

Yan, W., Wilson, C.C. & Haring, J.H. (1997): Effects of neonatal serotonin depletion on the development of rat dentate granule cells. *Brain Res. Dev. Brain Res.* **98,** 177–184.

Chapter 19

Mental retardation: definition and classification systems

Daria Riva, Arianna Usilla, Chiara Vago, Federica Aggio and Sara Bulgheroni

Department of Developmental Neurology, Fondazione IRCCS Istituto Neurologico 'C. Besta', via Celoria 11, 20133 Milan, Italy
driva@istituto-besta.it

Summary

In this chapter we outline the main diagnostic systems used to define and describe mental retardation. The principal classifications are described, along with the theoretical paradigm on which they are based, which enables them to be grouped into two main reference models: biomedical and bio-psychosocial. These two main systems are clearly complementary (and always have been) and they respond to different needs in different settings, so one cannot exclude the other, nor is one superior to the other.

All systems for classifying mental retardation are multiaxial and constantly consider the issue from different standpoints, making it necessary to use them in combination.

Mention is also made of how important it is to arrive at an aetiological diagnosis, as this can have enormous added value in terms of prognosis and treatment, and for a proper definition of the future prospects of an individual with cognitive impairment and related problems.

Introduction

The issue of definitions and classification systems is crucial in every field, and particularly in medicine, but it is even more fundamental in the neurobehavioural sciences, where defining also means finding words to describe the complexity of a pathological condition, characterized by a whole constellation of intellectual, neuropsychological, and psychiatric impairments, and where the pathological condition is expressed in more or less severe forms of functional disability. A proper definition is of crucial importance for the person concerned because it is used to assign them to one particular category rather than another, and it goes without saying that definition is an important responsibility in the diagnosis of mental retardation and its varying degrees of severity.

The definition is also crucial because it orients the current clinical, scientific, and social approaches to a patient at any given time and because it enables professionals in the field to use a common language.

It is also self-evident that an accurate definition allows the extent of a problem to be measured in an epidemiological sense. Merely establishing the precise number of subjects presenting the problem is not enough to enable plans to be made for the future management of the problem. The American Academy of Mental Retardation (AAMR) rightly places the emphasis on the importance of the support methods to use, and on their level of intensity, with a view to establishing adequate political and financial programming of the related needs.

The problem can thus be faced in its global sense by integrating a multidimensional diagnosis with the definition of the problem in terms of the resources needed to improve the patient's quality of life.

The definition of a problem relies on the fact that a definition attributes a meaning to the problem *per se* so that it can be generally understood, though the definition may not necessarily be shared by all the operators taking action in the field of a given problem. The definition of a person with mental retardation has changed over the years and various terms have been used, including weak-minded, slow-witted, subnormal, backward, oligophrenic, and so on.

However, the history of mental retardation goes back a long way, and as long ago as the 17th century, investigators such as Locke, Pinel, and Esquirol were seeking to distinguish mental retardation from other pathological conditions. The contributions from Geoget, Hoffbauer, and Prichard date from around 1820, and were followed in the mid 19th century by the early experiences of educational treatment applied by Itard and Seguin. During the course of the 19th century, stricter study methods were introduced and the period from 1905 onwards, and up until the 1960s, saw the introduction of intelligence tests. The first of these was designed by Binet and Simon, followed by those of Terman, Wechsler, and Raven, and mental retardation came to be defined on the strength of an assessment of the person's level of intelligence, quantified by means of the intelligence quotient (IQ).

The psychologist Edgar Doll (1941) is credited with one of the first definitions of mental retardation that considered aspects relating to social competence, the interruption of the patient's development, and the constitutional and incurable origins of the condition. The definition of the American Association of Mental Deficiency (AAMD) dates back to 1959, according to which mental retardation is characterized by a general intellectual functioning below the norm that begins during the developmental period and is associated with an impairment of adaptive behaviour (Heber, 1959).

In a revised version (Heber, 1961), an IQ of 85 was set as the threshold below which mental retardation could be diagnosed (that is, one standard deviation below the mean) and the inclusion of a 'borderline' category raised the proportion of people with mental retardation to approximately 16 per cent of the population (Smith, 1997). In the 1973 edition, the cut-off was lowered to an IQ of 70 (two standard deviations below the mean) and this reduced the prevalence of mental retardation from 16 per cent to 2.25 per cent. The 1977 version confirmed the previous model but attributed a greater relevance to the assessment of adaptive behaviour, a component further emphasized in the subsequent definition of 1983 according to which 'mental retardation refers to significantly subaverage general intellectual functioning existing concurrently with deficits in adaptive behaviour, and manifested during the developmental period' (Grossman, 1983).

With the contributions of Luckasson *et al.* (1992), the AAMR decided that mental retardation could be diagnosed even in a person with an IQ of 75, but we shall come back to this later on.

To further emphasize that establishing a definition is a dynamic process that evolves in parallel with numerous variables, and especially with the social attitudes of the times, it is worth noting that the term 'mental retardation' could be replaced in the near future by the term 'intellectual disability', for two fundamental reasons: the first is that the term *retardation* semantically implies the likelihood, or even the necessity, of a recovery; the second is that the term *disability* more extensively expresses the sum of the individual functioning impairments within a specific social context. The introduction of adaptive behaviour (Heber, 1959) as reflecting the social characteristics of the disability, intended as difficulty in adapting to the normal demands of daily living, consequently assigns less importance to the IQ and reduces the risks of false positives identified by a deficient IQ. Even as regards the definition of adaptive behaviour, however, there is no definitive consensus on its factorial structure, the best methods for its assessment, the accuracy of its measurement, or its real significance in day-to-day life.

By 'adaptive capacity', Greenspan (1999) and MacMillan *et al.* (2003) do not mean the person's practical capacities (which are not very clearly defined), but their capacity to make plans, to reach decisions, and to judge situations socially. We could add those capacities that, in the language of neuropsychology, go by the name of 'executive functions' – an umbrella term for a collection of interrelated functions that are responsible for a purposeful, goal-directed problem-solving behaviour.

Moving on to the specific issue of the classification systems, and bearing in mind our previous comments on the fact that such systems reflect not only the scientific approach adopted but also the way in which the problem is perceived in the existential and social context, we can place the classifications of mental retardation in two main categories:

The first refers to a *biomedical model*: this type of classification identifies and classifies not the person's problem, but the person's pathological condition. The various editions of the classification contained in the *Diagnostic and Statistical Manual of Mental Disorders* (DSM) and the various editions of the *International Classification of Diseases* (ICD) belong to this type of classification.

The second is based on the *bio-psychosocial model*, which identifies and classifies the person's problems in their existential and environmental complexity. This category includes the classification systems prepared by the AAMR, the International Classification of Impairments, Disabilities and Handicaps (ICIDH), and the International Classification of Functions (ICF).

Systems using the biomedical model

The systems in the first category transpose the medical model to a psychic problem, without considering the aetiopathogenesis, without establishing the psychosocial and ecological needs in an orderly and objective manner, and consequently without identifying the type of support suitable for responding to the above-mentioned needs.

These systems include the various DSM and the ICD classifications. They are structured on the basis of three variables: mental functioning, adaptive behaviour, and age of onset. The DSM and the ICD are substantially compatible in their approach, and also in the practical method of code assignment. The ICD is a product of the World Health Organisation (WHO), which was responsible for its development. Its 10th version was published in 1994 (WHO, 1994), and became the reference system for compiling hospital discharge records. The DSM is now in its fourth revised edition of 2000 and was drawn up by the American Psychiatric Association (APA, 2000).

The DSM-IV-TR defines mental retardation as the common final course of several pathological processes of the CNS, and uses three criteria for its diagnosis: (1) significantly below average intellectual functioning (generally two standard deviations below the mean); (2) concomitant impaired adaptive functioning in at least two areas (communication, self-care, home living, social/interpersonal skills, community resource use, attention to health and safety, self-direction, academic skills, work, and leisure activities); (3) onset before 18 years of age.

The DSM-IV-TR classification system is multiaxial and categorical, atheoretical as regards aetiology, and organized into five axes on the assumption of the multicomponent nature of mental disorders. Axis I concerns clinical syndromes and V codes (conditions not attributable to a mental disorder that are the focus of attention or treatment); axis II comprises developmental disorders and personality disorders; axis III includes physical disorders and conditions; axis IV concerns the severity of psychosocial and environmental stressors; and axis V is the global assessment of functioning.

The ICD-10 consists of tabular lists containing cause-of-death titles and codes (volume 1), inclusion and exclusion terms for cause-of-death titles (volume 1), a description, guidelines, and coding rules (volume 2), and an alphabetical index of diseases and the nature of injuries, external causes of injury, and a table of drugs and chemicals (volume 3). There is a clinical version, which also contains research criteria intended for the specialist (physicians, psychiatrists, developmental neuropsychiatrists, psychologists, and so on).

The criteria for classifying mental disorders are descriptive and phenomenological, and are consequently categorical. The ICD-10 classifies mental retardation on the strength of three criteria:
1) a condition of arrested or incomplete development of the mind;
2) impairment of cognitive, language, motor, and social abilities that contribute to the overall level of intelligence which becomes manifest during the developmental period (as IQ alone is not sufficient, a more extensive assessment of all the above-mentioned skills is needed);
3) impairment of adaptive behaviour.

This is also a multiaxial system, where axis I classifies the personality disorders, axis II the clinical and developmental disorders, axis III the mental retardation, and axis IV the psychosocial and environmental problems. The system does not include an axis for global functioning.

In the light of the above, the construct of the two systems is clearly very similar but not identical. The levels of severity are also similar between the two systems, with a discrepancy of five points for the DSM-IV-TR. Both classifications describe the main clinical signs of mental retardation, the associated signs, the course of the condition, and the criteria for its diagnosis. For both systems, the assessment is based on clinical evidence obtained by means of an accurate recording of numerous intellectual skills (strengths and weaknesses). The most obvious difference between the two systems is that the levels of social adaptive behaviour according to the ICD-10 are caused by the mental retardation, while for the DSM-IV-TR they accompany the mental retardation in a complementary relationship.

The bio-psychosocial model

The definitions of the AAMR, the ICDH, and the ICF refer to this model. In relation to the AAMR definition, Luckasson *et al.* (2002) used the DSM-IV-TR definition and defined mental retardation as currently subaverage general intellectual functioning, with concurrent deficits in adaptive behaviour and onset before 18 years of age. For this definition to hold, there are five issues to consider: the current impairment in intellectual functioning must be seen within the setting and community environments typical of the person's age and culture; cultural, linguistic, and communication differences, and sensorimotor and behavioural factors must be taken into account; strengths and weaknesses must coexist; it must be possible to prepare a report on how to develop the support required; and it must be possible to predict that the person's intellectual functioning could improve if adequate support is provided for a suitable period of time. The differences, compared with the DSM-IV-TR, include the IQ cut-off, which changes from 70 to 75, the reduced importance attributed to the degrees of severity, and the identification of the 'levels' of support needed to manage the mental retardation.

The novelty lies in the quantification of the support required (Luckasson et al., 2002), which is classified as intermittent, limited, extensive, or generalized. Thus the functioning of the individual with mental retardation is not just defined by the criteria for assessing the person's mental retardation and their adaptive functioning in certain areas; instead, the person's actual functioning is also defined by the type and intensity of the support they require. In short, the AAMR model shifts attention from the approach to the deficiency, towards the resources needed to provide support for the individual affected (Smith, 1997).

The second system is much less known. This is the ICIDH (WHO, 1980), a system that classifies the consequences of diseases and disabilities, focusing more on the social aspects, unlike the ICD-10. The paradigm is as follows: the disease or disorder (which represents the intrinsic condition) results in impairments – that is, in the limitation or loss of the ability to undertake a given activity (a visible exterior condition) – and this gives rise to the disability (a quantifiable and objective expression of the impairment), which in turn gives rise to the condition of social and environmental disadvantage.

The last and most recent classification system is the ICF, also produced by the WHO (WHO 2002), which has been calibrated on the paediatric population since 2006. The system is defined as a method for describing everything that is potentially describable in relation to life and existence in the world of human beings, in every corner of the earth, irrespective of any physical cultural, economic, or religious boundaries. As in the other two systems, the centre of gravity is represented by the individual, not by the disease or disability, so the individual becomes the subject, not the object of observation and, as subjects, individuals can express themselves in a space and time context.

In this system, mental retardation is defined as a disability that is the consequence or outcome of a complex relation between the individual's state of health and the personal and environmental factors that represent the real environment in which the individual lives. According to its authors, the ICF is consequently a model with a positive perspective, based on health and functioning parameters, in a complex, systemic and interconnected view, but using a language suited to various professions. In fact, the ICF system needs to be able to rely on a complementary system, such as the ICD family, to provide the mortality and morbidity data that the intellectual functioning data cannot do without. This means that an aetiological type of system such as the ICD-10 needs to be integrated with a functional type of system like the ICF, both of which have been issued by WHO.

Borderline cognitive functioning

It is important to focus on the particular condition of borderline intellectual functioning – that is, with an IQ between 71 and 84 – which puts a person in a category somewhere between normal, borderline, and mildly mentally retarded. This borderline category is the object of particular clinical attention in the DSM-IV-TR. Like all diagnostic situations or categories that cannot be clearly defined, mild cognitive dysfunction warrants careful attention, the application of sensitive diagnostic tools, and the use of different sources of information. Individuals belonging to this category are known as the 'forgotten generation', because the American administration has no dedicated measures for these people, who require specific strategies to provide a support system. Tymchuk *et al.* (2001) suggest first, the development of real-life models; second, the development of functional assessment systems; and third, an integrated system of measures. All this implies that a 'mild' cognitive disorder does not necessarily warrant 'mild' treatment measures, because awareness of their disability often makes it more difficult for people in this category to adapt, and their consequent reactive behaviour may be worse.

Conclusions

To sum up, we have discussed in this chapter the definition of mental retardation and the related classification systems, emphasizing the great complexity of these topics and the need to deal with mental retardation by practising a multicomponent approach. Analysing the various systems makes it clear that there are two different reference models: one refers to the pathological condition and attempts to define it, the other identifies the treatments required. It is clear that the systems are complementary and respond to different needs in different settings, and that one consequently does not exclude the other, nor is one better than the other. The definition systems refer to categorical diagnoses with complementary dimensional features (for example, the association with other diseases).

The classification systems that focus particularly on the disabilities derived from the disorder in various different settings are evolving in parallel with a greater social consideration for disabled people in general, bearing in mind that categorical definition systems have never lost sight of the person involved. In fact, the classification systems have always been multiaxial, constantly contemplating different approaches. The only difference now lies in the theoretical paradigm, and this makes it necessary to use the systems to complement one another.

Finally, it is worth emphasizing the importance of the aetiological diagnosis, the achievement of which can have great added value for prognosis and treatment, as well as for determining the future likelihood of neurocognitive impairment and associated problems.

References

American Psychiatric Association (2000): *DSM-IV-TR: diagnostic and statistical manual of mental disorders*, 4th ed., text revision. Washington, DC: American Psychiatric Publishing.

Doll, E.A. (1941): The essentials of an inclusive concept of mental deficiency. *Am. J. Ment. Defic.* **46**, 214–219.

Greenspan, S. (1999): What is meant by mental retardation? *Int. Rev. Psychiatry* **11**, 6–18.

Grossman, H.J. (1983): *Classification in mental retardation* (revised edition). Washington, DC: American Association on Mental Deficiency.

Heber, R. (1959): A manual on terminology and classification in mental retardation. *Am. J. Ment. Defic.* **64** (Monograph Suppl.).

Heber, R. (1961): *A manual on terminology and classification in mental retardation* (revised edition). Washington, DC: American Association on Mental Deficiency.

Luckasson, R., Coulter, D.L., Polloway, E.A., Reiss, S., Schalock, R.L., Snell, M.E., Spitalnik, D.M. & Stark, J.A. (1992): *Mental retardation: definition, classification and systems of support* (9th ed.). Washington, DC: American Association on Mental Retardation.

Luckasson, R., Borthwick-Duffy, S., Buntinx, W.H.E., Coulter, D.L., Craig, E.M., Reeve, A., Schalock, R.L., Snell, M.E., Spitalnik, D.M., Spreat, S. & Tassè, M.J. (2002): *Mental retardation: definition, classification and systems of support* (10th ed.). Washington, DC: American Association on Mental Retardation.

MacMillan, D.L., Siperstein, G.N. & Leffert, J.S. (2003): Children with mild mental retardation: a challenge for classification practices. In: *What is mental retardation?*, eds. H. Switzky & S. Greenspan, pp. 253–272. Washington, DC: American Association on Mental Retardation.

Smith, J.D. (1997): Mental retardation as an educational construct: time for a new shared view? *Educ. Train. Men. Retard. Dev. Disabil.* **20,** 179–183.

Tymchuk, A.J., Lakin, K.C. & Luckasson, R. (2001): *The forgotten generation: the status and challenges of adults with mild cognitive limitations.* Baltimore: Paul H. Brookes.

World Health Organisation (1980): *International classification of impairments, disabilities and handicaps. A manual of classification relating to the consequences of disease (ICIDH).* Geneva: WHO.

World Health Organisation (1994): *ICD-10: international statistical classification of diseases and related health problems: tenth revision.* Geneva: WHO.

World Health Organisation (2002): *International classification of functioning, disability and health: ICF.* Geneva: WHO.

Chapter 20

Neuropsychological profile of Williams syndrome

Stefano Vicari

IRCCS, Children's Hospital 'Bambino Gesù', and University LUMSA, piazza Sant'Onofrio, 00165 Rome, Italy
vicari@opbg.net

Summary

Neuropsychological research has allowed us to define different cognitive profiles among subjects with mental retardation of different aetiologies. For example, important claims have been made regarding the contrasting profiles of linguistic and cognitive performance observed in two genetically based syndromes, Williams syndrome and Down syndrome. Earlier studies suggested a double dissociation, with language better preserved than non-verbal cognition in children and adults with Williams syndrome, and an opposite profile in children and adults with Down syndrome. Overall, these observations seem to support the theoretical approach that considers the intellectual disorder in persons with mental retardation not as a mere slowing down of normal cognitive development, but as a picture characterized by a qualitative lack of homogeneity that confers specific peculiarities on each affected individual. Following this theoretical perspective – which suggests the need for strongly individualized rehabilitative treatment protocols adapted to the cognitive characteristics of each child – many recent studies have tried to define more satisfactorily the impaired cognitive capacities of individual cases, as well as their respective 'areas of strength' or relatively preserved abilities.
This chapter reviews the neuropsychological literature and presents recent data on cognitive performance in individuals with Williams syndrome. Possible neural substrates for these profiles are discussed.

Introduction

Williams syndrome is a rare genetic syndrome (the incidence is estimated to be 1 in 25,000 live births) caused by a microdeletion of the long arm of chromosome 7q11.23 (Ewart *et al.*, 1993; Frangiskakis *et al.*, 1996; Botta *et al.*, 1999; Bellugi & St. George, 2001). Children with Williams syndrome often have infantile hypercalcaemia, delays in growth and in psychomotor development, facial dysmorphism, congenital malformations (mostly in the cardiovascular system), and some degree of cognitive impairment (Arnold *et al.*, 1985; Bellugi *et al.*, 1990; Udwin & Yule, 1990).

Williams syndrome has received a great deal of attention recently because of its particular cognitive profile. Several investigators have noted that aspects of language development are relatively proficient, while visual-spatial processing ability, counting, planning, and implicit learning are severely impaired (Atkinson *et al.*, 2001; Bellugi *et al.*, 2001, Vicari *et al.*, 2001). This sort of cognitive dissociation becomes even more evident when the performance of children with Williams syndrome is compared not only with that of typically-developing children of the same mental age but also – and above all – with that of other children with mental retardation of a different type, for example Down syndrome (trisomy 21). Comparisons with the latter are especially interesting because the cognitive profile of children with Down syndrome seems to mirror that of Williams syndrome – for example, deficits in language ability often exceed impairments in visual-spatial abilities.

Several recent studies suggest, however, that the characterization of the cognitive profiles of children with Williams syndrome in terms of a dissociation between language and visual-spatial abilities is too simplistic. Studies from different laboratories have demonstrated a more complex neuropsychological profile in this population, with atypical development not only in the cognitive but also in the linguistic domain (Gosh *et al.*, 1994; Vicari *et al.*, 1996a; Volterra *et al.*, 1996; Pezzini *et al.*, 1999; Karmiloff-Smith *et al.*, 2003).

Linguistic abilities

In the language domain, comparative studies of adolescents with Williams syndrome and Down syndrome have shown that subjects with Williams syndrome were significantly more competent in terms of vocabulary, semantic fluency, morphological abilities, and narrative abilities (Bellugi *et al.*, 1990; Reilly *et al.*, 1990; Rubba & Klima, 1991; Bellugi *et al.*, 1996). More recent studies, however, report partially different results. A study by Klein & Mervis (1999) showed that receptive lexical abilities are equivalent for 9- and 10-year-old children when the two syndromes are matched for chronological and mental age. Another study involving large numbers of children with Williams syndrome and Down syndrome in the early stages of language development (Singer Harris *et al.*, 1997) found that both syndrome groups were substantially and equally delayed in the onset of language. However, children with Williams syndrome had a significant advantage over those with Down syndrome in the early stages of grammar. A study by Klein & Mervis (1999) on groups of very young children with Down syndrome and Williams syndrome, carefully matched for chronological age, confirmed language delay in both syndromes. However, in contrast to some of the results reported by Singer Harris *et al.* (1997), an expressive advantage in children with Williams syndrome relative to those with Down syndrome was apparent even at the age of 26 months.

Vicari *et al.* (2002) evaluated the linguistic abilities in Italian-speaking children with Williams syndrome and Down syndrome at a comparable global cognitive level (mean mental age 34 and 32 months, respectively; mean chronological age 58 and 67 months). A further control group was formed of typically-developing children matched for mental age. No dissociation was evident in the groups between lexical and cognitive abilities, but specific morphosyntactic difficulties emerged in both comprehension and production in children with Down syndrome. Children with Williams syndrome, albeit less compromised than those with Down syndrome, also showed difficulties in the sentence repetition task.

A complex but atypical linguistic profile in individuals with Williams syndrome also emerged in a more recent study conducted by Vicari *et al.* (2004), where they analysed both lexical comprehension and production abilities. The participants with Williams syndrome did not show particular difficulties in lexical comprehension, evaluated by the Peabody Picture Vocabulary Test, and they performed better than their controls (typically-developing children and children with Down syndrome, matched for mental age) when IQ was taken into account. In lexical production (the Boston Naming Test) a different picture emerged: children with Williams syndrome obtain similar results to Down syndrome children, but the Williams syndrome group performed significantly worse than typically-developing children even after IQ was controlled for. Results from the two morphosyntax tasks confirmed the heterogeneous Williams syndrome linguistic profile. In fact, although no differences were observed in grammatical comprehension between typically-developing children and the Williams syndrome participants, significant differences were obtained in phrase repetition (Williams syndrome children were less competent than typically-developing children).

On the word fluency test with semantic (CAT) and phonemic (FAS) cues, no differences were observed between Williams syndrome and typically-developing groups in CAT, but participants with Williams syndrome produced a larger number of words than typically-developing children in FAS.

These results showed that the linguistic abilities of toddlers with Williams syndrome are not above their cognitive level, and that language development in this special population is more deviant than delayed.

Visual-spatial abilities

In the visual-spatial domain a greater general difficulty in spatial constructive processing but relatively preserved visual-perceptual abilities – such as, for example, facial recognition – has been suggested in Williams syndrome (Bellugi et al., 1999a; Mervis et al., 1999; Pezzini et al., 1999; Bellugi & St George, 2001).

In an attempt to describe the biological bases of the spatial processing deficit, Atkinson et al. (1997) studied a group of 15 children with Williams syndrome and 30 with typical cognitive development. They administered tests traditionally held to be indices of the ability to process cortically the spatial *(dorsal cortical stream)* and visual characteristics *(ventral cortical stream)* of objects. The results showed that children with Williams syndrome were very deficient on tests involving the structures that are believed to rely on the dorsal stream for their correct execution, although the same children were in the norm on tests involving the processing of visual information. On the basis of Atkinson's studies (Atkinson et al., 1997; Atkinson et al., 2003), the spatial deficit observed by many investigators in children with Williams syndrome can reasonably be attributed to an impairment of the dorsal cortical stream, with relative sparing of the ventral stream. Consistent with this hypothesis, Vicari et al. (2006) documented a discrepancy in the performance level of visual and spatial perceptual and imagery tasks achieved by individuals with Williams syndrome. In line with the prediction of a specific deficit in the visual processing of spatial information, children with Williams syndrome performed as well as mental age-matched typically-developing controls in a visual perception test, but significantly worse on a judgment of line orientation test. Moreover, while subjects with Williams syndrome performed worse than their controls in both mental rotation tasks, no difference was found between groups in the mental colour comparison and animal tails tests, which required mentally visualising known objects but not spatially manipulating them (see Farran et al., 2001) for consistent results in individuals with Williams syndrome). Contrasting results were obtained by individuals with Down syndrome. Indeed, in both the perceptual and imagery tasks Down syndrome subjects performed significantly worse than typically-developing children when the visual configuration of the experimental material had to be processed. However, when the task involved processing spatial data, the performance of Down syndrome and typically-developing participants did not differ significantly.

It is interesting to note that, consistent with theories assuming a broad sharing of processing resources between visual-perceptual and mental imagery tasks (for example, Klein *et al.*, 2004), the performance of both groups of intellectually disabled persons was coherent in the perceptual and imagery tasks. In particular, Williams syndrome participants performed well in perceptual and visual-object imagery tasks (ventral stream) but poorly in perceptual and visual-spatial imagery tasks (dorsal stream).

Memory abilities

Studies from memory give us further information about cognitive and linguistic capabilities in Williams syndrome. Phonological short-term memory is usually at the level of the mental age (Udwin & Yule, 1990; Vicari *et al.*, 1996b) or higher than mental age (Mervis *et al.*, 1999). Furthermore, Wang & Bellugi (1994) and Jarrold *et al.* (1999) showed opposite patterns of memory span performance in children with Williams syndrome and Down syndrome – namely, a better verbal span in children with Williams syndrome and, conversely, better visual-spatial span in those with Down syndrome. Wang & Bellugi (1994) discussed these data in the light of a working memory model (Baddeley & Hitch, 1974; Baddeley, 1986) and suggested a better preservation of the articulatory loop in Williams syndrome but better preservation of the visual-spatial sketchpad (a system devoted to the processing of visual-spatial data) in Down syndrome.

Vicari *et al.* (1996a) investigated the contribution of phonological and semantic processes to verbal span in children with Williams syndrome. In particular, they explored phonological similarity and length and frequency effects in a verbal span task in groups of children with Williams syndrome and mental age-matched normal controls. The participants with Williams syndrome showed normal similarity and length effects in their performance, supporting the hypothesis of relatively preserved phonological competence in children with this syndrome. However, they found a reduced frequency effect in the verbal span in these participants compared with the group of normally developing children. Although both groups repeated high frequency words better than low frequency words, this effect was smaller in the Williams syndrome group. The reduced frequency effect in these children may be the result of a rigid use of phonological recoding strategy both for high and low frequency words. The dissociation between normal phonological encoding and the reduced contribution of lexical-semantic encoding mechanisms to word span in Williams syndrome is particularly interesting in the light of their pattern of linguistic abilities. As we have seen, several studies have shown that children with Williams syndrome have relatively impaired lexical-semantic abilities in the presence of well-preserved phonological processes (Volterra *et al.*, 1996; Grant *et al.*, 1997; Karmiloff-Smith *et al.*, 1997; Karmiloff-Smith *et al.*, 1998; Mervis *et al.*, 1999).

The marked difficulty that individuals with Williams syndrome have in spatial processing has also been explored in the memory domain. As reported above, it is well known that children with Williams syndrome perform worse than those with Down syndrome in the Corsi Block Tapping Test (Wang & Bellugi, 1994; Jarrold *et al.*, 1999). Recently Vicari *et al.* (2006) compared children with Williams syndrome and typically-developing children matched for mental age in a visual and spatial span test. The two tests involved studying the same complex, non-verbalizable figures and using the same response mode (pointing to targets on the screen). The crucial experimental variable was that in one case the position where the figure appeared on the screen had to be recalled; in the other, the physical aspect of the figure studied had to be recalled. The results showed a different performance profile in the two groups of children. Although the normal and Williams syndrome groups performed analogously in the visual span test, the spatial span performance of the Williams syndrome children was significantly worse than that of the controls.

Verbal and visual-spatial long-term memory has been investigated extensively in subjects with Williams syndrome in both explicit and implicit components (Vicari & Carlesimo, 2002). Explicit memory concerns intentional recalling or recognition of experiences or information. Implicit memory is manifested as a facilitation (that is, an improvement in performance) in perceptual, cognitive, and motor tasks, without any conscious reference to previous experiences. Explicit memory deficits in persons with mental retardation, and particularly with Williams syndrome, have also been extensively documented. For example, Vicari *et al.* (2005) investigated explicit long-term memory capacities for visual and spatial material in adolescents and young adults with Williams syndrome. They documented a level of learning comparable to that of typically-developing children matched for mental age on the visual-object test but a clearly lower level on the visual-spatial test. Interestingly, what mainly distinguished the performance of the typically-developing children from the Williams syndrome group on the visual-spatial task was the learning rate passing from the first to the third recognition trial. This finding is against a reductionist hypothesis postulating that deficient perceptual processing or working-memory maintenance of visual-spatial data is the origin of the long-term memory deficit in the Williams syndrome group. Indeed, while immediate recognition of only-once-studied items could also be heavily influenced by proficiency in the perceptual analysis and working-memory processing, the reduced performance improvement across successive learning trials seems a reliable index of the deficient ability to store new information in the long-term memory.

In conclusion, data on short- and long-term memory capacities are consistent with the results of several other studies which documented more difficulty on tests of spatial than visual processing in children with Williams syndrome (Bellugi *et al.*, 1999a; Bellugi *et al.*, 1999b; Mervis *et al.*, 1999; Pezzini *et al.*, 1999; Vicari *et al.*, 2006).

In the past few years, some experimental data have been reported on the possible extension to individuals with mental retardation of the dissociation between explicit and implicit memory processes so frequently described in brain-damaged adults with memory disorders. In relation to *repetition priming*, studies investigating facilitation in the identification of perceptually degraded pictures induced by previous exposure to the same pictures have consistently reported a comparable priming effect in individuals with mental retardation and typically-developing children matched for chronological or mental age (for a review, see Vicari & Carlesimo, 2002). However, a complex and somewhat contradictory pattern of results has emerged from studies investigating repetition priming for verbal material. Most of these studies were based on the stem completion procedure, in which subjects are requested to complete a list of stems (that is, the first three letters) with the first word that comes to mind. In this test, the priming effect is revealed by a bias in completing the stems with words that have been studied previously over unstudied words. Carlesimo *et al.* (1997) and Vicari *et al.* (2000; 2001) reported a priming effect with this procedure in various groups of individuals with mental retardation – aetiologically unspecified, Down syndrome, and Williams syndrome – comparable with mental age matched typically-developing children.

Less experimental work has been devoted to investigating the ability to learn visuo-motor or cognitive skills in mental retardation, and in Williams syndrome in particular. Vicari and co-workers suggested an intriguing difference in the skill-learning abilities between individuals with Down syndrome and Williams syndrome. In the first study (Vicari *et al.*, 2000), a group with Down syndrome showed the same rate of improvement as a group of mental age-matched typically-developing children across successive trials of the Tower of London Test and in a comparison of repeated *vs.* random blocks of a facilitated version of the Serial Reaction Time Test devised by Nissen & Bullemer (1987), which requires implicit learning of the sequential order of a series of visual events. However, in a second study, a group of children with Williams syndrome showed significantly reduced procedural learning compared with typically-developing children on both of these tests (Vicari *et al.*, 2001). These findings were confirmed in a very recent study (Vicari *et al.*, 2007), where implicit abilities of Williams syndrome, Down syndrome, and typically-developing children were directly compared (Fig. 1).

The two groups of individuals with mental retardation who participated in the study showed different patterns of procedural learning. First, and confirming some previous reports (Vicari *et al.*, 2001), children with Williams syndrome revealed poor implicit learning of the temporal sequence of events characterizing the repeated blocks in the Serial Reaction Time Test. In comparison with normal controls, Williams syndrome participants showed a reduction in reaction-time speeding when passing from repeated block II to repeated block V. Most importantly, the rebound effect – which so dramatically affects normal children's reaction times on passing from V (repeated) to VI (random) block – had only a marginal influence on the reaction times of Williams syndrome children. This shows that, while the reaction-time reduction of typically-developing children across the successive blocks of repeated sequences was largely mediated by learning the temporal sequence of events, in the Williams group speeding of manual responses was only the effect of practice, with no or little effect of sequence learning. Note that the reduced implicit learning observed in Williams syndrome cannot be explained by a basic difficulty in the processing of visual-spatial data or manual dexterity; indeed, the deficit persisted even when the performance scores on the spatial working memory and constructive tasks were taken into account.

In contrast to the Williams syndrome group, the rate of procedural learning of the participants with Down syndrome was comparable to that of their mental age-matched controls. Indeed, Down syndrome and typically-developing individuals showed parallel reaction time variations in the series of repeated blocks and, more importantly, when passing from V (repeated) to VI (random) block. Therefore, substantial preservation of skill-learning abilities in this genetic syndrome is confirmed (Vicari *et al.*, 2000; Krinsky-McHale *et al.*, 2003).

In long-term memory, individuals with Williams syndrome show different patterns in explicit and implicit memory domains. Though children with Williams syndrome usually do worse than typically-developing mental age controls in visual-spatial explicit memory tasks, in the implicit memory domain comparable results may be observed between the two groups in repetition priming tasks but not in procedural learning.

It is worth noting that the memory profile observed in Williams syndrome is not shared with other genetic syndromes that are also characterized by mental retardation. We have indeed reported a case of Down syndrome characterized by an impairment in explicit memory and a relative preservation of implicit memory.

Neurobiological perspectives

The cognitive profile we have described in individuals with Williams syndrome presumably results from some specific characteristics of their anomalous brain development. However, any attempt to identify which neuroanatomical structures are specifically involved in the cognitive impairment shown by people with Williams syndrome is speculative, and it must necessarily be based on qualitative comparisons of their deficit with that shown by patients with acquired brain lesions.

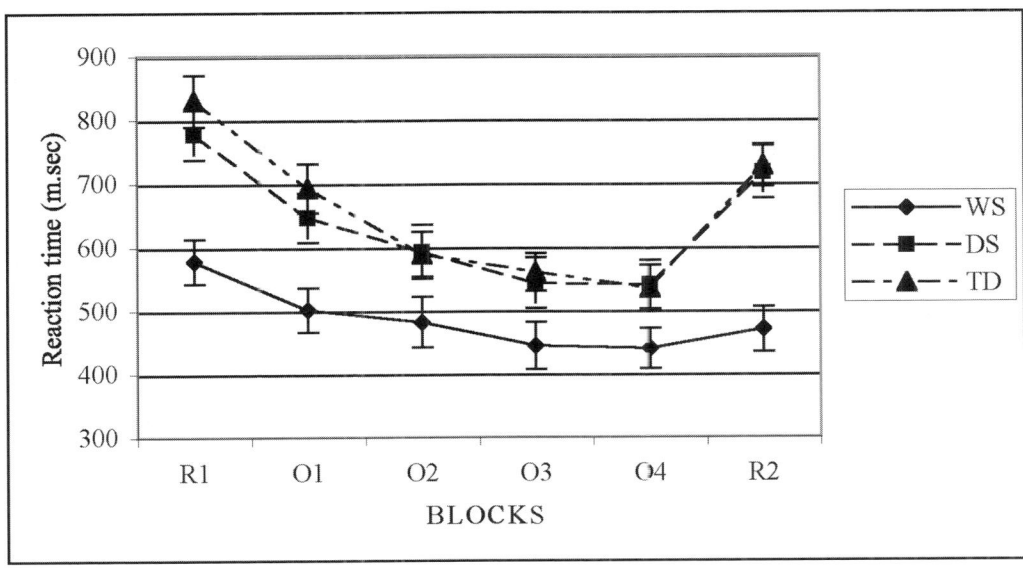

Fig. 1. Average reaction times and standard errors of Williams syndrome (WS), Down syndrome (DS) and typically-developing children (TD) on the serial reaction-time task.

In this regard, it is worth noting that brain development in children with Williams syndrome is characterized by marked atrophy of the posterior region of the brain as well as of the basal ganglia (Jernigan et al., 1993; Bellugi et al., 1999b). Though cerebellar volume is relatively preserved (Jernigan et al., 1993; Bellugi et al., 1999b), a neurochemical alteration (reduction of the neurotransmitter N-acetylaspartate) has been demonstrated in the cerebellum (Rae et al., 1998).

In contrast, in Down syndrome the frontal cortex is disproportionately reduced in volume, as are the limbic structures of the temporal lobe (including the uncus, amygdala, hippocampus, and parahippocampal gyrus) and cerebellar size. However, the brains of individuals with Down syndrome usually show relative preservation of the volume of subcortical areas such as the lenticular nuclei (Jernigan et al., 1993; Bellugi et al., 1999b).

The different neuropsychological profiles we have described between Williams syndrome and Down syndrome might depend upon differences within the cortical and subcortical structures observed in these syndromes. For example, in agreement with Fabbro et al. (2002), the deficient performance of subjects with Williams syndrome in a subset of linguistic tasks may be related to dysfunction of the basal ganglia involved in expressive language processing, while the deficient performance in Down syndrome may partially be explained in terms of impairment of the frontocerebellar structures involved in articulation and working memory, and the often reported hearing loss.

Moreover, several recent observations made using magnetic resonance imaging suggest a possible impairment of the dorsal cortical stream in Williams syndrome. For example, Reiss et al. (2000) documented reduced representation of the posterior areas (parietal and occipital) in subjects with Williams syndrome compared with age-matched controls. The dorsal areas of the parietal cortex are markedly involved in the mediation of spatial processing; in contrast, the temporal ventral (and perhaps frontal) areas intervene in working memory for objects and faces and, more generally, in the processing of visual material (Courtney et al., 1996; Nelson et al.,

2000). Therefore, a deficit of the dorsal stream in children with Williams syndrome may play an important role in their reduced spatial abilities, including their reduced spatial span.

A further more recently described characteristic of the Williams syndrome brain is a reduced volume in the posterior regions of the corpus callosum (Tomaiuolo *et al.*, 2002; Luders *et al.*, 2007). This hypoplasia of the corpus callosum may cause defective callosal transfer of information, resulting in insufficient integration and coordination of the activity of the two cerebral hemispheres. On the basis of all these observations, the possible role played by the reduced posterior regions of the brain and the corpus callosum in the visual-spatial difficulties in individuals with Williams syndrome is, although speculative, very suggestive.

Finally, the different implicit memory profiles shown by the various aetiological groups of individuals with mental retardation presumably results from some specific characteristics of their anomalous brain development. Recent neuroimaging studies (Galaburda & Bellugi, 2000; Schmitt *et al.*, 2001) have attempted to document the presence of particular morphological cerebral characteristics to explain the distinct cognitive and behavioural profiles observed in people with mental retardation, especially in known genetic syndromes. In relation to implicit memory, both neuropsychological (Molinari *et al.*, 1997) and functional neuroimaging data (Van Der Graaf *et al.*, 2004) assign a critical role to the basal ganglia and cerebellum in the implicit learning of visuo-motor skills. Brain development of individuals with Williams syndrome is characterized by remarkable atrophy of the basal ganglia (Jernigan & Bellugi, 1990), while the morphology of the cerebellum is generally normal (Wang *et al.*, 1992). Further, a neurochemical alteration (reduction of the neurotransmitter N-acetylaspartate) has been reported in the cerebellum of individuals with Williams syndrome (Rae *et al.*, 1998). In contrast, the brains of subjects with Down syndrome show severe cerebellar hypoplasia with normal morphology of the basal ganglia (Jernigan *et al.*, 1993). In the light of these data, we can tentatively conclude that the deficient maturation of visuo-motor skill learning in Williams syndrome is related to the deficient maturation of the striatal circuits known to be critical for this ability.

Studies conducted in genetic syndromes describing their neuropsychological profiles in relation to specific brain characteristics are just beginning. However, it seems a fascinating topic and a route to the better understanding of the biological nature of behaviour and of the cognitive and linguistic differences observed in people with mental retardation.

Conclusions

Williams syndrome is characterized by a complex neuropsychological profile, with some abilities being more impaired than others. In particular, language (and specifically morpho-syntax), lexical production, spatial manipulation of information at different levels of processing (perceptual, short-term, and explicit long-term memory), and implicit long-term memory are usually impaired. Lexical comprehension, visual perception, and visual and verbal short- and long-term memory are relatively preserved. This cognitive pattern is sustained by a particular form of brain development, with reduced volumes in subcortical areas such as the lenticular nuclei as well as in the posterior (parietal and occipital) cortical grey matter.

From a theoretical point of view, the results of the experimental reports reviewed in this chapter are relevant to students working in the fields of both normal cognitive development and neuropsychological outcome following cerebral damage. The former can compare 'normal' cognitive development with that of individuals with Williams syndrome in an attempt to dissociate distinct functional components of the cognitive and linguistic systems on the basis of discrepant developmental trends. The latter can attempt to apply the same theoretical and experimental approaches already used in the investigation of neuropsychologically disordered adults to the deficits shown in Williams syndrome to gain new insights into the neural substrate and the basic mechanisms of normal and pathological cognitive development. From a practical point of view, these data can provide invaluable information for educational psychologists and teachers for planning rationally grounded interventions to alleviate the learning difficulties and social maladjustment of these individuals.

Acknowledgments: The financial support of Telethon-Italy (grant No. E.C. 685) is gratefully acknowledged.

References

Arnold, R., Yule, W. & Martin, N. (1985): The psychological characteristics of infantile hypercalcaemia: a preliminary investigation. *Dev. Med. Child Neurol.* **27,** 49–59.

Atkinson, J., King, J., Braddick, O., Nokes, L., Anker, S. & Braddick, F. (1997): A specific deficit of dorsal stream function in Williams syndrome. *Neuroreport* **8,** 1919–1922.

Atkinson, J., Shirley, L., Braddick, O., Mason, A. & Braddick F. (2001): Visual and visuospatial development in young children with Williams syndrome. *Dev. Med. Child Neurol.* **43,** 330–337.

Atkinson, J., Braddick, O., Anker, S., Curran, W., Andrew, R., Wattam-Bell, J. & Braddick, F. (2003): Neurobiological models of visuospatial cognition in children with Williams syndrome: measures of dorsal-stream and frontal function. *Dev. Neuropsychol.* **23,** 139–172.

Baddeley, A.D. (1986): *Working memory.* Oxford: Oxford University Press.

Baddeley, A.D. & Hitch, G. (1974): Working memory. In: *The psychology of learning and motivation,* ed. G.H. Bower, pp. 47–90. New York: Academic Press.

Beery, K. (1997): *Developmental tests of visual-motor integration.* Parsippany, NJ: Modern Curriculum Press.

Bellugi, U. & St. George, M. (2001): *Journey from cognition to brain to gene. Perspectives from Williams syndrome.* Cambridge, MA: MIT Press.

Bellugi, U., Bihrle, A., Jernigan, T., Trauner, D. & Doherty, S. (1990): Neuropsychological, neurological and neuro-anatomical profile of Williams syndrome. *Am. J. Med. Genet.* (Suppl.), **6,** 115–125.

Bellugi, U., Bihrle, A., Neville, H., Jernigan, T. & Doherty, S. (1996): Language, cognition and brain organization in a neurodevelopmental disorder. In: *Developmental behavioural neuroscience,* eds. M. Gunnar & C. Nelson. Hillsdale, NJ: Erlbaum.

Bellugi, U., Mills, D., Jernigan, T., Hickok, G. & Galaburda, A. (1999a): Linking cognition, brain structure, and brain function in Williams syndrome. In: *Neurodevelopmental disorders,* ed. H. Tager-Flusberg, pp. 111–136. Cambridge, MA: MIT Press.

Bellugi, U., Lichtenberger, L., Mills, D., Galaburda A. & Koremberg, J.R. (1999b): Bridging cognition, the brain and molecular genetics: evidence from Williams syndrome. *Trends Neurosci.* **22,** 197–207.

Bellugi, U., Lichtenberger, L., Jones, W., Lai, Z. & St. George, M. (2000): The neurocognitive profile of Williams syndrome. I: a complex pattern of strengths and weaknesses. *J. Cogn. Neurosci.* **12** (Suppl.1), 7–29.

Bellugi, U., Koremberg, J.R. & Klima, E.S. (2001): Williams syndrome: an exploration of neurocognitive and genetic features. *Clin. Neurosci. Res.* **1,** 217–229.

Botta, A., Sangiuolo, F., Calza, L., Giardino, L., Potenza, S., Novelli, G. & Dallapiccola, B. (1999): Expression analysis and protein localization of the human HPC-1/syntaxin 1A, a gene deleted in Williams syndrome. *Genomics* **15,** 525–528.

Carlesimo, G.A., Marotta, L. & Vicari, S. (1997): Long-term memory in mental retardation: evidence for a specific impairment in subjects with Down's syndrome. *Neuropsychologia* **35,** 71–79.

Courtney, S.M., Ungerleider, L.G., Keil, K. & Haxby, J.V. (1996): Object and visual working memory activate separate neural systems in human cortex. *Cereb. Cortex* **6,** 39–49.

Ewart, A.K., Morris, C.A., Atkinson, D., Jin, W., Sternes, K., Spallone, P., Stock, A.D., Leppert, M. & Keating, M.T. (1993): Hemizygosity at the elastin locus in a developmental disorder, Williams syndrome. *Nat. Genet.* **5,** 11–16.

Fabbro, F., Alberti, A., Gagliardi, C. & Borgatti, R. (2002): Differences in native and foreign language repetition task between subjects with Williams and Down syndromes. *J. Neurolinguistics* **15,** 1–10.

Farran, E.K., Jarrold, C. & Gathercole, S.E. (2001): Block design performance in the Williams syndrome phenotype: a problem with mental imagery? *J. Child Psychol. Psychiatry* **42,** 719–728.

Frangiskakis, J.M., Ewart, A.K., Morris, C.A., Mervis, C.B., Bertrand, J., Robinson, B.F., Klein, B.P., Ensing, G.J., Everett, L.A. & Green, E.D. (1996): LIM-kinase-1 hemizygosity implicated in impaired visuospatial constructive cognition. *Cell* **86,** 59–69.

Galaburda, A.M. & Bellugi, U. (2000): Multi-level analysis of cortical neuroanatomy in Williams syndrome. *J. Cogn. Neurosci.* **12,** 74–88.

Gosh, A., Stading, G. & Pankau, R. (1994): Linguistic abilities in children with Williams-Beuren syndrome. *Am. J. Med. Genet.* **52,** 291–296.

Grant, J., Karmiloff-Smith, A., Gathercole, S.E., Paterson, S., Howlin, P., Davies, M. & Udwin, O. (1997): Phonological short-term memory and its relationship to language in Williams syndrome. *Cogn. Neuropsychiatry* **2,** 81–99.

Jarrold, C., Baddeley, A.D. & Hewes, A.K.(1999): Genetically dissociated components of working memory: evidence from Down and Williams syndrome. *Neuropsychologia* **37,** 637–651.

Jernigan, T.L. & Bellugi, U. (1990): Anomalous brain morphology on magnetic resonance images in Williams syndrome and Down syndrome. *Arch. Neurol.* **47,** 529–533.

Jernigan, T.L., Bellugi, U., Sowell, E., Doherty, S. & Hesselink, J.R. (1993): Cerebral morphologic distinction between Williams and Down syndromes. *Arch. Neurol.* **50,** 186–191.

Karmiloff-Smith, A. (1998): Development itself is the key to understanding developmental disorders. *Trends Cogn. Sci.* **2,** 289–298.

Karmiloff-Smith, A., Grant, J., Berthoud, I., Davis, M., Howlin, P. & Udwin, O. (1997): Language and Williams syndrome: how intact is 'intact'? *Child Dev.* **68,** 246–262.

Karmiloff-Smith, A., Tyler, L.K., Voice, K., Sims, K., Udwin, O., Howlin, P. & Davis, M. (1998): Linguistic dissociations in Williams syndrome: evaluating receptive syntax in on-line and off-line tasks. *Neuropsychologia* **36,** 343–351.

Karmiloff-Smith, A., Brown, J.H., Grice, S. & Paterson, S. (2003): Dethroning the myth: cognitive dissociations and innate modularity in Williams syndrome. *Dev. Neuropsychol.* **23,** 227–242.

Klein, B.P. & Mervis, C.B. (1999): Contrasting patterns of cognitive abilities of 9- and 10-year-olds with Williams syndrome or Down syndrome. *Dev. Neuropsychol.* **16,** 177–196.

Klein, I., Dubois, J., Mangin, J.F., Kherif, F., Flandin, G., Poline, J.B., Denis, M., Kosslyn, S.M. & Le Bihan, D. (2004): Retinotopic organization of visual mental images as revealed by functional magnetic resonance imaging. *Brain Res. Cogn. Brain Res.* **22,** 26–31.

Krinsky-McHale, S.J., Devenny, D.A. & Silverman, W.P. (2003): Implicit memory in aging adults with mental retardation with and without Down syndrome. *Am. J. Ment. Retard.* **108,** 219–233.

Luders, E., Di Paola, M., Tomaiuolo, F., Thompson, P.M., Toga, A.W., Vicari, S., Petrides, M. & Caltagirone, C. (2007): Effects of Williams syndrome on callosal thickness in scaled and native space. *Neuroreport* **18,** 203–207.

Mervis, C.B., Morris, C.A., Bertrand, J. & Robinson, B.F. (1999): Williams syndrome: findings from an integrated program of research. In: *Neurodevelopmental disorders,* ed. H. Tager-Flusberg, pp. 65–110. Cambridge, MA: MIT Press.

Molinari, M., Leggio, M.G., Solida, A., Corra, R., Misciagna, S., Silveri, M.C. & Petrosini, L. (1997): Cerebellum and procedural learning: evidence from focal cerebellar lesions. *Brain* **120,** 1753–1762.

Nelson, C.A., Monk, C.S., Lin, J., Carver, L.J., Thomas, K.M. & Truwit, C.L. (2000): Functional neuroanatomy of spatial working memory in children. *Dev. Psychol.* **36,** 109–116.

Nissen, M.J. & Bullemer, P. (1987): Attentional requirements of learning: evidence from performance measures. *Cogn. Psychol.* **19,** 1–32.

Pezzini, G., Vicari, S., Volterra, V., Dilani, L. & Ossella, M.T. (1999): Children with Williams syndrome: is there a unique neuropsychological profile? *Dev. Neuropsychol.* **15,** 141–155.

Rae, C., Karmiloff-Smith, A., Lee, M.A., Dixon, R.M, Grant, J., Blamire, A.M., Thompson, C.H., Styles, P. & Radda, G.K. (1998): Brain biochemistry in Williams syndrome: evidence for a role of the cerebellum in cognition. *Neurology* **51,** 33–40.

Reilly, J., Klima, E.S. & Bellugi, U. (1990): Once more with feeling: affect and language in atypical populations. *Dev. Psychopathol.* **2,** 367–391.

Reiss, A.L., Eliez, S., Schmitt, J.E. & Straus, E. (2000): Neuroanatomy of Williams syndrome: a high-resolution MRI study. *J. Cogn. Neurosci.* **12,** 65–73.

Rubba, J. & Klima, E.S. (1991): Preposition use in a speaker with Williams syndrome: some cognitive grammar proposals. *Center for Research in Language Newsletter* **3,** 3–12.

Schmitt, J.E., Eliez, S., Warsofsky, L.S., Bellugi, U. & Reiss, A.L. (2001): Corpus callosum morphology of Williams syndrome: relation to genetics and behavior. *Dev. Med. Child Neurol.* **43,** 155–159.

Singer Harris, N.G., Bellugi, U., Bates, E., Jones, W. & Rossen, M. (1997): Contrasting profiles of language in children with Williams and Down syndromes. *Dev. Neuropsychol.* **13,** 345–370.

Tomaiuolo, F., Di Paola, M., Caravale, B., Vicari, S., Petrides, M. & Caltagirone, C. (2002): Morphology and morphometry of the corpus callosum in Williams syndrome: a magnetic resonance imaging analysis. *Neuroreport* **13,** 1–5.

Udwin, O. & Yule, W. (1990): Expressive language of children with Williams syndrome. *Am. J. Med. Genet.* (Suppl. **6,** 108–114.

Van Der Graaf, F.H., De Jong, B.M., Maguire, R.P., Meiners, L.C. & Leenders, K.L. (2004): Cerebral activation related to skills practice in a double serial reaction time task: striatal involvement in random-order sequence learning *Brain Res. Cogn. Brain Res.* **20,** 120–131.

Vicari, S. (2006): Motor development and neuropsychological patterns in persons with Down syndrome. *Behav. Genet* **36,** 355–364.

Vicari, S. & Carlesimo, G.A. (2002): Children with intellectual disabilities. In: *Handbook of memory disorders,* eds A. Baddeley, B. Wilson & M. Kopelman, pp. 501–518. New York: John Wiley & Sons.

Vicari, S., Carlesimo, A., Brizzolara, D. & Pezzini, G. (1996a): Short-term memory in children with Williams syndrome: a reduced contribution of lexical-semantic knowledge to word span. *Neuropsychologia* **34,** 919–925.

Vicari, S., Brizzolara, D., Carlesimo, A., Pezzini, G. & Volterra, V. (1996b): Memory abilities in children with Williams syndrome. *Cortex* **32,** 503–514.

Vicari, S., Bellucci, S. & Carlesimo, G.A. (2000): Implicit and explicit memory: a functional dissociation in persons with Down syndrome. *Neuropsychologia* **38,** 240–251.

Vicari, S., Bellucci, S. & Carlesimo, G.A. (2001): Procedural learning deficit in children with Williams syndrome *Neuropsychologia* **39,** 665–677.

Vicari, S., Caselli, M.C., Gagliardi, C., Tonucci, F. & Volterra, V. (2002): Language acquisition in special populations a comparison between Down and Williams syndromes. *Neuropsychologia* **40,** 2461–2470.

Vicari, S., Bellucci, S. & Carlesimo, G.A. (2003): Visual and spatial working memory dissociation: evidence from a genetic syndrome. *Dev. Med. Child Neurol.* **45,** 269–273.

Vicari, S., Bates, E., Caselli, M.C., Pasqualetti, P., Gagliardi, C., Tonucci, F. & Volterra, V. (2004): Neuropsychological profile of Italians with Williams syndrome: an example of a dissociation between language and cognition? *J. Int. Neuropsychol. Soc.* **10,** 862–876.

Vicari, S., Bellucci, S. & Carlesimo, G.A. (2005): Visual and spatial long-term memory: differential pattern of impairments in Williams and Down syndromes. *Dev. Med. Child Neurol.* **47,** 305–311.

Vicari, S., Bellucci, S. & Carlesimo, G.A. (2006): Evidence from two genetic syndromes for the independence of spatial and visual working memory. *Dev. Med. Child Neurol.* **48,** 126–131.

Vicari, S., Verucci, L. & Carlesimo, G.A. (2007): Implicit memory is independent from IQ and age but not from aetiology: evidence from Down and Williams syndromes. *J. Intell. Disabil Res.* (in press).

Volterra, V., Capirci, O., Pezzini, G., Sabbadini, L. & Vicari, S. (1996): Linguistic abilities in Italian children with Williams syndrome. *Cortex* **32,** 663–677.

Volterra, V., Longobardi, E., Pezzini, G., Vicari, S. & Antenore, C. (1999): Visuo-spatial and linguistic abilities in a twin with Williams syndrome. *J. Intell. Disabil. Res.* **43,** 294–305.

Wang, P.P. & Bellugi, U. (1994): Evidence from two genetic syndromes for dissociation between verbal and visual-spatial short-term memory. *J. Clin. Exp. Neuropsychol.* **16,** 317–322.

Wang, P.P., Hesselink, J.R., Jernigan, T.L., Doherty, S. & Bellugi, U. (1992): Specific neurobehavioral profile of Williams syndrome is associated with neocerebellar hemispheric preservation. *Neurology* **42,** 1999–2002.

Chapter 21

Neuropsychology of mental retardation: fragile X syndrome as paradigm of the cognitive-behavioural phenotype

Daria Riva, Arianna Usilla, Chiara Vago, Federica Aggio and Sara Bulgheroni

Department of Developmental Neurology, Fondazione IRCCS Istituto Neurologico 'C. Besta', via Celoria 11, 20133 Milan, Italy
driva@istituto-besta.it

Summary

The neuropsychology of mental retardation considers deficiencies of frontal executive functions as the core malfunction behind the pathological condition, whatever its origin, while the cognitive-behavioural phenotype is defined in an attempt to characterize the cognitive functioning specific to a person with mental retardation of a distinct aetiology. This chapter considers fragile X syndrome as a paradigm because it is the most common form of mental retardation on a hereditary basis and because it allows a strong phenotype-genotype correlation to be drawn in males and females with a complete mutation, as well as in premutated cases. The distinctive features of the syndrome – in addition to the deficient executive abilities (also seen in premutated subjects) – include a macroscopic dissociation between verbal and visuospatial abilities in favour of the former, an advantage of expressive language over receptive language, and particular behavioural disorders, the most common of which are autistic-like in males. The deficiencies comprising the core symptoms of the syndrome are correlated with the cerebral areas that process the functional impairments in which the protein coded by the mutation is deficient.

Introduction

According to the definition of the *Diagnostic and Statistical Manual of Mental Disorders* (DSM-IV-TR), mental retardation is a final outcome common to numerous processes involving the CNS and consequently it includes conditions that may differ greatly from one another. Its causes may be genetic (chromosomal, microdeletions, monogenic, and so on) or result from malformations or pre-/peri- or postnatal lesions, or in a sizable proportion of cases they may remain unknown (Wilska & Kasky, 2001). Each cause will clearly take effect according to different mechanisms and on different neurological targets (altering the coding of a protein, disrupting the timing of developmental mechanisms – synaptogenesis, myelinogenesis, synaptic pruning – of certain circuits or parts of circuits, and so on), thus interfering with the individual's development as a whole or in some specific area.

The neuropsychology of mental retardation is a difficult issue because of the complexity and heterogeneity of the condition, and the correspondingly complex and heterogeneous nature of the neuropsychological mechanisms underlying it.

The history of neuropsychological research began with studies on mental retardation seen as a single phenotype, which coincided with the definition of the deficiency, and evolved towards studies that have attempted to identify specific phenotypes correlating with the cause of the condition. Of course, the methodology of the two approaches differs substantially, moving away from using intellectual tests alone, towards highly complex assessments that demand an abundant and well differentiated battery of tests, a strong and up-to-date understanding of developmental neuropsychology, and a good dose of imagination.

It is important to emphasize, however, that even just administering a developmental scale or an intellectual test takes skill, a thorough understanding of the test and its intrinsic structure, careful administration, and a good capacity for interpretation. It is essential not to make the mistake of assuming that an apparently simple test is 'simple' in terms of the above-mentioned variables, because measuring intelligence is a difficult procedure and can only be done by an expert.

As for defining the single phenotype, developmental theories can be divided as follows: the developmental hypothesis, which identifies mental retardation as a delay in development (Zigler & Hodapp, 1986); the structural hypothesis, which assumes that the diversity of mental retardation lies in an altered structure of the mind and not just in its slower development (Zigler & Hodapp, 1986); and a hypothesis that combines those two – that is, one that considers the impaired structure and late development as inseparable from one another (Zigler & Hodapp, 1986). Meanwhile, studies on mental retardation based exclusively on the use of IQ tests have made it obvious that similar total IQs can emerge from quite different profiles identified by the single items (Vicari et al., 1992). Another important point is that these profiles are not homogeneous, but represent a set of strengths and weaknesses, even though the overall performances are always below the norm.

The unitary viewpoint and the approach that sees the different levels of performance in the various tests as indicative of a relative independence between the different domains of the mind can be traced back to two different ways of designating intelligence, and consequently also mental retardation: for the former, mental functioning is characterized by an inseparable integration of the processes, while for the latter the processes are separate and relatively independent of each other. These convictions give rise to two different models that refer to two separate theories. One is Anderson's general holistic theory (Anderson, 1986), according to which human cognition is unitary and the very essence of its functioning derives from its unitary nature. The other is Fodor's theory of modularism (Fodor, 1983), which describes the mind as a set of computational systems (or modules) that are more or less encapsulated, depending on how the theory is variously interpreted. Both these theories identify a central supervisory, control, or integration system that constitutes the most refined expression of human mental functioning.

Returning now to mental retardation, we might say that dealing with and examining these patients identifies a general core deficiency common to all of them and, if not a phenotype, at least an individual profile with particular strengths and weaknesses.

So what do the different forms of mental retardation have in common? There is a generally simplified cognitive functioning, with a more limited complexity of the mental operations and processing skills. This is the impression gained from direct experience and from the clinical assessment of patients with mental retardation, and it is formalized in the theories outlined below.

The Sternberg and Spear triarchic model (Sternberg & Spear, 1985) distinguishes the components of a cognitive action into, first, higher-level executive processes or metacomponents; second, performance components; and third, learning components. Having identified an objective, the executive components (or metacomponents) formulate a project, then they monitor it constantly, adapting the original project as necessary, and once the objective has been achieved, they store the behaviour (or part of it) for future recall in similar experiences. In other words, mental retardation would be an impairment or malfunction in our capacity to think about what we are doing (and consequently the functioning of those control or integration systems that the two previously mentioned theories have in common). So any impairment of such higher order components would lead to unintelligent behaviour, because it would result in a behaviour that is barely metacognitive and strategic. The qualifying aspect of intelligence is represented, on the other hand, by our ability to plan our behaviour to pursue a goal, and the more our project is efficient and parsimonious, the more intelligent our consequent behaviour will be.

According to another theory, the cognitive system is a system in equilibrium between automatic and voluntary processes, where the originality and novelty of the voluntary processes demand mental energy and self-awareness of functioning, while the automatic processes use up much less energy because they are the result of innate skills or frequent experiences that have made them automatic. Mental retardation would consequently be characterized by a more or less severe impairment of the voluntary processes and a greater reliance on innate patterns, with a more limited capacity for active, aware self-control, giving rise to a behaviour that is scarcely adaptive in cognitive terms (Ellis et al., 1989). A theory that encompasses both the previous points of view and also attempts to establish a neuro-anatomical developmental correlation is the Karmiloff-Smith theory of 'representational redescription' (Karmiloff-Smith, 1992), which is founded on two factors: the first refers to the progressive specialization and automation of innate capabilities; the second to the conscious redescription of these capabilities. The first factor is represented by the fact that each of us is born with a set of innate behavioural patterns essential to our survival (a good example lies in the fact that babies are born with reflex but effective behaviour that makes them turn their head only to the side on which their cheek is stimulated in order to suckle); these are available to us without having to be learnt. Later on, as the brain develops, these abilities tend to become more refined; they are implemented with a greater degree of specialization, and a database of possible behaviour patterns develops that is less influenced by the context and consequently more readily available for selection and combination in new processes and behaviour patterns. This specialization is not subconscious – the individual is capable of representing it and consequently of converting it from implicit to explicit. The parallel neural development evolves from the specialization of subcortical circuits – the processors of automatic elementary functions that naturally guide the individual towards human development – to the more complex cortical circuits, which are capable of higher order cognitive processes of which the individual is aware. Given a normal set of genes and conditions of normal environmental stimulation, the brain's hardware is thus induced to draw the greatest possible advantage from experience in a mutual modelling action, thus developing an extraordinary, almost unlimited amount of software. When this model is placed in a neurological context, any genetic mutation or lesion may affect the timing or the processes of synaptogenesis, myelinogenesis, synaptic pruning, migration, and so on, making the basic circuits inaccessible or less readily available. This consequently prevents the evolution towards the more complex circuits that can process such higher order functions as strategic control, metacognition, and self-awareness, abilities that all come under the umbrella term of frontal executive functions. In fact, the studies that have evaluated individuals with mental retardation using tests of frontal executive type have always found varying degrees of impairment (Aylward, 2002). Even assessments of mental retardation that rely on intelligence tests alone identify strengths and weaknesses in different individuals with mental retardation that reflect dissociations between different functions, or even within the same function. If these dissociations are consistent in successive assessments and are constantly associated with a given disorder, then they represent a cognitive behavioural phenotype (CBP). This term was introduced by Nyhan in 1971, who used it to describe the behaviour observed in Lesh-Nyhan syndrome. It identifies a characteristic pattern of motor, cognitive, linguistic, and social anomalies that are consistently associated with a given biological disorder and refer to recognizable and stable behaviour patterns (Flint & Yule, 1994).

To understand the meaning and the methods for interpreting the CBP, it is worth mentioning that even at a very early age the cerebral regions process different functions and, within these regions, certain functions are processed by specialized circuits. Hemispheric, intrahemispheric, and single-circuit specialisations become operational very early on, responding to a genetic programme characteristic of the species and of the individual concerned, and shaped by the environment. In this redundant evolution, moreover, some areas undergo a parallel and interdependent development (for example, the prefrontal areas and the cerebellum) (Riva, 1999).

We can consequently expect to find different phenotypes depending on the site and timing of the lesion, disorder, or genetic mutation responsible for the condition. For instance, in the case of pre-, peri-, or postnatal lesions, and infantile cerebral palsy in particular, attempts have been made to identify the distinctive cognitive-behavioural features of the most frequent forms, such as the congenital hemiplegias and diplegias. Malformations and brain tumours (with or without any associated neurotoxic therapy) can also be responsible for complex impairments on various levels and in various types of mental retardation, that basically correlate with the area/structure involved (or which is primarily affected by the neurotoxic treatment).

In children with genetic syndromes with known mutations or with a recognized syndrome, the identification of a specific behavioural phenotype affords an extraordinary natural experimental setting for studying intelligence and its genetic determinants.

Genotype-phenotype correlation studies in humans

The link between genes and behaviour can be explained as follows: the gene codifies for a protein that comes to form a part of regions, structures, and circuits that process cognitive and emotional behaviour. In reality, the problem is much more complex, because a given protein is represented extensively in the brain, not just in certain circuits.

The cognitive-behavioural phenotype of the fragile X syndrome

This syndrome can be seen as a paradigm because it is the most common form of mental retardation on a hereditary basis, and because it enables fairly clear phenotype-genotype correlation to be identified in cases (both male and female) with a complete mutation, and in carriers of both sexes. The syndrome affects 1/1,200 males and 1/2,500 females, and it is common knowledge that males are more severely affected than females. The phenotype is characterized by macrocephaly (cranial circumference above the 50th centile), an elongated face that becomes more apparent with time, a prominent jaw and long ears, laxity of the ligaments, soft connective tissue, and post-pubertal macroorchidism (testicular size more than

30 ml) (Simko et al., 1989). Females differ only slightly from normal, but 50 per cent of those affected intellectually have long ears and other, albeit milder, characteristic somatic features (Simko et al., 1989). Other associated disorders include mitral valve prolapse (80 per cent), scoliosis, joint laxity (73 per cent), recurrent otitis media (63 per cent), and epilepsy (20 per cent) (Simko et al., 1989).

Patients with fragile X syndrome usually belong to families with mental retardation, but the phenotypic somatic features are not seen in all cases and often only become manifest later in life, so they cannot be considered as justification for carrying out molecular tests. The gene involved *(FMR1)* is located on Xq27. The syndrome is the result of a marked expansion of an unstable trinucleotide, CGG, that induces downregulation of the gene's expression. Males with more than 200 repetitions always show the signs of the disease, while only one in two females with the same number of repetitions expresses the disease (Phadke, 2005). Healthy subjects have from 5 to 45 triplets; premutated (transmitting or carrier) males have between 55 and 200 triplets, and no signs of the disease, and they generate female offspring without the expansion, transmitting the premutation only to their daughters. Mothers with the premutation are at risk of having sons with either the premutation or the complete mutation. The premutation may increase in size when it is transmitted by a female carrier, and it may continue to expand in each subsequent generation. The premutated condition is not usually accompanied by the disorder, but it has been suggested that female carriers of the premutation are likely to have mild signs of the condition (Reiss et al., 1993). The male and female offspring of the daughters of carriers have between 200 and 2,000 triplets and the full-blown disorder. The expanded CGG triplet causes hypermethylation of the promoter region with the transcriptional suppression of the *FMR1* gene, which thus abolishes or reduces the output of fragile X mental retardation protein (FMRP).

This protein is expressed extensively in the neurons, but particularly in the cholinergic cells of the basal ganglia and hippocampus, and in the cerebellum. It regulates synaptic plasticity (Tamanini et al., 1997) and consequently plays a fundamental role in the development of the fetal brain and in the learning capacity of the mature brain. This protein does not seem to interfere with neurogenesis and neuron migration, but it does affect the late phase of synaptic pruning, consequently giving rise to an altered cerebral structuring. During development there are numerous small synapses distributed along the dendritic spines that subsequently become reduced in number, but larger, with small spines, while the immature pattern has been found in fragile X syndrome and in knockout mice with the mutation (Rudelli et al., 1985; Irwin et al., 2000).

Neuropsychological development

Males and females have different developmental profiles. Males have delayed development, hypotonia, and behavioural disorders: on average, they can achieve sitting position independently at 10 months of age and they can walk unassisted at 21 months. Their language development is more severely delayed: they utter their first words at 18 to 29 months and produce phrases at between 45 and 56 months (Freund, 1994).

Cognitive-behavioural phenotype of males with full mutation

Males with a full mutation have an average IQ typical of moderate-to-severe retardation, though this can vary from severe to borderline retardation (De La Cruz, 1985).

Their average IQ is 54 ± 15 (as opposed to 85 ± 15 in females), with a progressive decline from borderline – mild to moderate – severe as they grow older (from 8 to 15 years of age), which is particularly evident in males. According to a study on 144 families, the level of mental retardation relates to the quantity of FMRP (Pulsifer, 1996; Sundheim *et al.*, 2006).

The more specifically neuropsychological profile identifies a deficiency in frontal executive tests, with major dissociations represented by a better performance in the sphere of language than in the visuospatial skills. There are also dissociations within the sphere of language – that is, expressive language is more developed than receptive language and, though fluent, it reveals particular stereotypias and stalling. In fact, the expressive language is repetitive and often echolalic, tangential and cluttered, giving the impression of impairment of lexical access. There is also a marked loss of prosody. The maximum level of language development corresponds approximately to that of a 4 year old, which means that a diagnosis of fragile X syndrome has to be borne in mind when facing a child with delayed or disturbed language skills.

The non-verbal phenotype is represented by a deficit in spatial tests, recognizing faces, judging line orientation, and praxis in general.

Various psychiatric disorders are seen in mutated males, and in variable associations. They may be dysthymic or antisocial, have relational difficulties or reveal self-injurious behaviour (biting their hands/fingers), object sniffing, selective mutism, social phobia, Tourette syndrome or obsessive-compulsive disorders, attention-deficit hyperactivity disorder, hypersensitivity to sensory stimuli, and autistic-like behaviour. As concerns this last sign, mutated subjects with autism represent a specific subgroup. Among the various case series reported, a mean of 16 per cent of individuals with autism carry the mutation, with a prevalence of males over females of 6.5 to 4. Autism is more frequent in cases with the complete mutation. It is also worth adding here that the presence of autism is a negative prognostic indicator, though there is no correlation between autism and FMRP levels (Bailey *et al.*, 2001), as there is for mental retardation.

Although aetiological screening in autism now routinely includes searching for the fragile X mutation, a particularly expert and prolonged assessment can identify differences between fragile X-related and classic autism. Autistic children with the fragile X mutation are more aware of others, even though they resort to gaze aversion and avoidance behaviour, and their adaptive behaviour is fairly good for their age, unlike the often anguished inability of autistic children to adapt. This behaviour might consequently be interpreted as a situation of withdrawal due to anxiety, a 'go away closer' behaviour expressed through a set of mannerisms, often misdiagnosed as the stereotypias typical of autism (Dykens *et al.*, 1989).

Female phenotype with full mutation

The female phenotype is different from the male. Females with the premutation seem no different from the healthy members of their families. Only about 50 per cent of the cases have mild-to-moderate mental retardation (Rousseau *et al.*, 1994) and their development in the first year of life is normal. The mental retardation becomes evident only later and these girls do not experience the progressive cognitive decline described in males with the complete mutation.

The phenotype with mental retardation is also characterized in females by difficulties in frontal executive tests (Hagermann & Sobesky 1989; Mazzocco *et al.*, 1992; Borghgraef *et al.*, 1996; Jacala *et al.*, 1997).

The most frequent neuropsychological impairments are the same as in males, but less severe. There is a dissociation between the girls' verbal and non-verbal abilities, in favour of the former, and deficits in the attention domain and in visuospatial tests, including visual memory. Although it is one of the children's strengths, their language has a bizarre content and typically lacks prosodic intonation and fails to adhere to the rules of the pragmatics of communication (Pulsifer, 1996; Sundheim *et al.*, 2006).

Females without mental retardation are frequently diagnosed as having learning disorders, performing particularly poorly in arithmetic but doing quite well in reading and writing (Mazzocco *et al.*, 1993).

The most common psychiatric disorders are a marked shyness and introversion, with avoidance behaviour and anxiety, and motor disorders with signs in the schizophrenic spectrum, particularly the schizotype (Sobesky *et al.*, 1994). In females, a longer length of the CGG repeat coincides with a reduction in the level of FMRP and is associated with a greater severity of the psychiatric symptoms (Franke *et al.*, 1996).

Carriers

It is worth mentioning the characteristics of carriers, because mild neurocognitive and neuropsychological impairments combined with minor dysmorphic signs should arouse the suspicion of fragile X syndrome. Male carriers have minor somatic and neurocognitive signs, with a normal IQ or mild mental retardation, and the symptoms of cognitive malfunctioning typical of the complete mutation, albeit in a very mild form, but the deficit in the frontal executive tests is evident (Pulsifer, 1996; Sundheim *et al.*, 2006).

Female carriers usually have a normal IQ, with a discrepancy in favour of the verbal IQ and a mild degree of neuropsychological malfunctioning, here again with deficient results in the frontal executive tests (Pulsifer, 1996; Sundheim *et al.*, 2006).

Genotype-phenotype correlations

Let us now attempt to correlate the cognitive and behavioural symptoms of the syndrome with the genetic and anatomical characteristics.

Deficits in frontal executive tests

Neurofunctional studies in females (chosen because their condition is less severe) to assess the recruitment of the prefrontal cortex in performing executive tests have identified an impairment not only in activation but also in deactivation (that is, the ability to inhibit a given activity, which is again an ability of frontal executive type). As demonstrated in a study using the Stroop test, different degrees of inability in activation and deactivation of the prefrontal cortex are associated with different levels of FMRP (Tamm *et al.*, 2002).

Language disorders of mainly pragmatic type with lexical access difficulties associated with behavioural disorders of autistic type

In mutated subjects, the cerebellar vermis is smaller than in normal children or subjects with other developmental disorders. This size reduction seems to be due to an altered development rather than to atrophy (Reiss *et al.*, 1991). The lobes affected are the sixth and seventh, as described by Courchesne in a subgroup of subjects with autism (Courchesne *et al.*, 1988). These diminished dimensions of the cerebellar vermis also correlate with a lower IQ and stereotypical behaviour (Mazzocco *et al.*, 1998). To interpret these findings correctly, we have to remember that the cerebellum – and the vermis in particular – is believed to be a crucial partner in the processing of language, even in children, and this might explain both the peculiarity of fragile X syndrome patients' language and their difficulties in lexical access (Riva & Giorgi, 2000), as well as the trouble they have in placing the language components in the right order (Theobald *et al.*, 1987).

Visuospatial deficiencies

In normal individuals, high FMRP levels are found in the magnocellular layer of the lateral geniculate body, which is part of the parietal visual-dorsal stream. Mutated patients have a condition afflicting the magnocellular system without any concomitant malfunction of the parvocellular system. This malfunction would be responsible for the severely impaired visuospatial skills of mutated subjects, as the magnocellular system leads into the parietal visual-dorsal stream, which forms part of the central visual system that integrates higher-order visuomotor processes (Kogan *et al.*, 2004).

Conclusions

The neuropsychology of mental retardation identifies the common denominator of the pathological condition – whatever its origin – in impairments of higher-order metacognitive and frontal executive performance. The definition of the phenotype tends to characterize the specific cognitive functioning of an individual with mental retardation of a particular aetiology. From the clinical standpoint there is an obvious added value in studying distinctive impairments (also to help tailor any rehabilitation to the patient's needs). However, from the neurosciences viewpoint the correlation emerging between the mutation and the functional alteration is scarcely satisfactory, because it should be based on the fact that the mutation only affects a specific neuronal system (and no other), the constituents of which form a causal chain in which we should be able to identify the molecular components of a signal transduction pathway (Weeber *et al.*, 2002). In reality, the FMRP deficiency is expressed extensively in the neurons of the basal ganglia, hippocampus, and cerebellum, and the protein is represented throughout the brain because it regulates synaptic plasticity. As a result, the cognitive behavioural genotypic-phenotypic correlation holds, for the time being, for the regions in which the levels of the protein are low, and not with an altered molecular system.

References

Anderson, M. (1986): Understanding the cognitive deficit in mental retardation. *J. Child. Psychol. Psychiatry* **27**, 297–307.

Aylward, G.P. (2002): Cognitive and neuropsychological outcomes: more than IQ scores. *Ment. Retard. Dev. Disabil. Res. Rev.* **8**, 234–240.

Bailey, D.B., Hatton, D.D., Skinner, M. & Mesibov, G. (2001): Autistic behavior, FMR1 protein, and developmental trajectories in young males with fragile X syndrome. *J. Autism Dev. Disord.* **31**, 165–174.

Borghgraef, M., Umans, S., Steyaert, J., Legius, E. & Fryns, J.P. (1996): New findings in the behavioral profile of young FraX females. *Am. J. Med. Genet.* **9**, 346–349.

Courchesne, E., Yeung-Courchesne, R., Press, G.A., Hesselink, J.R. & Jernigan, T.L. (1988): Hypoplasia of cerebellar vermal lobules VI and VII in autism. *N. Engl. J. Med.* **26**, 1349–1354.

De La Cruz, F.F. (1985): Fragile X syndrome. *Am. J. Ment. Def.* **90**, 119–123.

Dykens, E.M., Hodapp, R.M., Ort, S., Finucane, B., Shapiro, L. & Leckman, J. (1989): The trajectory of cognitive development in males with fragile X syndrome. *J. Am. Acad. Child. Adolesc. Psychiatry* **28**, 422–428.

Ellis, N.R., Woodley-Zanthos, P., Dulaney C.L. & Palmer, R.L. (1989): Automatic-effortful processing and cognitive inertia in persons with mental retardation. *Am. J. Ment. Retard.* **93**, 412–423.

Flint, J.& Yule, W. (1994): Behavioral phenotypes. In: *Child and adolescent psychiatry*, 3rd edition, ed. M. Rutter, E. Taylor & L. Hersov, pp. 666–687. Oxford: Blackwell Scientific.

Fodor, J. (1983): *The modularity of mind. an essay on faculty psychology.* Cambridge, MA: MIT Press.

Franke, P., Maier, W., Hautzinger, M., Weiffenbach, O., Gänsicke, M., Iwers, B., Poustka, F., Schwab, S.G. & Froster, U. (1996): Fragile-X carrier females: evidence for a distinct psychopathological phenotype? *Am. J. Med. Genet.* **64**, 334–339.

Freund, L.S. (1994): Diagnosis and developmental issues for young children with fragile X syndrome. *Infants Young Child.* **6**, 34–45.

Hagerman, R.J. & Sobesky, W.E. (1989): Psychopathology in fragile X syndrome. *Am. J. Orthopsychiatry* **59**, 142–152.

Irwin, S.A., Galvez, R. & Greenough, W.T. (2000): Dendritic spine structural anomalies in fragile-X mental retardation syndrome. *Cereb. Cortex* **10**, 1038–1044.

Jakala, P., Hanninen, T., Ryynänen, M., Laakso, M., Partanen, K., Mannermaa, A.& Soininen, H. (1997): Fragile-X: neuropsychological test performance, CGG triplet repeat lengths, and hippocampal volumes. *J. Clin. Invest.* **15**, 331–338.

Karmiloff-Smith, A. (1992): *Beyond modularity. A developmental prospective on cognitive science.* Cambridge, MA: MIT Press.

Kogan, C.S., Boutet, I., Cornish, K., Zangenehpour, S., Mullen, K.T., Holden, J.J., Der Kaloustian, V.M., Andermann, E. & Chaudhuri A. (2004): Differential impact of the FMR1 gene on visual processing in fragile X syndrome. *Brain* **127**, 591–601.

Mazzocco, M.M., Hagerman, R.J., Cronister-Silverman, A. & Pennington, B.F. (1992): Specific frontal lobe deficits among women with the fragile X gene. *J. Am. Acad. Child. Adolesc. Psychiatry* **31**, 1141–1148.

Mazzocco, M.M., Pennington, B.F. & Hagerman, R.J. (1993): The neurocognitive phenotype of female carriers of fragile X: additional evidence for specificity. *J. Dev. Behav. Pediatr.* **14**, 328–335.

Mazzocco, M.M., Baumgardner, T., Freund, L.S. & Reiss, A.L. (1998): Social functioning among girls with fragile X or Turner syndrome and their sisters. *J. Autism Dev. Disord.* **28**, 509–517.

Phadke, S.R. (2005): Fragile X syndrome. *Orphanet Enciclopedia*.

Pulsifer, M.B. (1996): The neuropsychology of mental retardation. *J. Int. Neuropsychol. Soc.* **2**, 159–176.

Reiss, A.L., Freund, L., Tseng, J.E. & Joshi, P.K. (1991): Neuroanatomy in fragile X females: the posterior fossa. *Am. J. Hum. Genet.* **49**, 279–288.

Reiss, A.L., Freund, L., Abrams, M.T., Boehm, C. & Kazazian, H. (1993): Neurobehavioral effects of the fragile X permutation in adult women: a controlled study. *Am. J. Hum. Genet.* **52**, 884–894.

Riva, D. (1999): Le lesioni cerebrali focali. In: *Manuale di neuropsicologia dell'età evolutiva*, ed. G. Sabbadini, pp. 484–504. Bologna: Zanichelli.

Riva, D. & Giorgi, C. (2000): The cerebellum contributes to higher functions during development: evidence from a series of children surgically treated for posterior fossa tumours. *Brain* **123**, 1051–1061.

Rudelli, R.D., Brown, W.T., Wisniewski, K., Jenkins, E.C., Laure-Kamionowska, M., Connell, F. & Wisniewski, H.M. (1985): Adult fragile X syndrome. Clinico-neuropathologic findings. *Acta Neuropathol. (Berl.)* **67**, 289–295.

Rousseau, F., Heitz, D., Tarleton, J., MacPherson, J., Malmgren, H., Dahl, N., Barnicoat, A., Mathew, C., Mornet, E., Tejada, I., Maddalena, A., Spiegel, R., Schinzel, A., Marcos, J.A.G., Schorderet, D.F., Schaap, T., Maccioni, L., Russo. S., Jacobs, P.A, Schwartz, C. & Mandel, J.L. (1994): A multicenter study on genotype-phenotype correlations in the fragile X syndrome, using direct diagnosis with probe StB12.3: the first 2,253 cases. *Am. J. Hum. Genet.* **55**, 225–237.

Simko, A., Hornstein, L., Soukup, S. & Bagamery, N. (1989): Fragile X syndrome: recognition in young children. *Pediatrics* **83**, 547–552.

Sobesky, W.E., Hull, C.E. & Hagerman, R.J. (1994): Symptoms of schizotypal personality disorder in fragile X women. *J. Am. Acad. Child. Adolesc. Psychiatry* **33**, 247–255.

Sternberg, R.G. & Spear, L.C. (1985): A triarchic theory of mental retardation. *Int. Rev. Res. Ment. Retard.* **13**, 301–325.

Sundheim, S.T.P.V., Myers, R.M. & Voeler, K.K.S. (2006): Mental retardation. In: *Pediatric neuropsychiatry*, ed. C.E. Coffey, R.A. Brumback, D.R. Rosenberg & K.K.S. Voeller, pp. 151–161. Baltimore: Lippincott Williams & Wilkins.

Tamanini, F., Willesmen, R., van Unen, L., Bontekoe, C., Galjaard, H., Oostra, B.A. & Hoogeveen, A.T. (1997): Differential expression of fmr1, fxr1 and fxr2 proteins in human brain and testis. *Hum. Mol. Genet.* **6**, 1315–1322.

Tamm, L., Menon, V., Jhonston, C.K., Hessl, D.R. & Reiss, A.L. (2002): fMRI study of cognitive interference processing in females with fragile X syndrome. *J. Cogn. Neurosci.* **14**, 160–171.

Theobald, T.M., Hay, D.A. & Judge, C. (1987): Individual variation and specific cognitive deficits in the fragile X syndrome. *Am. J. Med. Genet.* **28,** 1–11.

Vicari, S., Albertini, G. & Caltagirone, C. (1992): Cognitive profiles in adolescents with mental retardation. *J. Intellect. Disabil. Res.* **36,** 415–423.

Weeber, E.J., Levenson, J.M. & Sweatt, J.D. (2002): Molecular genetics of human cognition. *Mol. Intervent.* **2,** 376–390.

Wilska, M.L. & Kasky, M.K. (2001): Why and how to assess the aetiological diagnosis of children with intellectual disability/mental retardation and other neurodevelopmental disorders: description of the Finnish approach. *Eur. J. Pediatr. Neurol.* **5,** 7–13.

Zigler, E. & Hodapp, R.M. (1986): *Understanding mental retardation.* Cambridge: Cambridge University Press.

Achevé d'imprimer par Corlet, Imprimeur, S.A.
14110 Condé-sur-Noireau
N° d'Imprimeur : 105993 - Dépôt légal : novembre 2007
Imprimé en France